Work and the Eye

Publisher: Caroline Makepeace
Development editor: Myriam Brearley
Production controller: Chris Jarvis
Desk editor: Claire Hutchins
Cover designer: Alan Studholme

Work and the Eye

Second edition

Rachel V. North BSc MSc PhD
FCOptom

Senior Lecturer, Department of Optometry and Vision Sciences
Cardiff University, Cardiff, UK

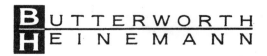

OXFORD AUCKLAND BOSTON JOHANNESBURG MELBOURNE NEW DELHI

Butterworth-Heinemann
Linacre House, Jordan Hill, Oxford OX2 8DP
225 Wildwood Avenue, Woburn, MA 01801-2041
A division of Reed Educational and Professional Publishing Ltd

℞ A member of the Reed Elsevier plc group

First published 1993
Second edition published 2001

British Library Cataloguing in Publication Data
North, Rachel V.
  Work and the eye. – 2nd ed.
  1. Optometry 2. Industrial hygiene 3. Eye – Protection
  I. Title
  617.7′5

Library of Congress Cataloguing in Publication Data
North, Rachel V.
  Work and the eye/Rachel V. North. – 2nd ed.
  p. ; cm.
  Includes bibliographical references and index.
  ISBN 0 7506 4172 X
  1. Industrial ophthalmology. 2. Eye – Wounds and injuries. I. Title.
  [DNLM: 1. Eye Injuries – prevention & control. 2. Accidents, Occupational – prevention
  & control. 3. Occupational Health. WW 525 N866w 2001]
  RE825 .N67 2001
  617.7–dc21   00–068889

ISBN 0 7506 4172 X

Data manipulation by David Gregson Associates, Beccles, Suffolk
Printed and bound in Great Britain, by Martins the Printers, Berwick-upon-Tweed

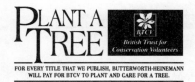

Contents

Preface

This textbook aims to provide a single source of information for those concerned with the field of occupational optometry. However, it is a subject that requires constant review, and since the first edition of this book there have been a number of changes. New regulations regarding eye protection have been published. European Standards have been issued relating to eye protectors, replacing some of the previous British Standards. A new edition of the CIBSE Code for interior lighting has been published. There is also an increased incidence of sports-related eye injuries, which frequently result in severe ocular damage. It is therefore important for sports players, especially those participating in racket sports, to be made aware of the need to wear appropriate eye protection. In addition, there have been revisions to some of the vision standards advised for various occupations. Therefore, this second edition aims to bring the subject up to date.

It is hoped that this textbook will continue to be of interest not only to undergraduate and practising optometrists, but also to health and safety officers, occupational hygienists, occupational nurses and others involved in eye care.

Rachel V. North

Acknowledgements

I would like to express my sincere thanks again to all those who have given assistance in the writing of this book. In particular, I am indebted to John Grundy BSc FBCO, Professor M. Millodot OD PhD FAAO FBCO and Dr David Woolf BSc PhD MCOptom for their comments, suggestions and corrections of the manuscript. I also wish to thank the AOP, HMSO and BSI for their assistance and permission to copy sections of their standards and regulations, and the Chartered Institution of Building Services Engineers, the Electricity Association Services Ltd and Thorn Lighting for the many tables and figures extracted from their publications.

1 Visual performance

There are many varied and complex types of work in industry today. Any professional engaged to advise on visual performance would need, in the first instance, to visit the place of work to gain a full understanding of the task(s) and obtain a precise knowledge of its demand(s) upon the employee. The goal is to minimize stress on the visual system, which will result in an efficient and safe visual performance. In addition to the assessment of the work place and the tasks involved, an assessment of individual capabilities is required to determine whether the visual abilities match the visual requirements of the job. If not, one of two things can happen: first, changes can be made to the work place; or secondly, direct assistance can be given to the employee – for example, in the form of spectacles or magnifiers.

The ability to perform most tasks depends on many visual and non-visual variables, and the factors that influence the visual performance are:

- The visual capability of the individual
- The visibility of the task
- Psychological and general physiological factors.

It is not within the scope of this text to deal with the third group of factors in depth, although psychological and general physiological factors (such as motivation, intelligence, general health, etc.) should not be forgotten, because they can all influence the visual performance. This chapter will deal with the first two variables, visual capability and the visibility of the task.

VISUAL CAPABILITIES

A knowledge of the capabilities and limits of the visual system is essential so that tasks can be designed to allow maximum performance and a minimum number of errors. A task that requires the visual system to operate at its limit may cause general stress, asthenopia, and decreased performance and efficiency. Far too often, insufficient attention is given to determining the visual capabilities of a person and to ensuring that he or she is capable of seeing adequately in relation to the demands of a particular task.

The functions of the visual system can be divided into four broad groups:

1. Detection
2. Recognition
3. Colour discrimination
4. Depth perception.

The functions and factors that influence the above visual parameters have been described thoroughly in many books (see Further reading), and they are the main sources used to compile this chapter.

Detection

The functions involved in the detection of objects include the following:

- Visual field
- Head and eye movements
- Light perception
- Visual adaptation
- Flicker frequency
- Contrast sensitivity.

Visual field

The stationary eye can detect a visual stimulus within an area extending 60° superiorly, 70° inferiorly, 95° temporally and 60° nasally. The total horizontal visual field extends to 190°, 145° being the monocular visual field, and with a 120° binocular overlap (Weston, 1962). The sensitivity of the retina to a stimulus varies; the retina is least sensitive at the periphery and most sensitive at the fovea.

Detection of a visual stimulus will depend on its size, distance, colour, and the background illumination. Different occupations make different demands on the visual field. Some tasks, such as VDU work, make little demand on the peripheral visual field but a lot on the central visual field. Other tasks such as driving or flying, where safety is a major concern, require full visual fields.

Individuals with monocular vision are at a disadvantage both because they have a reduced visual field and because they do not have the binocular overlap to compensate for the blind spot. Consequently they have an absolute scotoma within their field of view. It is important to allow for the length of time that individuals have been monocular, and therefore the time that they have had to adapt to the loss of visual field, as well as to the loss of stereopsis. For example, in Sweden a person who has lost the vision in one eye is barred from driving for 1 year, to allow time for adaptation.

Age influences the extent of visual field; the lateral visual field declines after the age of 35 years (Burg, 1968). The restriction of the field is thought to be partly due to senile enophthalmos, a sinking of the globe within the orbit. Drance *et al.* (1967) also found an age-related loss of visual field, particularly in the superior field. They found a decrease in sensitivity of 1 dB per decade averaged over the total visual field. Haas *et al.* (1986) found that age appeared to influence the sensitivity of the upper half of the visual field to a greater extent than the lower half, and the periphery and the centre were found to be more affected than the pericentric area. The sensitivity was found to decrease, on average, by 0.58 dB per decade.

Visual fields may be unintentionally restricted by a heavy library-type of spectacle frame, opaque side shields on safety spectacles, or the lens type. Any person requiring full visual fields for an occupation or task should be provided with spectacle frames and lenses of a type that least restrict the field of view.

Head and eye movement

Detection ability is enhanced by both head and eye movements. Eye movements are controlled by four neurological systems (Robinson, 1968):

1. Saccadic
2. Smooth pursuit
3. Vestibular
4. Vergence.

The visual environment may be sampled by fast conjugate eye movements (400–600°/s) known as saccades, which locate an object of interest on the fovea. Fixation of the object is maintained by slow pursuit movements for objects that are moving at less than 45°/s. Corrective saccades are required to follow objects moving at speeds greater than 45°/s. The stabilization of the eyes with regard to the environment during head and body movements is the function of the vestibular system. The vergence system allows accurate fixation of the object of regard located at any distance in the visual field, and hence it acts as a range-finding system, which can interact with the other systems.

The extent of the horizontal and vertical eye movements is in the range of 45–50° either side of the primary position, but head movements generally occur when the eye movement exceeds 15°. Therefore, a person reading at a desk will lower their head rather than depress the eyes (Weston, 1962).

Tasks requiring frequent changes in direction of gaze can be visually fatiguing and cause discomfort. This is most likely to occur when the eyes are near the limit of their range. In addition, there will be different amounts of accommodation and convergence required for different viewing distances. Visual discomfort is therefore more likely to occur in people with poor convergence and fusion when viewing near tasks. A presbyopic worker wearing a bifocal prescription may have to adopt an unnatural head posture when the viewing distance is either at or above eye level. An example would be a pilot's instrument panel, some of which is above head level and requires the head to be tilted back to an unnatural angle to see through the near vision segment of the bifocal. Care should therefore be taken when prescribing for the presbyope; the type of lens and the height and size of the near addition segment must be appropriate for the task.

Light perception and visual adaptation

The visual system can operate over a very large range of luminances due to the actions of the photoreceptors – the rods and cones. At luminances below 10^{-6} cd/m^2 there is insufficient light for the visual system to operate. The rods function at luminance levels between 10^{-6} and 10^{-3} cd/m^2, which is referred to as scotopic vision. An intermediate state exists where both the rods and cones operate at levels between 10^{-3} and 3 cd/m^2; this is mesopic vision. Above luminances of 3 cd/m^2, the rods are completely saturated and only the cones function; this is photopic vision (Boyce, 1981).

The spectral responses of the rods and cones are different; the peak sensitivity for cones occurs at 555 nm and that for rods at 505 nm. The spectral response of the eye will change as luminance shifts from scotopic to photopic conditions, and this is known as the Purkinje shift. Colours are not visible under scotopic conditions, as only the rods are functioning. Colour is gradually recognized as the luminance level is increased, until full colour vision is acquired under photopic conditions.

Absolute threshold

The absolute threshold represents the smallest amount of light that gives rise to a visual sensation. The threshold will depend on the spectral nature of the light, which increases from white to red to violet (Gunkel and Gouras, 1963). The absolute threshold is found to increase with age. This is thought to be partly due to senile miosis and greater absorption of the crystalline lens, which reduce the amount of light reaching the retina. The latter is proportional to the pupil area, and therefore as the pupil size decreases with age, the amount of light reaching the retina will also decrease. There will also be a greater absorption of blue light within the crystalline lens as it yellows with age, resulting in a more marked increase in the blue light threshold when compared to other wavelengths.

Dark adaptation

Retinal sensitivity can increase by 100 000 times after half an hour in a dark room. This remarkable sensitivity to the detection of light is called dark adaptation, i.e. change in absolute threshold with time. The process has three phases:

1. A rapid phase involving neural mechanisms
2. A medium-length phase of adjustment of the pupil size
3. A slow phase due to the regeneration of the photosensitive pigments.

The regeneration of the cone pigments is faster than that of the rods, being approximately 2 minutes and 8 minutes respectively. Adaptation is rapid if the initial and final adaptation luminances are both in the photopic range, as only the cones are involved. If the initial luminance level is in the scotopic range then adaptation takes longer, as it involves pigment regeneration of both the rods and cones.

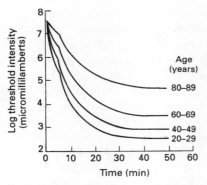

Fig. 1.1 *Dark adaptation as a function of age. The threshold intensity is measured in micromillilamberts (after McFarland et al., 1960).*

The adaptation process is influenced by such factors as size and colour of the adapting and test fields, initial and final luminance of the test field, and the area of retina stimulated.

Age will also influence the dark adaptation process (Domey and McFarland, 1961; Jackson *et al.*, 1999). The dark adaptation curves for increasing ages lie parallel to one another, and the threshold increases (Figure 1.1). The dark adaptation is slower with age, and the same level of sensitivity is not achieved. The intensity of the light stimulus has to be doubled for each 13 years of age (Domey and McFarland, 1961). The slowing of the rod-mediated dark adaptation is attributed to the delayed rhodopsin regeneration, and the amount of time taken to reach within 0.3 log units of baseline scotopic sensitivity increases by 2.76 min/decade (Jackson *et al.*, 1999). These changes in the rod-mediated dark adaptation may be partly responsible for the fact that many elderly drivers feel unsafe driving at night.

Differential threshold

When the eye has adapted to a new luminance level, it can then function to distinguish or detect objects. The ability of the eye to detect a stimulus can be described in terms of the smallest increment of luminance (ΔI) that can be detected from a uniform background luminance (I). This is known as the differential threshold, and ΔI is usually directly proportional to $I(\Delta I/I = 1/100)$; this is the Fechner Law (Davson, 1990). Once again, other factors that will influence the differential threshold include the size and colour of the object, state of adaptation of the eye, and duration of

exposure. The differential threshold also increases with age, as does the effect of glare upon the differential threshold (Wolf, 1960). This is thought to be partly due to the scattering of light by the ocular media, which occurs with age (Weale, 1961).

The ability to see well at low levels of illumination is not a common requirement of many occupations. However, it is particularly important in tasks such as driving, flying or sailing at night, or photographic darkroom work.

Flicker frequency

If the frequency of a flickering light is steadily increased, a point will be reached where the light appears to be steady. The frequency at which the flicker ceases is known as the critical fusion frequency (CFF). It can be taken as a measure of the temporal resolving power of the visual system. The CFF depends on many factors, including size, colour and luminance of the stimulus; the area of the retina being stimulated; and the duration of the flashes. The CFF increases with the size and luminance of the flickering stimulus, and it is generally higher in the peripheral than in the central retinal regions. Fluorescent lights and movie films flicker but we are unaware of it, because they are designed to flicker at a rate above the CFF. Some reports suggest a decrease in the CFF after 50 years of age, and hence lights that are seen to be flickering by a younger person may be seen as fused/steady by an older person (Brozek and Keys, 1945; Weale, 1965). This is believed to be partly due to an increase in the persistence of stimuli in the nervous system with age (Axelrod, 1963; Botwinick, 1978).

Contrast sensitivity

Contrast sensitivity is the ability to detect border contrast, and is the reciprocal of the minimum perceptible contrast. It is an evaluation of the detection of objects, usually presented as sinusoidal gratings, of varying spatial frequencies and of variable contrast. The acuity for gratings is specified by spatial frequency in cycles/degree. When the spatial frequency is plotted as a function of the contrast between the bars forming the grating, the plot is termed the contrast sensitivity function. The contrast sensitivity is the reciprocal of the contrast threshold; contrast $= L_{max} - L_{min}/L_{max} + L_{min}$ where L_{max} and

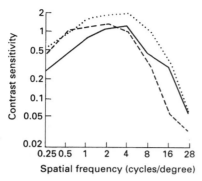

Fig. 1.2 *Contrast sensitivity functions for different age groups (———) 8–15 years, (·····) 18–39 years and (- - -) 45–66 years. The contrast sensitivity is the reciprocal of the contrast threshold. Contrast* = $L_{max} - L_{min}/L_{max} + L_{min}$, *where* L_{max} *and* L_{min} *are the maximum and minimum luminances (cd/m²) in the grating display, respectively (after Arundale, 1978; reproduced by kind permission of the British Medical Association).*

L_{min} are the maximum and minimum luminances (cd/m²) in the grating display respectively.

It is generally accepted that the contrast sensitivity improves with age up to the thirties, and Figure 1.2 shows that the 18–39 years age group is optimal at all frequencies. The 45–66 years age group is similar up to 0.5 cycles/degree, and then the contrast sensitivity decreases, especially in the 4–20 cycles/degree range (Arundale, 1978). If the contrast sensitivity is measured as a function of retinal illumination, the sensitivity difference is reduced but not eliminated. (A visual acuity of 6/6 is equivalent to 30 cycles/degree.) Binocular thresholds are lower than monocular ones, and this is most marked for high frequencies. As the environment and the tasks performed within it are not composed of high contrast objects alone, but also of those of medium and low contrast, it is often suggested that contrast sensitivity is a better assessment of a person's visual capabilities to perform tasks such as driving.

Recognition

Static acuity
Static visual acuity is the capacity for seeing distinctly the details of a stationary object. Quantitatively, it is represented in two ways: first, as the reciprocal of the minimum angle of resolution, in minutes of arc; and secondly, as the Snellen fraction.

The usual method of specifying visual acuity (VA) is by using letters, which are expressed as a Snellen fraction. The Snellen letter is constructed on an equal-sided grid, so that each limb width is one-fifth of the letter height. The letter size is expressed as a Snellen fraction in the form 6/6, 6/9, 6/12, etc., where the numerator is the test distance in metres and the denominator is the distance at which the letter subtends 5 min of arc. Normal visual acuity by this notation is 6/6, which means that a letter of 5 min of arc with a limb separation of 1 min of arc can be resolved at 6 m.

A new chart for recording visual acuity has been designed to overcome some of the problems of the traditional Snellen Chart. It was originally designed by Bailey and Lovie (1976), and is now accepted as the test of choice for research and is being used increasingly in clinical practice. There are five letters on each line, and each line of letters increases in a constant ratio of 1.26 (0.1 log unit steps). The visual acuity is recorded in terms of log MAR score (MAR = minimum angle of resolution). A Snellen acuity of 6/6 is equivalent to a logMAR of zero ($\log_{10} 1 = 0$), and 6/60 is equivalent to 1 ($\log_{10} 10 = 1$). Each line has a score of 0.1, and each letter has a score of 0.02; therefore, if two letters were missed on the 6/6 line the score would be 0.04.

There are numerous factors – physical, physiological, and psychological – that can influence the ability of the visual system to see details. These include luminance, contrast, the spectral nature of light, the size and intensity of the surrounding field, the region of the retina stimulated, the distance and size of the object, the time available to see the object, glare, a foggy/steamy atmosphere, the refractive error, pupil size, age, attention, IQ, boredom, the ability to interpret blurred images, general health, and emotional state (Riggs, 1965; Westheimer, 1987). Some of the major factors are discussed below.

Distance of the task
Naturally, the distance of the task from the observer and the size of the detail of the task affect the retinal image size, and hence the visual acuity required to distinguish it. The distance of the task also determines the level of accommodation and convergence and the degree of uncorrected refractive error or phoria that may be tolerated. Working distances may be classified

as: far (> 2 m), intermediate-to-near (< 2 m and > 30 cm), and very near (< 30 cm) (Grundy, 1988). Examples of tasks involving far working distances include driving a vehicle and flying an airplane; intermediate-to-near tasks include secretarial work, VDU operating and lathe operating; and very near tasks include sewing, micro-electronics assembly work and watch repairing.

The amount of accommodation decreases with age, and generally after their mid-forties workers require a spectacle prescription to focus near objects clearly and comfortably. As the range of accommodation reduces with age, the range of clear vision through the various near vision additions becomes smaller. Table 1.1 shows the range of clear vision obtainable by the emmetrope (or ametrope with corrected distance vision) through the various additions according to the patient's usable accommodation (Grundy, 1987). It must be remembered that it shows the average amount of accommodation for the various ages, and that there is natural variation between individuals and accommodation is also influenced by general health and certain medications. The amount of accommodation that can be exerted for a prolonged period of time is one-half the total accommodation available (Millodot and Millodot, 1989), and Table 1.1 takes this into account when stating the amount of usable accommodation.

Table 1.1 can be used to indicate the most effective combination of powers of prescriptions to provide clear vision at all the required distances, and it also shows that it is not always possible to fulfil the needs of the presbyope with a 'normal' prescription. For example, consider the visual requirements of a 45-year-old VDU operator who needs to see the VDU screen at 70 cm and the documents at 35 cm. The amplitude of accommodation is $+3.50$ dioptres (D) for a 45-year-old, and the amount that can be exerted for a prolonged period of time is half that (i.e. $+1.75$ D). Inspection of the 'age' column of Table 1.1 shows that $+1.25$ D addition will give clear vision from 33.33 to 80 cm, and so the visual requirements will be satisfied. If, however, the operator is older (e.g. 55 years), it is not possible to view the required distances with a single addition. The 55-year-old will have $+1.50$ D of accommodation, of which $+0.75$ D is usable. To focus the screen at 70 cm an addition of $+0.75$ or $+1.00$ D could be used, but the document at 35 cm will not be seen

clearly with either. To focus at 35 cm an addition of $+2.25$ D is required, and therefore a lens that incorporates these powers must be selected.

It must be remembered that the ageing eye takes longer to relax accommodation when looking from near to far. This usually gives rise to complaints of temporary blurred vision when looking from a near task to some objects of attention in the distance. Also, if the working distance is very close, base in prism may be required to take the strain off the convergence system.

Size of task

The size of the critical detail of the task needs to be taken into account so that the angle subtended at the eye, and hence the visual acuity necessary to perform the task comfortably and efficiently, can be calculated. The retinal image size of any object is inversely proportional to its distance from the eye. Therefore objects may differ greatly in physical dimensions but form similar retinal image size due to the fact that they are viewed at different distances. So, whilst the visual acuity may be the same, the demands made upon accommodation and convergence may be different. A very small object may have to be placed very close for the detail to be large enough to be resolved, but this will require good accommodation and convergence.

The angle subtended at the eye, and hence the visual acuity required, can be calculated mathematically (Figure 1.3):

$$\text{Tan visual angle} = \frac{\text{size of critical detail}}{\text{working distance}} = \frac{x}{d}$$

or graphically using a Nomogram (see Figure 2.1). Table 1.2 shows the optimum visual acuity required for the different visual angles (Grundy, 1988). The visual acuity necessary should be approximately twice that of the minimum calculated (Grundy, 1981) so that the individual is not working at their limit. If the visual angle is less than 3 min of arc, then it may be worthwhile considering magnification to increase the angular subtense of the task at the eye. This is particularly useful in the electronics industry. Magnification may be provided by hand- or stand-magnifiers (which may have built-in illumination), monocular or binocular loupes, or more complicated devices such as microscopes, telescopes, and binoculars for distant objects or projection devices.

Table 1.1 Range of clear vision (cm) with reading prescriptions (reproduced by kind permission of J.W. Grundy and *Optometry Today*, 1987)

Age (years)		40	42	45	48	50	52	55	60	65
Amplitude of accommodation (D)		4.50	4.00	3.50	3.00	2.50	2.00	1.50	1.00	0.50
Usable accommodation (D)		2.25	2.00	1.75	1.50	1.25	1.00	0.75	0.50	0.25
Range of clear vision (cm)										
Power of add (D)	Plano	44.4 / Infinity	50.0 / Infinity	57.1 / Infinity	66.6 / Infinity	80.0 / Infinity	100.0 / Infinity	133.3 / Infinity	200.0 / Infinity	400.0 / Infinity
	+0.50	36.4 / 200.0	40.0 / 200.0	44.4 / 200.0	50.0 / 200.0	57.1 / 200.0	66.7 / 200.0	80.0 / 200.0	100.0 / 200.0	133.3 / 200.0
	+0.75	33.3 / 133.3	36.4 / 133.3	40.0 / 133.3	44.4 / 133.3	50.0 / 133.3	57.1 / 133.3	66.7 / 133.3	80.0 / 133.3	100.0 / 133.3
	+1.00	30.8 / 100.0	33.3 / 100.0	36.4 / 100.0	40.0 / 100.0	44.4 / 100.0	50.0 / 100.0	57.1 / 100.0	66.7 / 100.0	80.0 / 100.0
	+1.25	28.6 / 80.0	30.8 / 80.0	33.3 / 80.0	36.4 / 80.0	40.0 / 80.0	44.4 / 80.0	50.0 / 80.0	57.1 / 80.0	66.7 / 80.0
	+1.50	26.7 / 66.7	28.6 / 66.7	30.8 / 66.7	33.3 / 66.7	36.4 / 66.7	40.0 / 66.7	44.4 / 66.7	50.0 / 66.7	57.1 / 66.7
	+1.75	25.0 / 57.1	26.7 / 57.1	28.6 / 57.1	30.8 / 57.1	33.3 / 57.1	36.4 / 57.1	40.0 / 57.1	44.4 / 57.1	50.0 / 57.1
	+2.00	23.5 / 50.0	25.0 / 50.0	26.7 / 50.0	28.6 / 50.0	30.8 / 50.0	33.3 / 50.0	36.4 / 50.0	40.0 / 50.0	44.4 / 50.0
	+2.25	22.2 / 44.4	23.5 / 44.4	25.0 / 44.4	26.7 / 44.4	28.6 / 44.4	30.0 / 44.4	33.3 / 44.4	36.4 / 44.4	40.0 / 44.4
	+2.50	21.1 / 40.0	22.2 / 40.0	23.5 / 40.0	25.0 / 40.0	26.7 / 40.0	28.6 / 40.0	30.8 / 40.0	33.3 / 40.0	36.4 / 40.0
	+2.75	20.0 / 36.4	21.1 / 36.4	22.2 / 36.4	23.5 / 36.4	25.0 / 36.4	26.7 / 36.4	28.6 / 36.4	30.8 / 36.4	33.3 / 36.4
	+3.00	19.1 / 33.3	20.0 / 33.3	21.1 / 33.3	22.2 / 33.3	23.5 / 33.3	25.0 / 33.3	26.7 / 33.3	28.6 / 33.3	30.8 / 33.3
	+3.25	18.2 / 30.8	19.1 / 30.8	20.0 / 30.8	21.1 / 30.8	22.2 / 30.8	23.5 / 30.8	25.0 / 30.8	26.7 / 30.8	28.6 / 30.8
	+3.50	17.4 / 28.6	18.2 / 28.6	19.1 / 28.6	20.0 / 28.6	21.1 / 28.6	22.2 / 28.6	23.5 / 28.6	25.0 / 28.6	26.7 / 28.6

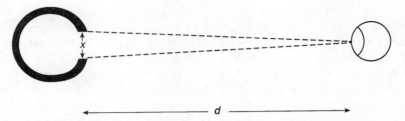

Fig. 1.3 *Angular size of the critical detail (d, working distance; x, size of critical detail).*

Table 1.2 Visual acuity and angular size of critical detail (reproduced by kind permission of J.W. Grundy and Butterworth–Heinemann, 1988)

	Angular size of critical detail (minutes of arc)	Minimum VA required	Optimum VA required	
Large	10.0	6/60	6/30	N20
Medium	6.0	6/36	6/18	N12
Small	3.0	6/18	6/9	N6
Very small	1.5	6/9	6/4.5	N3
Minute	0.75	6/4.5	Magnification + good VA required	

The near point equivalents refer to a viewing distance of 40 cm. VA, visual acuity.

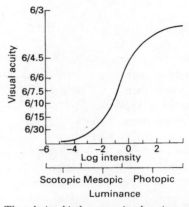

Fig. 1.4 *The relationship between visual acuity and luminance (measured in millilamberts) (König's data replotted by Hecht, 1934).*

Luminance and contrast

Two major factors that influence visual acuity are luminance and contrast. The influence of luminance upon visual acuity is shown in Figure 1.4. The capacity of the visual system to resolve details increases with increasing luminance, although there is a level beyond which visual acuity does not increase; in fact it may diminish due to disability glare. Contrast has a maximal effect on visual acuity at low levels of illumination, but a minimal effect at high levels.

Age

There is a small decline in visual acuity with age. The general causes are cataract, macular degeneration and glaucoma, particularly in the over-70 years age group (Grey *et al.*, 1989). However, visual acuity is not normally affected during the working lifetime (Figure 1.5).

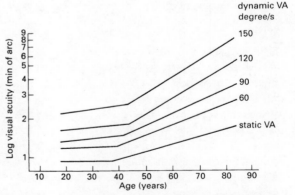

Fig. 1.5 *Static and dynamic visual acuities as a function of age. (After Hills, 1975; Crown copyright is reproduced with the permission of the Controller of HMSO.)*

Time available

The time available to view the letters etc. will influence the visual acuity measured. It has been estimated that a person can transmit up to 10 bits/s (a bit is a unit of information) of visually displayed information. This is a very small amount of information, when it is estimated that the human sensory system has a capacity to transmit millions of bits/s. Therefore it is not the input of the visual system that limits the visual performance, but the processing, decision-making and motor output. Letters can usually be recognized in under a second and, obviously, the better the illumination and the larger the letter, the faster the recognition time.

Refractive error

It is generally agreed that in early childhood the normal eye is hypermetropic. Later, the refraction shifts towards emmetropia until the early twenties. The refraction then stays relatively stable until the forties, when a hypermetropic shift may occur. In the later years there may be a myopic shift, known as index myopia, which occurs due to nuclear sclerosis of the crystalline lens. The astigmatism also changes with age. Most children have astigmatism 'with the rule', i.e. the vertical meridian of the cornea is steeper than the horizontal. This changes throughout life so that the majority of people in later life show 'against the rule' astigmatism, i.e. the horizontal meridian of the cornea is steeper than the vertical. The greatest change in astigmatism occurs between the ages of 30 and 50 years (Weale, 1963).

An ametropic person generally requires a spectacle prescription. However, for certain tasks it may be beneficial to leave the eyes uncorrected. For example, uncorrected myopes have been found to be far more efficient at their hosiery task than hyperopes, as they did not have to accommodate to see the task detail. Various surveys over the years have shown that many people have uncorrected or insufficiently corrected refractive errors that may affect visual acuity, efficiency and comfort (Ungar, 1971; Grundy, 1984; Anon, 1996). Often it is presbyopic workers whose visual efficiency is reduced, as they require a near vision addition that they fail to have updated regularly.

Vernier acuity

The type of visual acuity discussed so far has been form acuity – the ability to discriminate between two small parts of an object. However, in some occupations line detail is required – for example, the use of micro- meters or precision gauges requires the discrimination of a break in contour or alignment – i.e. vernier acuity. The visual system is extremely sensitive to these details, and it is approximately one-twentieth of the corresponding angle for details to be resolved in form acuity (Grundy, 1988). If the form acuity for a certain distance is known, then it is relatively easy to calculate the equivalent visual angle for vernier acuity and the actual size that may be resolved, and *vice versa*. Misalignments of segments of a divided line of approximately 3 s of arc can be detected at moderately high levels of illumination, whereas the minimum angle of resolution is between 30 and 60 s of arc (Westheimer, 1987).

Dynamic visual acuity

The visual system can not only detect moving objects, but also discriminates and identifies the object. Dynamic (kinetic) visual acuity is the term used to define the acuity based on a moving target. The discrimination of detail of a moving object depends upon the ability of the eyes to remain fixated on it. At slow speeds the acuity is nearly the same as for static tests, but as the speed is increased the dynamic visual acuity decreases. Head movements are required for target speeds of above 60°/s, otherwise there is a marked drop in acuity. Dynamic visual acuity is not directly related to static visual acuity. It is influenced by target angular velocity, target exposure time, luminance, contrast, extent of visual field, paramacular visual acuity, method of tracking head and eye movements, reaction time, learning factors and fatigue (Ludvigh and Miller, 1958; Fergenson and Suzansky, 1973). A progressive decline in dynamic visual acuity has been shown to occur with age (see Figure 1.5; Burg, 1966; Reading, 1968). Younger people are better at tracking fast moving objects than older. This is partly due to an increase in the latent period of onset of a following eye movement as age increases (Sharpe and Sylvester, 1978; Spooner *et al.*, 1980).

Dynamic visual acuity is believed to be a more reliable measure of a person's ability to perform such tasks as driving or inspection tasks on a conveyor belt than the conventional static test.

Colour discrimination

Under photopic conditions, the human visual system has a highly developed colour sense. The sensation of colour is subjective, but it can be analysed in terms of three attributes; hue, saturation and luminous intensity. It has been estimated that a person with normal colour vision can discriminate millions of detectably different colours. These estimates are based upon comparison of colours placed adjacent to one another, but for absolute judgements only about 30 colours can be identified reliably (Bishop and Crook, 1961). The fine colour discrimination of the visual system is such that it can discriminate most colours whose wavelengths differ by less than 5 nanometres (nm).

Colour discrimination depends upon:

- The state of adaptation of the retina
- The region of the retina stimulated
- Simultaneous contrast
- Successive contrast.

Colour vision extends 20–30° from the fovea. Beyond this the ability to discern colour is lost, as is the case in scotopic conditions. The ability to discriminate a colour from its background will be influenced greatly by the respective colours. This is especially the case when the luminance contrast between the object and its background is very small, so that colour contrast is the only method of discrimination. The colour of an object can also be perceived differently depending on the colour of the background. This is known as simultaneous contrast, when the colour of the object tends towards the complementary colour of the background – for example, a grey spot viewed against a red background will appear greenish. Similarly, a person may complain of coloured afterimages due to prior exposure to another colour. This is known as successive contrast, where the after-image tends towards the complementary colour of the initial exposure – for example, after viewing an ocular fundus through a red-free filter (i.e. a green filter), a reddish after-image is seen.

Colour-defective vision may be congenital or acquired. The most common type is congenital, which affects more men (8 per cent) than women (0.5 per cent) (Voke, 1980). Three types of defective colour vision are usually recognized; anomalous trichromatism, dichromatism and monochromatism. The last is total colour blindness, in which there is a perception of luminance but not of colour. Anomalous trichromatism is a form of defective colour vision in which the three primary colours (red, green and blue) are necessary to see any colour, but the proportions of

each primary are not the same as those required by a normal. Dichromatism is a form of colour vision deficiency in which all colours can be matched by a mixture of only two primary colours.

In protanomaly, a high proportion of red is needed when mixing red and green to match a yellow, whereas in deuteranomaly a high proportion of green is needed; the latter case being the most common type of congenital colour defect. Tritanomaly is where an abnormally high proportion of blue is needed when mixing blue and green to match a given blue-green stimulus. Protanopia is a condition in which only two hues are seen; below 495 nm all radiations appear bluish, whereas above it they all appear yellowish. Hence the colours confused will be reds, oranges, blue-greens and greys. Deuteranopia is a condition in which red and green are confused; the longer wavelengths appear yellow and the shorter wavelengths appear blue. Tritanopia is a very rare condition in which blue and yellow are confused; the reds, bluish greens and greens are seen clearly.

Colour is commonly used to code information, and hence the correct identification of colours may be very important for efficient work. It is also used with hazard warnings and safety messages. For example, the contents of fire extinguishers, pipelines, electric cable and microelectronic components are all colour-coded. Colour coding can also be used in sorting tasks and filing systems, as it can reduce search times and improve efficiency. Tasks involving the judgement of colour can be divided into four classes (Cole, 1973):

1. Those requiring comparative judgements of colour, as when precise matches of colour are made or subtle colour differences need to be appreciated – e.g. mixing dye stuffs to match a sample.
2. Those requiring connotative recognition of colour, as when colour is used to code information – e.g. signal lights.
3. Those requiring denotative colour recognition, where colour is used to identify an object – this is often used in filing systems or in sorting tasks.
4. Those requiring aesthetic colour judgements, where colours are selected for their harmonious effects or evocative qualities – e.g. interior decorating, the advertising industry.

Guidelines have been given concerning the suitability of people with colour vision defects for certain occupations, see Appendix A (Voke, 1980).

Depth perception

The visual system can effectively judge the distance of objects using both monocular and binocular cues, the latter being the most sensitive measure. A perception of depth can be achieved by a monocular subject from the following cues: geometric perspective, aerial perspective, interposition, distribution of light and shade, interpretation of size, and parallax. The binocular cues to depth are stereopsis (by utilizing the small angular disparity between the two eyes) and convergence.

Obviously depth perception is not necessary for all tasks, but stereopsis is of vital importance for jobs utilizing stereoscopic viewing instruments (e.g. aerial contour photography and binocular microscopy) and for other jobs such as fork-lift truck operators, crane drivers and pilots. Hofstetter and Bertsch (1976) found that stereopsis does not decline between 8 and 46 years of age, but beyond 46 years it does appear to decline (Bell *et al.*, 1972). Brown *et al.* (1993) found that stereopsis reduced from about 16 s of arc in the under 60 years age group to 27 s of arc in the 60–70 years age group. Wright and Wormald (1992) found that only 27 per cent of their study group over the age of 65 years had full stereopsis as assessed by the Frisby stereotest.

Depth perception can be affected by such factors as uncorrected refractive errors, uncompensated muscle balances, amblyopia, anisometropia and squints. At low levels of illumination depth perception is of a very low order, which may be a problem for some occupations (e.g. photographers who need to cut photographic papers or pour chemical solutions in a dark room). In such circumstances, extra care needs to be taken to avoid accidents (Grundy, 1988).

Also of great importance for maximum visual comfort when performing a task is the stability of binocular vision, especially for near tasks. Stress may be caused by an uncompensated excessive horizontal or vertical phoria. Heterophorias can be induced by prolonged periods of work. Some studies have reported an increase in esophoria after sustained fixation at near (Stenhouse-Stewart, 1945; Ehlrich, 1987). Stress may also be caused by deficiencies in the fusional reserves or due to a low near point of convergence when near tasks are being carried out.

The advantages of binocular vision over monocular vision are:

- the presence of stereopsis
- improved visual acuity
- a lower absolute threshold
- a closer near point of accommodation
- an enlarged field of peripheral vision
- slightly brighter perception of objects.

VISIBILITY OF TASKS

The ability to perform a task safely, efficiently and comfortably depends upon its visibility as well as on the visual capabilities of the employee. Naturally, the better the visibility, the easier it is to perform the task. The factors that influence the visibility of a task are:

- The size of the task
- The distance of the task
- Illumination
- Contrast
- Colour
- The time available to view the task
- The movement of the task
- Glare
- The atmospheric conditions.

How these factors affect visibility has been investigated by many researchers using different methods. One method is indirect; the influence of lighting, contrast, size of task, etc. upon job performance is assessed by measuring, for example, speed and accuracy. The simplest of the factors to adjust is the illumination, and therefore many studies have investigated its influence. The aim is to establish the range of lighting conditions that permits an improvement in job performance. With any study, either in a real environment or laboratory simulated conditions, certain factors must be taken into account and controlled if possible, e.g. motivation, methods of payment of employees, and type of work (and therefore level of visual difficulty of the task). There are other problems that are encountered in studies in the real environment (Henderson and Marsden, 1972):

- It is difficult to define the contrast in a task by reflectances from the detail and background

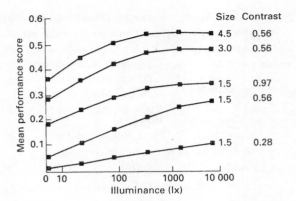

Fig. 1.6 *Mean performance scores for Landolt ring charts (after Weston, 1945).*

because it is rare for the surfaces to be perfectly matt

- The exposure time can be hard to control – the viewing time allowed for many tasks is not externally controlled
- The size of the task can be variable and can be altered by the employee moving closer to the task and hence increasing the angular subtense at the eye.

One study in particular has influenced the lighting codes of Britain. Weston (1945) assessed the effects of illumination upon a self-paced scanning task. The observers viewed an array of 256 Landolt rings, the gaps of which were randomly arranged in one of eight directions, and they were asked to cancel all the rings with a gap in a specific orientation. The total time taken and the number of errors made, along with the number of appropriate rings missed, were recorded. Allowing for the time required for physically cancelling the rings, it was then possible to give a value of performance in terms of speed and accuracy. The test was repeated using different levels of illumination, different contrasts between the rings and their background, and different ring sizes. The results are presented in Figure 1.6, which shows the mean performance for different contrast, size and illumination producing relative visual performance curves. Four main conclusions can be drawn from the results:

1. Increasing the illumination produces an increase in performance, but this follows the law of diminishing returns – i.e. smaller and smaller
2. The point of the maximum performance is

different for rings of different sizes and contrast – the smaller the size and the lower the contrast, the higher the level of illumination at which maximum performance occurs
3. Larger improvements in performance can be achieved by changing the task size or contrast than by increasing the illumination
4. Increasing the illumination does not make it possible to perform a visually difficult task (i.e. one of small size and poor contrast) to the same level as a visually easy task.

Although the findings above do, in principle, apply to all tasks, the relationship between illumination on the task and performance achieved will vary according to the type of task. In summary, the effect of illumination upon task performance will vary according to:

- The visual difficulty of the task
- The extent to which the visual part of the task determines the overall performance.

The greater the visual difficulty, the greater the effect of the illuminance, whereas in a task such as audiotyping (where there is only a small visual component) the effect of illuminance upon the overall task performance will be small.

To determine the optimum illumination levels for a task the contrast and size need to be measured and, as mentioned, it is not easy to measure the contrast of a practical task. Weston therefore developed a simplified method, which avoided measuring the task contrast. He used 0.9 reflectance to give one contrast curve, which meant that only the size needed to be measured. This provided the basis for the illumination standards in the CIBSE Code (1994). These recommendations apply to tasks of normal contrast and reflectance. If, however, the contrast or reflectances are low, or if mistakes are made due to wrong perception and these are likely to be dangerous or costly, the recommended illumination should be increased.

Studies by Blackwell and Blackwell (1971, 1980) concerning the visibility of tasks have influenced the American codes for lighting. The initial experiments carried out investigated the threshold detection of static disc targets, and later experiments involved the detection of dynamic targets. The dynamically presented targets were believed to create conditions more similar to a practical task.

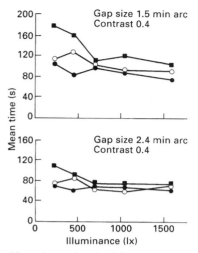

Fig. 1.7 *Mean times taken for different age groups examining Landolt ring charts.* ● *16–30 years;* ○ *31–45 years;* ■ *46–50 years (reproduced by kind permission of P. R. Boyce and The Chartered Institution of Building Services 1973).*

Older individuals require more light than younger ones to perform a similar task. This is partly due to the fact that, with increasing age, senile miosis and lowered transmission of the ocular media (especially the crystalline lens) reduce the light reaching the retina and also increase the light scatter. There is a three-fold reduction in the amount of light reaching the retina of a 60-year-old compared to that of a 20-year-old (Weale, 1961). The scattering of light means that glare becomes more of a problem with age, especially after the age of 40 years (Wolf, 1960; Reading, 1968; Paulson and Sjostand, 1980). Studies were carried out by Weston (1949), who investigated the effect of age upon visual performance at various lighting levels. The results showed a decrease in visual performance with age, but the performance of the older workers improved as the illumination was increased. A study by Boyce (1973) on a larger number of workers has also confirmed these findings for similar static tasks. The mean time taken by different age groups to read Landolt C charts of different size, contrast and illumination was measured. When the performance of older workers is compared with younger ones, the difference between the groups diminishes as the illumination is increased (Figure 1.7). While older workers generally gain more from an increase in illumination, it is unclear whether the same level of performance can be achieved by all ages by simply increasing the illumination.

Boyce (1973) found no significant difference between the age groups at the highest illuminances used (up to 10 000 lx).

The effect of veiling reflections and the complexity of the task have a significant impact on job performance. Veiling reflections are due to light from a high luminance surface (such as a luminaire) being reflected from a specular surface that is being viewed. These veiling reflections cause a reduction in performance due to the decreased contrast created on the task by the superimposed reflections.

The ability to discriminate colours is particularly influenced by age and illumination. It has been shown that with age there are more errors in hue discrimination in the blue-green and red regions (Verriest *et al.*, 1962). Similar effects have been found by Boyce and Simons (1977), who also found that the older age group made more errors in sorting the hues in the FM 100 hue test and that the number of errors decreased with increasing illumination.

The time available to see the task is important; too short a time exposure will reduce the visibility, especially if the task is moving.

Atmospheric conditions in such industries as foundries and mining, where there may be dust, smoke, or steam, will reduce visibility due to the absorption of light.

It is worthwhile mentioning that workers with poor visual acuity may also benefit from increased lighting levels (Silver *et al.*, 1980; Julian, 1984) and from more magnification to increase the retinal image size. As the majority of people with visual impairment are past the retirement age, the work that they undertake is mainly of a domestic nature. People with macular degeneration, a common cause of low visual acuity in the elderly, do benefit from an increase in illumination level (Sloan 1969; Sloan *et al.*, 1973), and their visual acuity was found to increase with an increase of luminance of the task up to 300 cd/m^2. A high level of illumination may also allow people to read continuous text without the aid of a magnifier, or with less magnification than normally required at lower levels of illumination. People with a loss of peripheral vision are more difficult to help, as the problem that they experience is of orientation and location of objects. Of most benefit to these workers is the provision of good contrast between objects and the background; for example, door frames and door handles should be a different colour to the door itself, and the edge of a step should also be highlighted – e.g. by a white strip on a dark step (Jay, 1980). The use of different colours, sizes, and shapes may also be useful to distinguish different containers. Objects are also more easily detected if a plain rather than patterned background is used (Sicurella, 1977).

To summarize, the illumination, size and contrast of the critical detail of the task have a marked influence upon job performance. However, other factors must not be forgotten, such as veiling reflections, complexity of the task and motivation. Whilst lighting is one of the easiest factors to adjust to improve visibility, it must be remembered that a greater increase in visibility may be achieved by altering the contrast or the size of the task. Also, the idea that the higher the level of lighting the better the visibility is not always the case, as visibility may be reduced by disability glare.

Visibility meters

The principle of visibility meters is to reduce the visibility of a task to threshold and then relate the amount of reduction to a measure of visibility. Visibility meters can be used in several ways:

- To assess the relative visibility of a task and compare it to a standard condition
- Once the level of visibility is established, to assess how much illumination is required to make the task as visible as the standard
- To immediately assess the effects of illumination, contrast, colour and polish of objects on the visibility.

Some meters reduce the visibility of the task to threshold by increasing the amount of veiling luminance and simultaneously decreasing the luminance from the task. This means that the overall luminance at the observer's eye does not change, nor does the state of adaptation of the eye (see Figure 1.8). A variable beam splitter can be used to achieve this effect. The visibility meter designed by Eastman (1968) uses a glass plate with varying amounts of chromium alloy vaporized on it for this. The veiling luminance is provided by either the task background or by a standard reflecting surface placed beside the task. Other meters use an internal light source to provide the veiling luminance.

Practical lighting installations do not generally produce completely diffuse illumination, and it is therefore necessary to have a measure of the extent

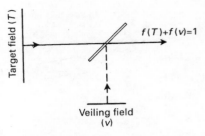

Fig. 1.8 *Visibility meter. $f(T)$ fraction of total luminance from the target field reaching the observer's eye; $f(v)$ fraction of total luminance from the veiling field reaching the observer's eye, $f(T) + f(v) = 1$. (After Eastman, 1968.)*

to which lighting conditions differ from reference conditions. The contrast-rendering factor (CRF) is a measure of the relative visibility under actual lighting conditions compared with the relative visibility under reference lighting conditions. (Reference lighting can be defined as that provided by an intergrating sphere where light is incident equally from all directions.) The CRF can be measured by viewing a task through a visibility meter. The task is first viewed under the actual lighting conditions, and the visibility is reduced to threshold by increasing the veiling luminance. The relative visibility of the target can be calculated:

$$\text{Relative visibility} = \frac{\text{Total luminance}}{\text{Luminance from target field}}$$

The relative visibility of the same task is measured under reference lighting conditions with the same adaptation luminance at the person's eye. The CRF can then be calculated and will have a value between zero and one; the nearer the CRF is to 1, the closer the actual conditions are to the reference conditions.

A simple and inexpensive visibility indicator that can be used to determine whether lighting levels for near vision tasks are adequate has been designed by Grundy (1989) (Figure 1.9). It is a card with dots of decreasing size and three different contrast levels (high, medium, and low). It can be used to compare the visual performance under lighting conditions in an optometrist's practice to those at home or work. The visual capability is assessed by asking the person to look down each of the three columns of different contrast levels in turn, until the dots can no longer be seen. This should be carried out under the recommended lighting level with any near prescription

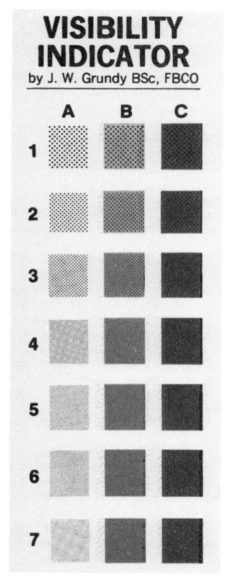

Fig. 1.9 *Visibility indicator (copyright J.W. Grundy, 1989).*

Table 1.3 Approximate levels of illumination (lux) that can be expected from 100-W and 60-W pearl bulbs (reproduced by kind permission of J.W. Grundy and *Optometry Today*, 1989)

	Distance (cm)							
	30	40	50	60	70	80	90	100
60-W bulb	900	500	320	225	165	125	100	80
100-W bulb	1800	1000	640	450	330	250	200	160

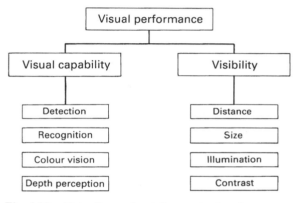

Fig. 1.10 *Major factors that influence visual performance.*

home, it may be that the illumination level is inadequate and that an additional light source will improve the visibility.

required, and in the same position and at the same distance as the task to be assessed. If a light meter is not available to measure the illumination level, an approximate guide as to the level, which may be provided by a 60- and 100-watt bulb in a simple reflector such as an anglepoise, is given in Table 1.3 (Grundy 1989). A note is made on the card where the dots can no longer be seen, and the test is then repeated by the person in the work or home situation. If the visibility is poorer at work or at

SUMMARY
Many factors influence visual performance, and Figure 1.10 summarizes the major ones. These are factors inherent in both the observer and the task itself. For maximum visual performance, the task and the worker should be assessed so as to match the requirements of the task with the visual capabilities of the worker.

REFERENCES
Anon (1996) Survey shows 16% of all UK drivers fail number-plate test. *Optom Today*, **Oct 21**, 10.

Arundale K. (1978) An investigation into the variation of human contrast sensitivity with age and ocular pathology. *Br J Ophthalmol*, **62**, 213–215.

Axelrod S. (1963) Cognitive tasks in several modalities. In *Processes of Aging*, Vol. 1 (eds Williams, R.H., Tibbits C. and Donahue W.). Atherton, New York, pp. 132–145.

Bailey I.L. and Lovie J.E. (1976) New design principles for visual acuity letter charts. *Am J Optom Physiol Opt*, **53**, 740–745.

Bell B., Wolf E. and Bernholz D. (1972) Depth perception as a function of age. *Aging Hum Dev*, **3**, 77–81.

Bishop H.P. and Crook M.H. (1961) Absolute identification of colour for targets presented against white and coloured backgrounds. USAF WADC Report 60-611. In *Vision and its Protection. A Symposium on Visual Efficiency and Eye Protection at Work* (eds Wigglesworth E.C. and Cole B.L.). Australian Optometrical Publishing Company, Sydney, Chapter 1.

Blackwell O.M. and Blackwell H.R. (1971) Visual performance data for 156 normal observers of various ages. *J Illum Eng Soc*, **1**, 3–13.

Blackwell H.R. and Blackwell O.M. (1980) Population data for 140 normal 20–30-year-olds for use in assessing some effects of lighting upon visual performance. *J Illum Eng Soc*, **9**, 158–74.

Botwinick J. (1978) *Aging and Behaviour*, 2nd edn. Springer, New York.

Boyce P.R. (1973) Age, illuminance, visual performance and preference. *Ltg Res Technol*, **5**, 125–139.

Boyce P.R. (1981) *Human Factors in Lighting*. Applied Science Publishers, London.

Boyce P.R. and Simons R.H. (1977) Hue discrimination and light sources. *Ltg. Res. Technol*, **9**, 125–140.

Brown B., Yap M.K.H. and Fan W.C.S. (1993) Decrease in stereoacuity in the 7th decade of life. *Ophthal Physiol Opt*, **13**, 138–142.

Brozek J. and Keys A. (1945) Changes in flicker fusion frequency with age. *J Consult Psychol*, **9**, 87–90.

Burg A. (1966) Visual acuity as measured by dynamic and static tests. *J Appl Psychol*, **6**, 460–466.

Burg A. (1968) Lateral visual field as related to age and sex. *J Appl Psychol*, **52**, 10–15.

CIBSE (1994) *Code for Interior Lighting*. The Chartered Institution of Building Services Engineers, Lighting Division, London.

Cole B.L. (1973) The handicap of abnormal vision. In *Vision and its Protection. A Symposium on Visual Efficacy and Eye Protection at Work* (eds Wigglesworth E.C. and Cole B.L.). Australian Optometrical Publishing Company, Sydney, pp. 37–43.

Davson H. (1990) *Davson's Physiology of the Eye*, 5th edn. Macmillan Press, London.

Domey R.G. and McFarland R.A. (1961) Dark adaptation as a function of age and individual prediction. *Am J Ophthalmol*, **51**, 1262–1268.

Drance S.M., Berry V. and Hughes A. (1967) Studies on the effect of age on the central and peripheral isopters of the visual field in normal subjects. *Am J Ophthalmol*, **63**, 1667–1672.

Eastman A.A. (1968) A new contrast threshold visibility meter. *J Illum Eng Soc*, **63**, 36–40.

Ehrlich D.L. (1987) Near vision stress: vergence adaptation and accommodative fatigue. *Ophthal Physiol Optics*, **7**, 353–357.

Fergenson P.E. and Suzansky J.W. (1973) An investigation of dynamic and static visual acuity. *Perception*, **2**, 343–356.

Fletcher R.J. (1961) *Ophthalmics in Industry*. Hatton Press, London, Chapter 5.

Grey R.H.B., Burns-Cox C.J. and Hughes A. (1989) Blind and partial sight registration in Avon. *Br J Ophthalmol*, **73**, 88–94.

Grundy J.W. (1981) Visual efficiency in industry. *Ophthal Opt*, **21**, 548–552.

Grundy J.W. (1984) When your car could break down through a visual defect. *Ophthal Opt*, **Feb 4**, 77–80.

Grundy J.W. (1987) A diagrammatic approach to occupational optometry and illumination. *Optom Today*, **Aug 1**, 503–508.

Grundy J.W. (1988) Prescribing and patient management: occupational and recreational considerations. In *Optometry* (eds Edwards K. and Llewellyn R.). Butterworths, London, pp. 475–485.

Grundy J.W. (1989) A visibility indicator. *Optom Today*, **Nov 20**, 6–10.

Gunkel R.D. and Gouras P. (1963) Changes in scotopic visibility thresholds with age. *Arch Ophthalmol*, **69**, 4–9.

Haas A., Flammer J. and Schneider U. (1986) Influence of age on the visual fields of normal subjects. *Am J Ophthalmol*, **101**, 199–203.

Hecht S. (1934) Vision II. The nature of the photoreceptor process. In *A Handbook of General Experimental Psychology* (ed. Murchinson C.). Clark University Press, Worcester, MA.

Henderson S.T. and Marsden A.M. (eds) (1972) *Lamps and Lighting*, 2nd edn. Edward Arnold, London.

Hills B.L. (1975) Some studies of movement perception, age and accidents. Report SRi 37, Department of the Environment, TRRL, Crowthorne, Berkshire.

Hofstetter H.W. and Bertsch J.D. (1976) Does stereopsis change with age? *Am J Optom Physiol Optics*, **53**, 644–667.

Jackson G.R., Owsley C. and McGwin G. (1999) Aging and dark adaptation. *Vision Res*, **39**, 3975–3982.

Jay P.A. (1980) Fundamentals. In *Light for Low Vision*, Proceedings of the Symposium held at University College, London on 4th April 1978 (ed. Greenhalgh R.). Partially Sighted Society, Doncaster, pp. 13–29.

Julian W.G. (1984) Variation in near visual acuity with illuminance for a group of 27 partially sighted people. *Ltg Res Technol*, **16**, 34–41.

Ludvigh E. and Miller J.W. (1958) Study of visual acuity during the ocular pursuit of moving test objects. 1. Introduction. *J Opt Soc Am*, **48**, 799–802.

McFarland R., Domey R.G., Warren A.B. and Ward D.C. (1960) Dark adaptation as a function of age. 1. A statistical analysis. *J Gerontol*, **15**, 149–154.

Millodot M. and Millodot S. (1989) Presbyopia correction and the accommodation in reserve. *Ophthal Physiol Optics*, **9**, 126–132.

Paulson L.E. and Sjostand J. (1980) Contrast sensitivity in the presence of a glare light. *Invest Ophthalmol Vis Sci*, **19**, 401–406.

Reading V.M. (1968) Disability glare and age. *Vision Res*, **8**, 207–214.

Riggs L.A. (1965) Visual acuity. In *Vision and Visual Perception* (ed. Graham C.H.). Wiley, New York, pp. 321–349.

Robinson D.A. (1968) The oculomotor control system: a review. *Proc IEEE*, **56**, 1032–1049.

Sharpe J.A. and Sylvester T. (1978) Effect of aging on horizontal smooth pursuit. *Invest Ophthalmol Vis Sci*, **17**, 465–468.

Sicurella V.J. (1977) Colour contrast as an aid for visually impaired persons. *Vis Impair Blind*, **71**, 252.

Silver J.H., Gould E.S., Irvine D. and Cullinan T.R. (1980) Visual acuity at home and in eye clinics. *Ophthal Opt*, **20**, 4.

Sloan L.L. (1969) Variation of acuity with luminance in ocular diseases and anomalies. *Doc Ophthalmol*, **20**, 384.

Sloan L.L., Habel A. and Feiock K. (1973) High illumination as an auxiliary reading aid in diseases of the macula. *Am J Ophthalmol*, **76**, 745–757.

Spooner J., Sakala S. and Bahol R. (1980) Effect of aging on eye tracking. *Arch Neurol*, **37**, 575–576.

Stenhouse-Stewart D.D. (1945) Some observations on a tendency to near point esophoria and possible contributory factors. *Br J Ophthalmol*, **29**, 37–42.

Ungar P. (1971) Sight at work. *Work Study*, **March**, 46–48.

Verriest G., Vandevyvere R. and Vanderdonck R. (1962) Nouvelles reserches se rapportant a l'influence du sexe et de l'age sur la discrimination chromatique ainsi qu'a la signification practique des resultants du test 100 hue de Farnsworth Munsell. *Res d'Optique*, **41**, 499.

Voke J. (1980) *Colour Vision Testing in Specific Industries and Professions*. Keeler, London.

Weale R.A. (1961) Retinal illumination and age. *Trans Illum Eng Soc*, **26**, 95–100.

Weale R.A. (1963) *The Ageing Eye*. Lewis, London.

Weale R.A. (1965) On the eye. In *Aging, Behaviour and the Nervous System* (eds Welford A.T. and Birren J.E.). C.C. Thomas, Springfield, IL, pp. 307–25.

Westheimer G. (1987) Visual acuity. In *Adler's Physiology of the Eye. Clinical Application*, 8th edn. CV Mosby Co., St Louis, MS, pp. 415–428.

Weston H.C. (1945) *The Relationship between Illumination and Visual Performance*. Industrial Health Research Board Report No. 87. HMSO, London.

Weston H.C. (1949) On age and illumination in relation to visual performance. *Trans Illum Eng Soc (Lond)*, **16**, 281.

Weston H.C. (1962) *Sight, Light and Work*, 2nd edn. Lewis, London.

Wolf E. (1960) Glare and age. *Arch Ophthalmol*, **64**, 502–514.

Wright L.A. and Wormald R.P.L. (1992) Stereopsis and aging. *Eye*, **6**, 473–476.

FURTHER READING

Boyce P.R. (1981) *Human Factors in Lighting*. Applied Science Publishers, London.

Henderson S.T. and Marsden A.M. (eds) (1972) *Lamps and Lighting*, 2nd edn. Edward Arnold, London.

Moses R.A. and Hart W.M. (eds) (1987) *Adler's Physiology of the Eye. Clinical Application*, 8th edn. CV Mosby Co., St Louis, MS.

Overington I. (1976) Vision and Acquisition. *Fundamentals of Human Visual Performance, Environmental Influences and Applications in Instrumental Optics*. Pentech Press, London.

Rosenbloom A.A. and Morgan M.W. (eds) (1986) *Vision and Aging. General and Clinical Perspectives*. Professional Press Books, New York.

Sekuler R., Kline D., and Dismukes K. (eds) (1982) *Aging and Human Visual Function*. Alan Liss Inc., New York.

Weale R.A. (1963) *The Ageing Eye*. Lewis, London.

2 Vision screening

The general purpose of any vision screening programme is to detect those people who have defective vision but who do not present with symptoms that result in them seeking optometric attention. Every occupation has specific visual requirements that must be met to perform tasks efficiently, safely and with comfort. Therefore the main aim of vision screening is to detect those people whose visual ability is below the standard required. Vision screening programmes are generally carried out either by government organizations, such as education authorities and the armed forces, or by employers. For instance, vision screening is commonly used to identify young children with defective vision, which can affect their progress at school.

There are a surprisingly high number of people with defective vision. The need for vision screening has been clearly demonstrated by the results of several surveys, which have shown that on average one-third of employees in industry have visual defects and are, therefore, presumed to be operating less efficiently (Rousell, 1979; Grundy, 1986). In fact, a study by Grundy (1984) found that 40.87 per cent of the employees whose task was to inspect piston rings for flaws were referred for full eye examination after a vision screening. The main reason for referral was found to be defective near vision. In general, the employees were unaware of their visual deficiencies and had never considered that their vision might not have been adequate for the task. A more recent voluntary eye screening service for drivers found that 16 per cent of all drivers failed the number-plate test. A total of 8000 drivers were screened at 24 Granada Service stations throughout the UK (Anon, 1996).

The prevalence of vision defects in school children increases with age, and has been reported to be about 30 per cent at 14 years of age (Walters, 1984). A more recent study has shown that 19.6 per cent of children screened had some form of visual defect (excluding colour vision deficiences), of whom 66 per cent were unaware of any problem (Thomson and Evans, 1999).

It would therefore appear from these few studies that vision screening is indeed a worthwhile exercise.

ADVANTAGES TO INDUSTRY OF VISION SCREENING

Bailey (1973) and Collins (1983) concur in their assessment of the advantages to industry of vision screening. These can be summarized as follows:

1. Better selection of personnel. Visual ability can be used in the selection of new employees or the transfer of employees to a task they can perform efficiently.
2. Identification of employees with visual disabilities. These may be due to an uncorrected refractive error or ocular pathology. If the visual problems cannot be corrected, then employees can be transferred to a task they would be visually capable of performing efficiently.
3. Improved employee–employer relationships.
4. Improved visual efficiency can result in:
   - increased productivity
   - fewer accidents and therefore reduced insurance costs
   - reduced absenteeism, as the task is less visually fatiguing.
5. Easier settlement of compensation claims.

Given that an employer decides in favour of a vision screening programme, what steps need to be taken? First, visual standards for the various tasks must be established. This may be a relatively straightforward procedure or, if the task is unique or highly complex, it may involve detailed analysis and assessment. Secondly, the method of screening must be selected, along with the appropriate tests. For advice on these matters, a professional person such as an optometrist can be consulted.

ESTABLISHING OCCUPATIONAL VISUAL STANDARDS

There are two methods of determining the appropriate visual standard for a particular occupation; by the use of predetermined visual standards, or by the establishment of the relationship between visual ability and job performance/competence.

Predetermined visual standards

Lists of standards of vision for various occupations may be found in the *Association of Optometrists Members' Handbook* and other optical diaries. Some standards are listed in Appendix D, including those for such occupations as visual display unit operators, private motorists and pilots. Different tasks require different visual capabilities. For example, train drivers must be able to recognize certain colours, whilst crane drivers need good depth perception. The standards listed can also be applied to occupations that are considered to have comparable visual requirements.

Relating visual ability to job competence

While it is quite simple to establish employees' visual ability, relating this to their job competence is more complicated. There is no satisfactory method of grading job competence, due to non-visual factors (such as age, intelligence, attitude, motivation, manual dexterity and motor reaction times) influencing the assessment. Bailey (1973) drew up a five-step programme for establishing the vision standard:

1. Choose a method for grading job competence.
2. Analyse the visual factors required for the task (see Visual Task Analysis, below).
3. Decide on criteria for visual competence, e.g. VA 6/9 or better, and stereopsis.
4. Screen the vision of two groups of employees, age- and sex-matched if possible, who are judged to be:
   - job competent
   - job incompetent.
5. Compare their grading of visual competence to job competence. If the appropriate vision standard has been chosen, then the majority of the visually incompetent should fall into the job-incompetent group.

Table 2.1 Occupational analysis (reproduced with kind permission of J.W. Grundy and *Optometry Today*, 1987)

Name and general description of the task	
Working distances	a. Far (beyond 200 cm) b. Intermediate (200–55 cm) c. Near (55–30 cm) d. Very near (Less than 30 cm)
Size of detail	a. Large (Angular size of critical detail over 10′) b. Medium (5′–10′) c. Small (3′–5′) d. Very small (2′–3′) e. Extremely small (1′–2′) f. Minute (less than 1′)
Main working positions	a. Sitting b. Standing c. Moving d. Mixture
Size of working areas (in which critical vision is required)	a. Large b. Medium c. Small
Head movements	a. Side to side b. Up and down c. Mixture
Direction of gaze	a. Ahead b. Up. c. Down d. Side e. Mixture
Changes in direction of gaze	a. Frequent b. Occasional c. Seldom
Movement of the task	a. Stationary b. Slow movement c. Fast
Potential danger	a. High risk b. Medium risk c. Low risk
Special accuracy or care	a. Required b. Limited requirements c. Not required
Binocular vision and stereoscopic requirements	a. Required b. Not important c. Monocular vision adequate
Colour vision requirement	a. Good colour discrimination required b. Limited requirements acceptable c. Not required
Visual fields	a. Good field required b. Fair field acceptable c. Not important
Visibility (i.e. the relationship between the size of detail, working distances, contrast, and time available for viewing the task)	a. Good b. Fair c. Poor
Type of lighting in use, its adequacy and suitability	
Eye protection requirements	a. Required b. Not required
Hazard(s)	a. Basic b. Impact 2 c. Impact 1 d. Molten metal e. Dust f. Gas g. Chemicals h. Radiation i. Laser j. Other

Grading job competence can be done in a number of ways, and Bailey (1973) suggests:

- Supervisor rating
- Quality and quantity of production
- Accident frequency
- Absenteeism
- Employee turnover
- Wages (if on piece-rate).

Visual task analysis

Before the vision screening can be carried out, there must be an analysis of the visual tasks involved in the occupation concerned. Analysing the visual factors required for the task is of crucial importance, and ideally any analysis should be carried out at the place of work (e.g. factory or office). Factors such as distance and size of the critical detail of the task should be assessed, along with need for colour discrimination, depth perception, body, head and eye posture, field of vision, eye movements required, and the contrast and illumination of the task. From the subsequent analysis, the important visual factors can be identified.

There are occasions when on-site analysis is not possible. A logical method for determining the visual factors required for a particular task has been proposed by Grundy (1987) and is designed to act as a simple reference guide for use by optometrists in a consulting room (Table 2.1).

From the knowledge of the distance and size of the critical detail of the task, the visual acuity necessary to discriminate the smallest detail can be determined.

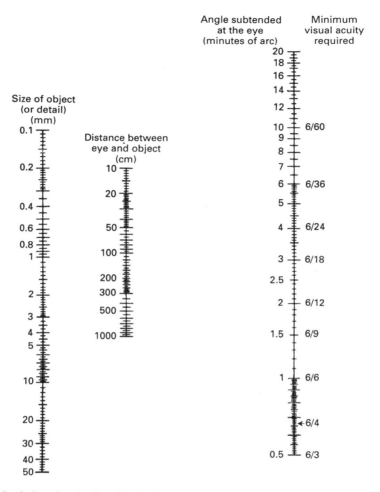

Fig. 2.1 *Nomogram for finding the visual angle subtended by objects of which the size and distance are known (after Weston, 1962).*

This can be calculated easily from a simple graphical method using a Nomogram, shown in Figure 2.1. For example, a task has a critical detail of 0.6 mm and it is viewed at 70 cm. When a straight line is drawn through these values, it will intercept the right-hand scale to indicate that the corresponding visual angle is 3.0 min of arc and the minimum visual acuity required is 6/18. It is important to remember that the values given are a measure of the resolving power of the eye, and higher standards are required for the task to be carried out for prolonged periods of time. It has been suggested that the visual acuity necessary for a demanding task should be approximately twice the minimum value (Grundy, 1981). Therefore, in the above case a visual acuity of 6/9 is advised. The employee can often move closer to the task, increasing the angular subtense at the eye, but this depends on the amount of accommodation and convergence available. The older presbyopic employee, who has a reduced amount of accommodation, may need an intermediate and a near prescription, depending on the distance of the task.

After analysis of the visual task, which allows the important visual factors to be determined, a standard can be set by one of the following methods:

- Choosing a standard believed to be necessary to work efficiently and safely, e.g. VA 6/12, distinguish principal colours. This can be tested by relating visual competence to job competence as described previously.

- Insisting on the normal level of visual capabilities for each factor chosen, e.g. VA 6/6, normal colour vision. This approach would exclude some who were capable of performing the task comfortably.

METHODS OF VISION SCREENING

Three techniques for screening vision may be used:

1. Modified clinical technique (MCT)
2. Instrument screeners
3. Computer programs.

Modified clinical technique

This method of screening is carried out by qualified personnel, e.g. optometrists, who assess the visual functions considered to be particularly important to job performance. The screening examination may therefore consist of any of the following (Bailey, 1973; Collins, 1983; Bennett and Rabbetts, 1984):

1. *History and symptoms.* This is particularly useful, as the history of a squint or amblyopic eye may be noted and this may reduce unnecessary referral. The presence of eyestrain when performing certain tasks can also be assessed.
2. *Visual acuity at any distance.* The measurement can be taken at the exact distance required, with the appropriate size of letters or task.
3. *External eye examination and ophthalmoscopy.* This allows detection of pathology of the eye that may otherwise go unnoticed. Ocular diseases do not always cause a reduction in vision that results in the person seeking medical attention.
4. *Retinoscopy.* This permits the precise degree of hyperopia or myopia to be assessed objectively. It will also indicate whether or not poor vision is due to the fact that spectacles are required.
5. *Amplitude of accommodation.* The result of this test will indicate whether the person can focus clearly and comfortably on a near task. Spectacles will generally be required by the older presbyopic person to see the task clearly.
6. *Binocular vision assessment.* This can include a cover test at the viewing distance required, motility, near point of convergence and stereopsis.

To avoid eyestrain, binocular vision needs to be stable and these tests will indicate whether the binocular functions are under stress for a particular task. The presence of a squint or phoria will be detected by the cover test.

7. *Visual field.* This can be assessed quite simply by a confrontation test to determine whether there is any marked reduction, such as a homonymous hemianopia or quadrantic defects. The central visual field can be assessed using an Amsler Chart. When held at 30 cm, this chart covers the central 10° of the field either side of fixation.
8. *Colour vision.* This can be assessed rapidly using tests such as the Ishihara pseudo–isochromatic plates, the City University test or the Saturated D-15. The Ishihara plates can be used to detect congenital colour vision defects, and the City University test and Saturated D-15 will detect acquired defects. However, if the task requires very fine discrimination of colours, then a more thorough test (such as the FM100 Hue) may be used. For further details regarding colour vision testing in industry and other professions, see Voke (1980) and Birch (2001).

Advantages and disadvantages of the MCT

Advantages of the MCT for vision screening include:

- Flexibility – tests can be selected depending on visual functions considered to be important for the task, and the tests can be performed at the appropriate distance
- The ability to assess the type and magnitude of any refractive error
- The possible detection of ocular pathology
- The detection of squint
- There will be very few false referrals.

Disadvantages include:

- Expense – it is an expensive method of screening due to the use of professional personnel such as optometrists
- It is time-consuming.

Instrument vision screeners

There are many different instrument vision screeners available, but most are basically modified stereoscopes. The eyepiece lenses are arranged so that their prismatic components simulate the viewing of a distant object, and the near vision is simulated by moving the targets closer, decreasing the separation between the half stereograms, or changing the lens power (i.e. introducing negative lenses).

The screeners usually have internal lighting, and the targets are mounted either on a rotary drum or separately on cards, which are changed manually or by remote control. The types of tests commonly included in the instrument screeners are:

- Visual acuity – distance and near (occasionally intermediate)
- Heterophoria – horizontal and vertical at distance and near
- Stereopsis
- Fusion
- Colour vision
- Fogging test
- Visual field
- Astigmatism.

Visual acuity

There are two methods used to assess the visual acuity, which is generally measured at distance and near:

1. Conventional letter charts, e.g. Illiterate Es
2. Specially designed optotypes, i.e. checkerboard targets (Figure 2.2). Some of the optotypes used measure detectability and not the actual resolving power of the eye. This can be an advantage in some cases; for example, if the work involves the inspection of materials for holes or flaws, then a detectability test is a more suitable measurement of visual acuity.

Regardless of the type of target used for visual acuity assessment, the results must be repeatable and provide valid measures. Results of several studies show that the distance visual acuity measures are repeatable, i.e. a high correlation is found between test and retest scores. Bailey and Cole (1968) investigated the validity of eight different vision screeners by comparing Snellen acuity measurements with those found from the screeners. They found that all but one of the screeners gave valid measures of the distance acuity.

Heterophoria

Many vision screeners include a test to measure the horizontal and vertical phorias. The test is generally based upon a dissociation technique, which can be used for distance and near measurements. Figure 2.3 shows an example of a horizontal and vertical phoria test. There is unfortunately a tendency for the distance

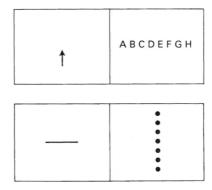

Fig. 2.3 *Horizontal and vertical phoria test targets.*

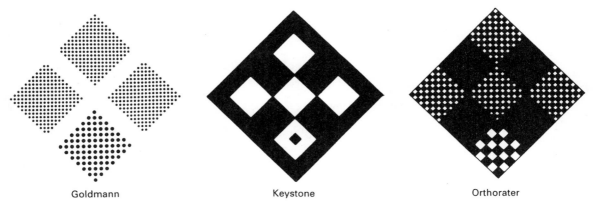

Goldmann   Keystone   Orthorater

Fig. 2.2 *Optotypes (courtesy of D.B. Henson and Butterworth-Heinemann, Oxford, 1983).*

phoria measured by the screeners to be relatively more esophoric than that found by conventional testing methods. This is due to the known proximity of the targets, which induces convergence (i.e. proximal convergence). The phoria test will also detect the presence of suppression as only one target will be seen, e.g. the arrow and not the letters.

Stereopsis

Most of the instruments include a test of stereopsis, in which one of a series of targets presented to each eye is seen with a small retinal disparity. The observer reports which target appears to stand out, and with a series of such tests, each with a different size disparity, the stereo-acuity can be measured. Failure of the stereopsis test may be due to suppression or an uncorrected refractive error, or to the artificially simulated viewing conditions. Therefore, it cannot automatically be assumed that the observer has no (or poor) stereopsis if they fail the test. The person should be referred for further investigation, when alternative tests can be used.

Fusion

Some instruments include a fusion test to assess the binocularity of the observer. This test presents similar targets to each eye but each has a control, i.e. one part of the target is only seen by the right eye and one part of the target is only seen by the left eye. For example, the Rodenstock screeners present a circle to each eye, with a vertical line seen above the circle by one eye and a vertical line seen below the circle by the other. If the observer has fusion, one circle will be seen with a vertical line above and below the circle. If the observer has double vision, two circles will be seen. The fusion test will also detect suppression, as only one target will be seen.

Colour vision

A series of isochromatic plates are included in most of the vision screeners to assess whether the observer has normal or defective colour vision. Unfortunately, due to the small number of plates used, the difficulty in accurate printing of the plates and the fact that tungsten lighting is often used instead of natural daylight, the sensitivity of the test is low. It would seem more sensible to screen those who require

colour vision separately, using the full set of isochromatic plates (Henson, 1983). Some screeners test colour vision by the correct naming of colours.

Rodenstock vision screeners have a different test to screen for red and green colour vision defects. The test disc includes six bipartite test fields (i.e. each test field is divided into an upper and lower half). The observer has to state if the colour of the upper and lower test fields appear the same or different.

Fogging tests

These tests are used to detect hyperopic observers. Positive lenses are incorporated, which will blur or fog the target viewed by an emmetrope, e.g. $+1.50\,D$ (Rodenstock R11, R12), $+1.75\,D$ (VS-II Vision Screener). A hyperope will find that the target is clear, or see it more clearly than an emmetrope, depending upon the magnitude of the refractive error and object distance.

Visual field

The extent of the horizontal visual field is assessed by one of two methods:

1. A perimeter attachment, which is manually rotated about a point located on top of the screener (e.g. Rodenstock Screeners). The target is brought from behind the observer's head while he or she fixates a central point, and the extent of peripheral vision is indicated on a dial.
2. An electronic perimeter, which has light-emitting diodes (LEDs) inset in a horizontal arc, either within the instrument (e.g. Keystone VS-II Vision screener) or in a separate attachment that can be placed on top of the instrument (e.g. Visiotest). The LEDs are illuminated by a push-button control, and their positions usually extend from 85° temporally to 45° nasally. Figure 2.4 shows the compact Keystone VS-II Vision Screener with the remote control unit. This operates the LEDs, which are positioned between the eyepieces and recessed in the temple areas of the headrest.

The Ergovision Vision Screener provides a more extensive test of the visual field. It presents each eye with 10 luminous dots; four points in the central area, four points for the peripheral area, and two points for the extent of the horizontal field.

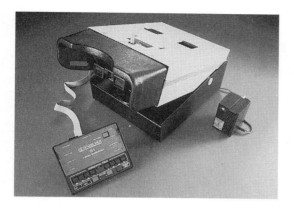

Fig. 2.4 *The Keystone VS-II Vision Screener (courtesy of Warwick Evans Optical Co. Ltd).*

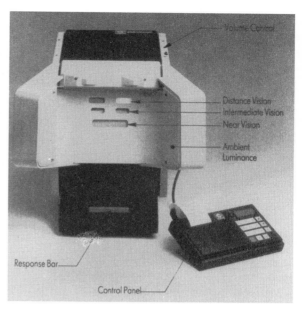

Fig. 2.5 *The Ergovision Vision Screener (courtesy of Essilor Ltd).*

Astigmatism

Only a few screeners include a test for astigmatism (e.g. Topcon Screenoscope). These tests consist of a fan of lines with the observer having to state whether any appear blurred or if they are all clear, and the number of clear lines seen on the fan may also be counted.

Two additional tests, very important for drivers, are featured in the Keystone Driver Vision Screener Model 2; distance visual acuity and stereopsis measurement under low illumination.

The Keystone and Rodenstock instruments offer a wide range of tests, and are used by many organizations. The Ergovision Vision Screener incorporates many additional tests as well as the conventional ones (Figure 2.5). New tests have been included to gather data on such factors as dynamic visual acuity, variable contrast acuity, visual fatigue and dazzle recovery time. The instrument uses a voice synthesizer to carry out the standard tests, and the results are printed out at the end of the programme. All the tests can also be carried out at three different lighting levels: 15, 150 and 300 cd/m^2. It is intended not only for diagnostic tests, but also for studying vision in the working conditions. The wide range of tests should allow visual examinations that are considered more closely matched to the task.

The Binoptometer (Figure 2.6) is a vision screener that overcomes the problem of proximal convergence. The tests are presented in free space, i.e. are seen against a distant wall, and hence eliminate proximal effects. This screener is currently available in

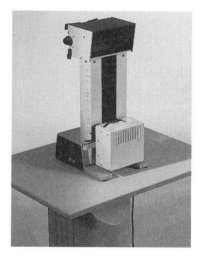

Fig. 2.6 *Binoptometer (courtesy of Oculus).*

Europe, and is produced by Oculus. Additionally, tests can be carried out at any distance from infinity to 0.3 m due to the optical design, which is similar to that of a Badal Optometer.

A summary of some of the tests included in the currently available vision screeners is given in Table 2.2. For precise details, see the manufacturers data. Lists of suppliers are included in Appendix B.

Table 2.2 Summary of some of the currently available vision screeners

Screener / Tests	Rodenstock			Keystone		Essilor		Optec 2000	Titmus II Vision Tester	Topcon Screenoscope SS-3	Oculus Binoptometer
	R10	R11	R12	VS II VS	Driver DVS II	Visiotest	Ergovision				
Acuity type	Checkerboard, Illiterate E, Numbers, Landolt C	Checkerboard, Illiterate E, Numbers, Pictures	Checkerboard, Illiterate E, Numbers, Landolt C	Numbers, Illiterate E	Numbers + low illumination	Letters Numbers	Letters Numbers	Checkerboard, Illiterate E, Landolt C	Landolt C	Illiterate E Landolt C	Landolt C
Phoria (H&V, D& 7N)	Yes	Yes	Yes	Yes	Yes at distance	Yes	Yes	Yes	Yes	Yes	Yes
Fusion	Yes	Yes	Yes	Yes	No	No	Yes	Yes	No	No	Yes
Stereopsis	Yes	Yes	Yes	Yes	Yes + low illumination	Yes	Yes	Yes	Yes	Yes	Yes
Colour vision	Yes	Yes	Yes	Yes	Yes	Yes	Yes	Yes	Yes	No	Yes
Fogging lens	No	Yes	Yes	Yes	No	Yes	Yes	Yes	No	Yes	No
Visual field	Yes	Yes	Yes	Yes	Yes	Yes	Yes	Yes	Yes	Yes	No
Astigmatism	No	No	No	No	No	Yes	Yes	No	No	Yes	No
Target change	Manual	Manual	Manual	Remote control	Remote control	Manual	Automatic or remote control	Manual	Remote control	Manual	Manual
Test distances	Distance only for drivers	Distance and 40 cm	Distance, 55 cm and 33 cm	6 m, 66 cm and 37 cm	6 m	5 m and 33 cm	5 m, 66 cm and 33 cm	6 m and 35 cm 76–50 cm with five lens sets	6m and 37 cm 1 m to 50 cm with five lens sets	5 m and 30 cm Lenses for intermediate	Infinity to 30 cm
Comments	For drivers	For children	For industry, VDU	VDU test Head position sensor	For drivers	VDU lens kit for 50 cm tests	Extra tests, e.g. visual fatigue, glare recovery, dynamic VA Three light levels	Slide sets for industry, medical, international use Head position sensor	Low light level Head position sensor Job standard manual	Job standard manual	VDU and driver test discs

Some tests are interchangeable between screeners, e.g. adult, industrial & driver discs

Advantages and disadvantages of instrument vision screeners

Advantages of instrument vision screeners include (Bailey, 1973):

- Operation by lay technicians
- Speed of screening
- They are always available for use
- Maintenance costs are low
- It is a cheap method of screening.

Disadvantages of instrument vision screeners include:

- The lack of flexibility of tests and testing distance, especially for those screeners where the targets are on a rotary drum
- They do not detect ocular pathology unless inferred by a reduction of visual acuity
- They cannot detect squints
- The awareness of the actual target distance may induce proximal accommodation and convergence, even when distance viewing conditions are simulated, and this can affect the visual acuity measurement and induce a relative esophoria at distance
- There can be unnecessary referral by a lay operator of people with amblyopia or a squint.

Computer programs for vision screening

Computer programs are available that can be used to screen the vision of VDU operators. The City University Vision Screening program can either be used in the consulting room or on site. When used on site, the system provides a direct assessment of the visual performance under the actual working conditions. It includes assessment of seven different tests of visual function, including visual acuity, search tasks, oculomotor balance, fixation disparity and central visual fields (Thomson, 1994; Figure 2.7). Visual acuity is measured using an illiterate E target monocularly and binocularly. Two search tasks have been included to assess if clear single vision can be sustained; the first task is to locate a single broken circle (C) hidden among a series of circles, and the second task requires the observer to count the number of times that a certain digit occurs within in an array of numbers. The latter task requires the observer to make a series of precise eye movements and maintain clear single vision. The oculomotor balance tests

require the observer to wear red–green goggles to dissociate the eyes. One test displays a red line and a green scale on the screen, and the observer reports the number that the line passes through. The fixation disparity test is based on the Mallett test, and the observer views an OXO target through the red–green goggles. A red and green marker located on either side of the X are seen monocularly with each eye. The presence or absence of fixation disparity is recorded. The central visual fields are assessed using a multiple stimulus screening strategy. The program also includes a questionnaire to determine any problems that VDU users may experience. The results of both the questionnaire and the visual function tests are analysed, and a report is then provided giving advice and recommendations for each person.

Computerized vision screeners have also been designed for use in schools (Hatch, 1993; Thomson and Evans, 1999). Thomson and Evans (1999) have designed a prototype vision screening program that includes measurements of visual acuity and stereopsis, with colour vision being tested by selected Ishihara plates. Visual acuity is measured by a single line of letters surrounded by crowding bars being presented on the computer screen. The letter size is increased from $\log MAR = 0.1$ (6/7.5) until all the letters are read correctly, and the order of the letters is randomized in order to avoid learning effects. To assess the stereopsis, the child views the computer screen through red–green goggles. Four pairs of red and green circles are displayed, with one pair having a greater separation than the other three. The child is asked to indicate which one stands out more than the others. The test can assess stereoacuity levels of 110, 220 and 330 s of arc.

Choice of vision screening method

The ideal screening programme should:

1. Maximize screening success, i.e. correct referral and non-referral
2. Minimize screening errors, i.e. low over and under referral rate. In other words, the test needs good sensitivity and specificity.

The use of visual acuity measures alone as a method for screening children is not sensitive enough, especially when compared to the modified clinical technique (MCT) or use of instrument screeners

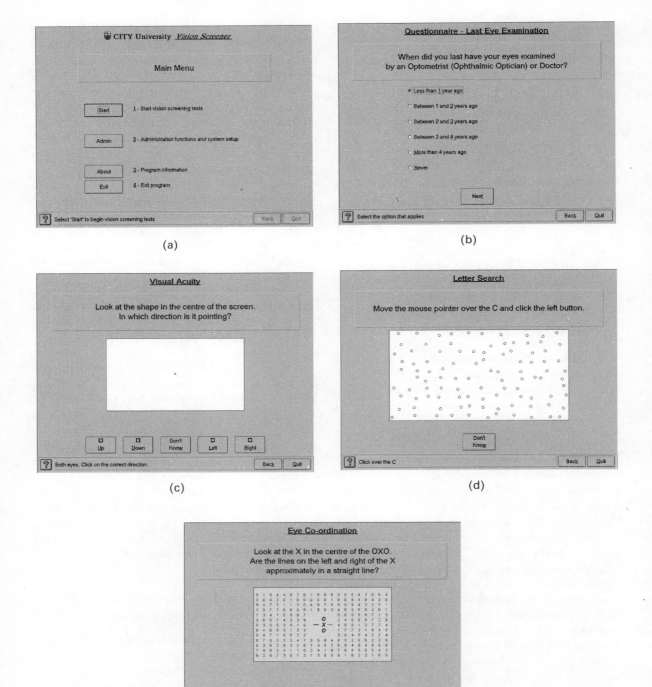

Fig. 2.7 *City University Vision Screener for VDU users – examples of the questionnaire and vision tests, including visual acuity, letter search and fixation disparity tests (reproduced courtesy of D. Thomson and City University).*

(Hatcher, 1976; Swarbrick, 1979; Worrall, 1981; Cohen *et al.*, 1983). When the MCT was compared to the use of instrument screeners or a battery of vision tests, it was found to be the most sensitive, with the lowest under- and over-referral rate (Peters *et al.*, 1959; Wick *et al.*, 1976; Wong, 1978; Cole and Robbins, 1981; Worrall, 1981). The newer computerized screeners have been shown to have a high sensitivity and specificity. Hatch (1993) used a computerized screener, known as the VTA/VERA, to test 602 school children between 6 and 13 years of age. When the results were compared with a full eye examination, the screener was found to have a sensitivity of 75 per cent and specificity of 93 per cent. The values found by Thomson and Evans (1999) compared well with these, being 96.1 per cent and 93.8 per cent for sensitivity and specificity respectively.

Instrument screeners are widely used for vision screening of adults, and are often the method of choice used in industry and by government organizations. However, it must be remembered that, whichever technique is used, it is only a screening test and not a substitute for a full ophthalmic examination.

REFERENCES

Anon (1996) Survey shows 16% of all UK drivers fail number-plate test. *Optom Today*, **Oct 21**, 10.

Association of Optometrists Members' Handbook. Association of Optometrists, 61 Southwark Street, London SE1 0HL.

Bailey I.L. (1973) Vision screening in industry: objective and methods. *Aust J Optom*, **56**, 70–85.

Bailey I.L. and Cole B.L. (1968) *Methods and Instruments for Screening Distance and Near Acuity*. Victorian College of Optometry, University of Melbourne, Australia.

Bennett A.G. and Rabbetts R.B. (1984) *Vision Screening, New Subjective Refractors and Techniques. Clinical Visual Optics*. Butterworths, London.

Birch J. (2001) *Diagnosis of Defective Colour Vision*. Butterworth-Heinemann, Oxford.

Cohen A.H., Lieberman S., Stolzberg M. and Ritty J.M. (1983) The NYSOA vision screening battery – a total approach. *J Am Optom Assoc*, **54**, 975–984.

Cole B.L. and Robbins H.G. (1981) The problems of screening children's vision. *Aust J Optom*, **64**, 193–196.

Collins M. (1983) *Occupational Public Health Optometry*. Department of Optometry, Queensland Institute of Technology, Brisbane, pp. 1–8.

Grundy J.W. (1981) Visual efficiency in industry. *Ophthal Opt*, **21**, 548–552.

Grundy J.W. (1984) When your car could break down through a visual defect. *Ophthal Opt*, **Feb 4**, 77–80.

Grundy J.W. (1986) A simple method of occupational vision requirements. *Optom Today*, **Oct 11**, 684–688.

Grundy J.W. (1987) A diagrammatic approach to occupational optometry and illumination.*Optom Today*, **Aug 1**, 503–508.

Hatch S.W. (1993) Computerised vision screening: validity and reliability of the VTA/VERA vision screener. *J Behavioural Optom*, **4**, 143–148.

Hatcher M.J. (1976) A kindergarten vision screening service. *Aust J Optom*, **59**, 198–201.

Henson D.B. (1983) *Optometric Instrumentation*. Butterworth-Heinemann Ltd, London, pp. 231–237.

Peters H.B., Blum H.L., Bettman J.W., Johnson, F. and Fellows, V. (1959) The Orinda vision study. *Am J Optom*, **36**, 455–469.

Rousell D. (1979) *Eye Protection*. Royal Society for the Prevention of Accidents Publication No.15126. RoSPA, Birmingham.

Swarbrick H.A. (1979) Vision screening in New Zealand schools. *Aust J Optom*, **62**, 374–382.

Thomson W.D. (1994) The City University Vision Screener for VDU users. *Br J Optom Disp*, **2**, 61–74.

Thomson W.D. and Evans B. (1999) A new approach to vision screening in schools. *Ophthal Physiol Opt*, **1**, 196–209.

Voke J. (1980) *Colour Vision Testing in Specific Industries and Professions*. Keeler Ltd, London.

Walters J. (1984) Portsea modified clinical technique: evaluation of an expanded optometric vision screening protocol for children. *Aust J Optom*, **67**, 212–220.

Weston H.C. (1962) *Sight, Light and Work*, 2nd edn. Lewis, London.

Wick B., O'Neal M. and Ricker P. (1976) Comparison of vision screening by lay and professional personnel. *Am J Optom Physiol Optics*, **53**, 474–478.

Wong S.G. (1978) Comparison of vision screening performed by optometrists and nurses. *Am J Optom Physiol Optics*, **55**, 384–389.

Worrall R.S. (1981) The Biopter vision test: use in school screening program. *Optom Monthly*, **72**, 10–13.

3 Incidence of ocular injuries and their prevention

INCIDENCE OF OCULAR INJURIES

Studies show that there is an unacceptably large number of eye injuries occurring in the UK (Canavan et al., 1980; Chiapella and Rosenthal, 1985; Wykes, 1988; MacEwen, 1989, Desai et al., 1996a). The visual impairment as a result of an eye injury may vary from a slight reduction in visual acuity to total blindness and, sadly, it appears that the majority of these injuries could have been prevented. While in the past eye injuries have been associated with industrial occupations, there are increasing numbers occurring in sports and leisure activities and at home.

Obviously the number of eye injuries caused by industrial accidents varies according to the level of industrialization in the area concerned. For example, a study in a heavily industrialized area (Wolverhampton, UK; Lambah, 1968) reported that 73.8 per cent of all eye injuries over a 10-year period occurred in industry, whereas only 15.4 per cent were reported in less industrialized Northern Ireland for a similar period (Canavan et al., 1980).

Canavan et al. (1980) carried out a survey into the causes and resultant types of ocular injury from 1967 to 1976. The causes of the ocular injuries of people admitted to the Royal Victoria Hospital, Belfast, in order of decreasing frequency, were as follows:

Cause of injury	Percentage
Children at play and sport	33.8
Road traffic accident	19.3
Industrial accident	15.4
Civil disturbance	9.1
Home accident	6.8

Table 3.1 Occupations of the patients when ocular injury occurred (reproduced by kind permission of A.P. Chiapelli and A.R. Rosenthal and the *British Journal of Ophthalmology*, 1985)

Occupation	No. of cases				
	All injuries	Burn	Contusion	Foreign body	Corneal abrasion
Press or machine tool operators	494	13	13	425	64
Motor vehicle or aircraft mechanic	147	10	7	111	18
Metal worker	145	7	4	111	27
Construction	131	16	6	82	37
Sheet metal worker	124	3	3	108	12
Electrician	104	5	3	77	24
General labourer	120	6	5	79	34
Welder	97	9	3	72	18
Bus, coach or lorry driver	76	4	5	46	23
Others in processing	51	4	1	23	8
Painter and decorator	44	7	1	23	17

Assault	6.8
Adult sport	4.8
Farm accident	4.0

Of the 2032 patients admitted, 1707 were male and 325 female The survey also recorded the type of ocular injury:

- Blunt injury – 49.2 per cent
- Perforating injury – 48.0 per cent
- Intra-ocular foreign body – 8.4 per cent.

Normal visual acuity was regained in 41.2 per cent of known cases, but many resulted in severe loss of vision. Perforation of the eye accounted for the majority of cases with severe loss of vision. Men younger than 36 years of age were subject to the highest percentage of injuries (77.4 per cent). Similar findings have subsequently been reported (Chiapella and Rosenthal, 1985; Wykes, 1988; MacEwen, 1989, Desai *et al.*, 1996a, 1996b). Desai *et al.* (1996b) found that the risk of having an eye injury requiring hospital admission is over nine times higher for men than woman between the ages of 15 and 64 years.

A common cause of perforating eye injuries used to be road traffic accidents in which the head impacted upon the jagged edges of the shattered windscreen. However, since the introduction of the compulsory wearing of seat belts in the UK in January 1983, there has been a significant decrease in this type of injury. Hall *et al.* (1985) found a 73 per cent reduction in such injuries; Cole *et al.* (1987), Johnson and Armstrong (1986) and Wykes (1988) have also noted similar reductions. The more recent introduction of airbags in cars has substantially reduced the overall rates of mortality and morbidity associated with accidents, but they have been reported to cause a variety of ocular injuries, ranging from orbital contusion to a ruptured globe (Duma *et al.*, 1996; Manchee *et al.*, 1997).

Another large UK study (Chiapella and Rosenthal, 1985) examined the clinical records of 6576 patients admitted to the eye casualty department at the Leicester Royal Infirmary during a 1-year period. While, again, the majority of patients were men in the 20–40 years age group, the main cause of eye injuries was foreign bodies. Table 3.1 shows the main occupations of the patients in whom the injuries occurred, with press and machine tool operators the most likely to suffer injury (32 per cent). However, it is important to remember that most of the occupations listed are known to have potential ocular hazards, and that eye protection should have prevented injury! The study suggests that eye protection was either inappropriate or was not being used correctly by the workers.

There are relatively few industrial processes that do not present an ocular hazard of some type. Despite the fact that legislation demands eye protection is worn

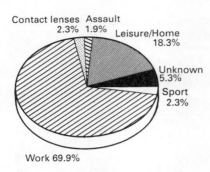

Fig. 3.1 *Causes of ocular injuries (reproduced by kind permission of C.J. MacEwen and the* British Journal of Ophthalmology, *1989).*

during hazardous tasks, many ocular injuries still occur. The exact number of these injuries is difficult to ascertain because there is no general consensus for collecting data, and injuries are often not reported unless they result in a loss of time from work. In 1993–1994, a total of 127 523 injuries occurred that led to employees requiring more than 3 days off work; of these, 2614 were eye injuries (Health and Safety Commission, 1994).

A study by MacEwen (1989) found that 70 per cent of all eye injuries presenting over a 1-year period at the Glasgow Eye Infirmary and the Western Infirmary casualty departments had occurred at work. A total of 5671 patients were seen from May 1987 to April 1988. Distribution of the various causes of injury is shown in Figure 3.1. The most common occupation at the time of injury was grinding/buffing, and 83 per cent of all those injured were not wearing the required eye protection. Interestingly, whilst most injuries occurred at work, the majority of the serious injuries in this study were due to sporting and leisure activities.

The most severe injuries are likely to occur to the young or elderly, either at home or during sports/leisure activities. A study from Scotland found that in a 1-year period from 1991 to 1992, a total of 428 patients suffered severe ocular injuries and were admitted to the ophthalmic units. Serious ocular trauma was most likely to occur at home (30.2 per cent), followed by the workplace (19.6 per cent) and sports/leisure (15.8 per cent) (Desai *et al.*, 1996a). Nearly a quarter of all injuries occurred as a result of using tools or machinery at home or work (24 per

cent). Again it was found that, where applicable, protective eyewear was only available for 48.6 per cent of patients, with only 19.4 per cent actually using it.

There have been reports of eye injuries occurring to workers within the chemical industry and to fire fighters (Jones and Griffith, 1992; Owen *et al.*, 1995). Both these reports emphasize the requirement for education regarding the need for eye protection to be worn.

Sport

The number of ocular injuries sustained during sport and leisure activities is on the increase. Not surprisingly, in the USA, the greatest number of injuries result from baseball, ice hockey and racket sports (Napier *et al.*, 1996). Hockey used to be a leading cause of eye injuries but the numbers have decreased since the introduction of the mandatory use of protective facemasks (Vinger, 1980), and this reduction by the use of eye protection can therefore serve as a model for other sports.

Racket sports are also responsible for many ocular injuries; this is not surprising, given the speed of the ball. A squash ball may reach speeds of 224 km/h (140 mph), a racket ball and tennis ball 192 km/h (120 mph), and a shuttlecock 232 km/h (145 mph). There is also the risk of the player being hit by the opponent's racket.

Squash became very popular in Australia in the 1970s, and this was reflected by the incidence of injuries; an amazing 32 per cent of all eye injuries admitted to the Royal Adelaide Hospital were received playing squash in the 30 months prior to November 1975 (Moore and Worthley, 1977). The very high potential for ocular injury in squash is due not only to the fact that the squash ball can be travelling at very high speed, but also because it is small enough to fit into the orbit.

In the UK, a study by Gregory (1986) examined the distribution of sports-related eye injuries (Table 3.2). Squash is the most common source, with soccer, badminton and tennis following closely behind. The majority of the injuries were to men, and 20 per cent of all patients were admitted to hospital.

Jones (1988) has reported that sport is becoming an increasingly important cause of severe eye injuries in the UK. In his year-long study of severe eye injuries

Table 3.2 Distribution of ocular injuries resulting from sports seen at the Sussex Eye Hospital (reproduced by kind permission of P.T.S. Gregory and the *British Journal of Ophthalmology*, 1986)

Sport	Total accidents	Hospital admissions	Male	Female
Squash	24	3	18	6
Soccer	19	7	19	0
Badminton	16	4	6	10
Tennis	11	1	9	2
Rugby	6	0	6	0
Cricket	5	0	4	1
Basketball	3	0	1	2
Hockey	3	0	2	1
Golf	2	1	2	0
Marbles	1	1	1	0
Karate	1	0	1	0
Lacrosse	1	0	0	1
Total	92	17	69	23

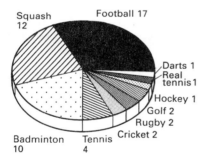

Fig. 3.2 *Number of sports related eye injuries (reproduced by kind permission of N.P. Jones and Eye 1988).*

admitted to the Manchester Royal Eye Infirmary, he found that racket sports accounted for half of the injuries (Figure 3.2). He also found that none of the patients had been wearing eye protection, and that they had no idea how to obtain it. Serious eye injuries to badminton players have also been reported by Kelly (1987), with damage being due to penetrating injuries from shattered glass spectacle lenses.

A 1-year study in Victoria, Australia, by Fong (1995) also found that sports injuries were likely to be more severe than those that occurred at work. A total of 6308 patients were treated for eye injuries in the hospital. The workplace accounted for 44 per cent

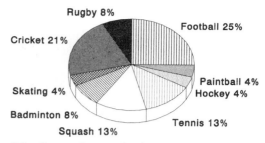

Fig. 3.3 *Causes of sports-related eye injuries (after Pardham et al., 1995).*

of all injuries and 19 per cent of severe injuries, whereas sports injuries accounted for only 5 per cent of all injuries but 19 per cent of severe ocular trauma. Many patients (67 per cent) were not wearing any form of eye protection, and if it had been worn over half the eye injuries could have been prevented.

A 1-year survey at Bradford Royal Infirmary by Pardham *et al.* (1995) found that racket sports were the commonest cause of sports-related eye injuries (Figure 3.3). The severity of the injuries was such that they all required follow-up treatment or admission. The results of a questionnaire regarding the knowledge of the university students about eye protectors for squash were also reported. Only 9 per cent of squash players wore eye protectors, which highlights the need for education about the potential hazards of racket sports and use of eye protectors.

A survey of all the squash clubs in the West Midlands also revealed the ignorance of the management and members about the hazards of their sport and the need for eye protection (David *et al.*, 1995). Of the clubs who responded, it was found that only 3 (6 per cent) sold eye protectors and that they all stocked the open/lensless type of eye guard, which is not recommended. Only one club supplied impact-resistant plastic lenses. None of the clubs provided any information warning their members of the potential ocular hazards.

It has been recommended that open eye guards should not be used because the ball changes its shape in motion and flattens, so that it can make eye contact through the eye guard. In addition, spectacle frames with hinges that open beyond 90° are not sufficiently rigid to prevent the frame from hitting the eye if a racket or ball strikes it (Easterbrook, 1981; Vinger, 1985; Napier *et al.*, 1996).

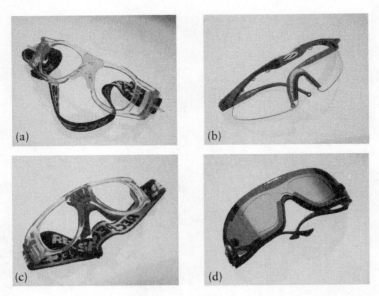

Fig. 3.4 *Examples of protective eye wear for racket sports (a–c), hockey (b, c) and mountain biking (b, d) (courtesy of the Norville Group Ltd).*

Unfortunately, there are cases where sportsmen suffer sight-threatening injuries of which they are unaware. A survey of 74 asymptomatic boxers showed that 58 per cent had a variety of ocular injuries, including traumatic cataracts and retinal tears (Giovinazzo *et al.*, 1987). It is difficult to provide eye protection for boxers, but the report concluded that a more rigorous control of the sport is required, including regular eye examinations. The introduction of a thumbless boxing glove would help to reduce some of the injuries.

There can be no doubt about the necessity for eye protection in sport, and the optometrist must be responsible for educating sportsmen and women about the potential hazards of their sport and the need for eye protection. It is particularly important that the monocular sports player is identified and advised accordingly (Napier *et al.*, 1996). Examples of protective eye wear for sports are shown in Figure 3.4.

The success of eye protectors in reducing ocular injuries has been demonstrated by the reduction in injuries to hockey players in the USA, as detailed by Vinger (1980). Eye protectors for racket sports have been developed in the USA and Canada and, apparently, no serious eye injury has been reported by a racket ball or squash player wearing the approved eye protectors (Easterbrook, 1988). In 1998, a British Standard for eye protection in squash was published (BS 7930, Part 1). This standard applies to eye protectors with polycarbonate oculars, and it includes prescription lenses. It should be noted that it does not apply to eye protectors designed for use over spectacles.

Accidents at home and to children

Many severe ocular injuries occur to children at play and in the home; such accidents are the major cause of blindness in the first two decades of life. Studies previously mentioned by MacEwen (1989), Desai *et al.* (1996b) and Fong (1995) found that a disproportionate number of serious eye injuries occurred to children. The survey in Australia by Fong (1995) found that 25

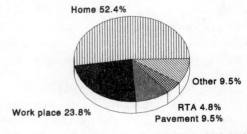

Fig. 3.5 *Places where severe ocular injury resulting in blindness occurred (VA < 6/60) (after Desai et al., 1996b).*

per cent of severe injuries occurred to young boys and teenagers less than 15 years of age.

Figure 3.5 shows the places where severe ocular injury resulting in blindness occurred (VA < 6/60; Desai *et al.*, 1996b). It can be seen that just over half of the blinding injuries occurred in the home (52 per cent), whilst the workplace accounted for 24 per cent.

La Roche *et al.* (1988) conducted an investigation into severe eye injuries in children. They found that young boys with perforating eye injuries accounted for the majority of cases involving severe loss of vision. Not surprisingly, the major cause of injury was due to objects being thrown (e.g. rocks, stones, snowballs etc.). BB gun pellets caused permanent loss of vision in almost half the cases seen (a BB gun is a type of air gun that fires ball–bearings). The report concluded that adult supervision could have prevented most cases of permanent visual loss. The authors also suggested that legislation restricting the use of BB guns should be passed, and that toy safety standards should be tightened. A programme of adult and child eye safety education should also be developed, and should include warnings of potentially hazardous toys, etc.

A similarly worrying report about eye injuries caused to children by guns was presented by Moore *et al.* (1987), who found that 70 per cent of ocular injuries caused by air guns occurred to the under 17 years age group. This emphasizes the need for parental control and education about the potential danger.

Hundreds of thousands of Americans have incurred eye injuries at home because they did not take safety precautions with potentially dangerous products (Randall, 1985). Some of the household products cited in many eye injury reports include oven cleaners, glue, disinfectants, nylon cord grass trimmers, chain saws, hair sprays, paints, insecticides and cleaning agents (e.g. ammonia, bleach). Lawn mowers are responsible for a staggering number of injuries; John *et al.* (1988) found that over a 10-year period from 1977–1987 they were responsible for 70 000 injuries every year, and 5 per cent of these involved the eyes.

There are numerous potentially hazardous products in every home, and injuries can occur from the most unlikely causes. For example, there have been reports of ocular injuries resulting from elasticated luggage straps and exploding eggs from microwave ovens!

PREVENTION OF INJURIES
Role of the optometrist/medical professions
In the USA, a national eye trauma system has been formed to combat the problem of eye injuries in general (Parver, 1988). This is composed of regional trauma centres with eye specialists always available to deal with severe ocular injuries. Data are also being collected to increase both the knowledge of ocular trauma so that treatment techniques can be improved, and understanding of the mechanisms and circumstances that result in ocular injury so that effective protection can be provided.

The optometrist has an important role to play in the prevention of eye injuries. In practice, a thorough history of patients should be taken and a detailed analysis of the visual requirements made. What are the patients' hobbies? Do they play sports? Do they enjoy gardening? Do they carry out DIY? Do they ride a motorcycle or bicycle? What is their occupation, and does this involve potential ocular hazards? From this information potential ocular hazards can be discussed, along with the need for eye protection where necessary (Woods, 1988). The need for protective lenses for the patient with an amblyopic eye should not be forgotten.

The optometrist may also help to reduce the number of injuries in industry by setting up eye protection programmes. The success of such a programme has been demonstrated by the Norfolk and Western Company in the USA, who were unhappy with the number of injuries suffered by their employees (Gross, 1982). The accidents appeared to be due to the lack of mandatory eye safety programmes, unwillingness to wear eye protection, and the unfortunate assumption by both the management and the employees that certain jobs were not potentially hazardous. Following the introduction of an eye protection programme for employees in the mechanical and engineering departments in 1980, there was a 78.4 per cent reduction in eye injuries over the next 3 years.

Perception of risk
It is well known that there is widespread wearer resistance to using eye protectors in hazardous industries (Farmer, 1982). This was clearly shown in the survey by MacEwen (1989), who found that, in 85 per cent of injuries that occurred at work, eye protection was not being worn when it should have been. There is concern that people do not take the available measures to protect

their health in general, and that health messages frequently do not achieve the desired effect. Various theories have been proposed to explain this attitude of indifference to health hazards. The Health Belief Model was put forward by Rosenstock *et al.* (1959), suggesting that a person's behaviour depended on various factors such as the degree of perceived risk, the perceived benefits of taking preventative measures, and the perceived barriers (e.g. inconvenience). A later model, the Dual Process Model, emphasizes the role of a person's experience based on past personal knowledge and the information from friends, colleagues, the media and his or her doctor (Levanthal *et al.*, 1983). Hence it concentrates on how an individual's 'perceptions' relevant to the Health Belief Model are formed. If the risk of receiving an eye injury is perceived as high, a person is more likely to wear an eye protector. It is suggested that an individual learns to appreciate risks through experiencing an injury either to themselves or to a friend (Powell *et al.*, 1971), and hence a worker who has not had such an experience will generally perceive the risk as being moderate. However, this is not always the case. In one study, a decreased perception of risk was found in workers who had survived (or who had seen others survive) eye injuries (Gervais, 1989). This study investigated the relationship between past experience of eye injuries in chemical industry workers and their attitude towards the use of safety spectacles. The publicizing of eye injuries as a warning might have a negative effect, as in some cases the worker will inform colleagues that 'it wasn't actually so bad'. In other cases the effect of near misses was useful, as there was a clear association between having eyesight saved by eye protection and perceived risk. Caution must therefore be exercised when publicizing eye injuries as a warning to workers. From the study, the following recommendations to promote eye safety were made:

1. Educational efforts should be directed at the younger employees, as they are less convinced about the risk they run when not wearing eye protection. Note that they often do not have the added benefit of improved vision through the use of prescription safety spectacles.
2. The publicizing of eye injuries must be considered carefully.
3. It may be beneficial to counsel workers after an eye injury to determine the perception of risk of their occupation. If their perception of risk is low, then efforts can be made to instruct them as to the hazards so that perhaps they will be more inclined to wear their eye protection.
4. Reasons for not wearing eye protection should be determined.
5. The possibility of compulsory wear should not be overlooked, but this should not be enforced in a heavy-handed manner.

Eye protection programme

In the past the safety of the employee was normally considered to be the employee's responsibility, and little liability was placed upon the employer. However, in more recent years the trend has been reversed and the employer is primarily responsible for the safety of the employees. This has led to claims for compensation, fines, and obligations to provide financial support during absence from work, as well as the cost of lost production. It has therefore become worthwhile for employers to invest in accident prevention programmes. The main aim of an eye protection programme is to identify potential ocular hazards and then eliminate or control them. This will not only fulfil legal obligations but will also have economic advantages (Collins, 1983). A reduction in eye injuries will result in a reduction of insurance and medical expenses, and there will be a reduction in lost production, work replacement and retraining costs for those who cannot continue in their previous job due to injury. An improvement in the employee/employer relationship may also result from the instigation of an eye protection programme. The importance of preventing the devastating effects that visual impairment causes to both the employee and their family should not be forgotten.

Naturally, the expenses incurred in developing such a programme will have to be evaluated. These will include the fee for a consultant to carry out the initial survey, and the cost of implementation. This may involve modifying manufacturing processes to either eliminate or control the hazards, which may be expensive. There is the cost of providing and maintaining eye protection for employees and, finally, there is the cost of employee education concerning the ocular hazards of their jobs and the use of eye protectors where necessary (Gross, 1982; Van Nakagawara, 1988).

The eye protection programme may consist of the

following parts (Lathey, 1973; Taylor, 1973; Wood, 1973; Gross, 1982; Van Nakagawara, 1988):

- Plant environment survey
- Vision screening
- Implementation of the programme
- Maintenance of the programme.

Plant environment survey

Initially, the potential hazards of the plant should be assessed. For example, there may be acids, flying particles from a lathe or radiation from welding against which the eyes need to be protected. The area of the plant and any particular dangerous tasks should be noted. Once the hazard has been identified, a method of eliminating or controlling it must be devised. Hazards may be eliminated at their source by modifying the design of the machinery or equipment and the layout of the work place. In some circumstances, non-hazardous materials may be used instead of the original hazardous ones. If the hazard cannot be eliminated, then it must be controlled or contained. Screens or splash guards may be fitted around machines; exhaust systems installed to remove dust, gases or fumes from the atmosphere; and water sprays used to reduce the problems of dust in the atmosphere (Collins, 1983). The wearing of eye protectors should be the last option. If eye protectors are required, then the areas where they should be worn must be clearly marked.

There is little doubt that poor lighting can be a contributory factor in some accidents. Lighting conditions should be assessed for the various tasks to check that they are appropriate for the job to be performed efficiently. In the UK, the CIBSE Code (CIBSE, 1994) gives recommended lighting levels for various tasks and industries, and this should be consulted.

Sites of emergency first aid equipment should be noted, and their placement and the need for any additional equipment assessed. For example, where chemicals are being used, a water fountain or shower unit should be installed to provide rapid dousing with water to dilute any chemicals accidentally splashed onto an employee.

Accident records from the factory first aid centre can be analysed to determine where and how ocular injuries have occurred. A note should always be made of whether eye protectors were being worn at the time of injury and, if not, whether they should have been. This information can be very useful in determining areas where injuries are likely to occur and in investigating their causes to prevent any further injuries.

Vision screening

The visual efficiency of the employees is one aspect that is often neglected. Various studies have shown that about one-third of employees have vision below the standard required for their occupation, and there has been a considerable amount of research supporting the relationship between accidents and defective vision. For example, one study cited by Grundy (1981) found that when vision screening was carried out in a large steel works, employees whose vision was below the standard required were found to have experienced on average 20 per cent more accidents than those who were visually efficient. Obviously, an employee whose vision is below standard is more likely to sustain self-injuries and to injure colleagues. Methods of assessing the visual efficiency of the employees may be carried out using a screening method, as described in Chapter 2. Vision screening can be carried out to detect those employees whose vision is not up to the standard required, and employees found to have a visual defect can then be referred to a qualified person for further investigation. Fortunately, the majority of cases can be corrected, given appropriate professional advice and correct treatment.

Implementation of the programme

It is important that the eye protection programme is carried out correctly; incorrect administration could result in a work environment that is more hazardous than that found initially. Depending on the findings of the plant survey, the following actions may be necessary:

1. Elimination or control of ocular hazards.
2. Provision of eye protectors, which must be personally issued to make sure that they fit correctly and are of the correct type for the task involved.
3. Clear marking of areas where ocular hazards exist, and where eye protection must be worn. These areas may be designated by lines painted on the floor, or by warning signs placed in pro-

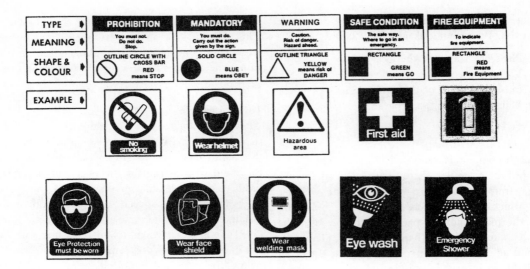

Fig. 3.6 *Safety signs (reproduced by kind permission of Signs and Labels Ltd, Stockport, Cheshire).*

minent positions. The Health and Safety (Safety, Signs and Signals) Regulations were introduced in 1996 to implement the European Safety Signs Directive (92/58/EEC), which has been designed to standardize safety signs. Safety signs and notices are divided into four categories, according to the type of message: (i) prohibition; (ii) mandatory; (iii) warning; and (iv) safe condition. Each category has its own distinctive shape and colour (Figure 3.6; BS 5378, 1980, Part 1). Provision must be made for eye protectors to be readily available for visitors to any hazardous areas.

4. Provision of first aid facilities, which should be set up so that immediate medical attention can be provided. All employees should be made aware of the first aid centres, which should be clearly signposted. Other emergency equipment that is required in hazardous work areas should be easily accessible – for example, water fountains in chemical factories.

5. Provision of lens cleaning stations, which should contain cleaning solutions, anti-fog solutions and clean cloths with which to wipe the eye protectors. Such stations are necessary to prevent cleaning with the first means available to the employee – often an oily rag, which will smear the lenses and make matters worse not

better. The employee may then remove the eye protectors to see more clearly, leaving the eyes unprotected.

6. Formation of a safety committee, which includes employee representatives.

7. Education of employees regarding the hazards involved in their jobs and the need for eye protection. Films, posters, and lectures, especially concerning the ocular consequences of failing to use eye protection, are very useful in emphasizing the importance of wearing eye protectors where necessary. There is a great need to motivate employees to wear their eye protection (Wigglesworth, 1970), and employees should be made aware of their legal obligations concerning the wearing of eye protectors. In the UK, the Royal Society for the Prevention of Accidents (RoSPA) provides safety films, posters and lectures, all of which are extremely useful.

Explanations of the initial symptoms that may be experienced when wearing eye protectors, especially by non-spectacle wearers, should be given. Problems such as a restricted field of view, reflection and aberrations from the lenses and magnification should be discussed.

Accident record sheets should be kept at the first aid centre. Anyone requiring treatment should have the following details recorded (Rooke *et al.*, 1980; Collins, 1983):

- How the injury occurred
- The cause of the accident
- Where the injury occurred
- Whether eye protection was being worn and if it should have been but was not, why not?
- The mechanical condition of the machine or tools used
- The apparent injury to the eye
- The time and date of the injury.

It is important to avoid suggesting blame in the questions. The above information is necessary for:

- Insurance purposes and to inform any claims for compensation by the employee
- Accident data collection and analysis
- A re-evaluation of the eye protection programme.

Maintenance of the programme
The maintenance of the programme is essential for continued safety and cost-effectiveness. It may involve:

1. Assessing new manufacturing processes and their potential hazards.
2. Continuing education and training for the employees.
3. Maintenance of lens cleaning and first aid facilities.
4. Vision screening, which should be carried out at regular intervals to maintain the necessary standard of vision.
5. Maintaining an active safety committee so that the employees can suggest methods of improving the safety of their environment.
6. Maintenance of stocks of replacement eye protectors. Employees should be informed as to the location of these supplies, which should be readily available. Any adjustments to the fitting of the eye protectors should be carried out by trained personnel to provide maximum comfort and protection. Frame heaters, screwdrivers, etc. should be available for the adjustment and maintenance of the eye protectors.
7. Recognition of employee achievements regarding their efforts to maintain and create a safer environment.

SUMMARY

There are still far too many eye injuries occurring, which can have devastating consequences. They not only occur at work but also at home or during leisure activities, and more frequently affect men. Sadly, an alarmingly high number of children receive eye injuries. There is a need for people to be made aware of the potential ocular hazards and the necessity to wear eye protection. The optometrist can play an important educational and clinical role in the provision of eye protection. Advice can be given regarding the visual abilities and safety of the employees in relation to the particular job requirements. Assessing the working conditions and, where necessary, making recommendations for improvement are also part of the optometrist's role in preventive eye care.

REFERENCES

BS 5378 Part 1 (1980) Safety signs and colours – specification for colour and design. British Standards Institution, London.

BS 7930 Part 1 (1988) Specification for eye protectors for racket sports – Part 1: Squash. British Standards Institution, London.

Canavan Y.M., O'Flaherty J., Archer D.B. and Elwood J.H. (1980) A 10-year survey of eye injuries in Northern Ireland 1967–76. *Br J Ophthalmol*, **64**, 618–625.

Chiapella A.P. and Rosenthal A.R. (1985) One year in an eye casualty clinic. *Br J Ophthalmol*, **69**, 865–870.

CIBSE (1994) *Code for Interior Lighting*. The Chartered Institution of Building Services Engineers, London.

Cole M.D., Clearkin L., Dabbs T. and Smerdon D. (1987) The seat belt law and after. *Br J Ophthalmol*, **71**, 436–440.

Collins M. (1983) *Occupational Public Health Optometry*. Queensland Institute of Technology, Queensland.

David D.B., Shah P., Whittaker C. and Kirkby G.R. (1995) Ocular protection in squash clubs – time for a change. *Eye* **9(5)**, 575–577.

Desai P., MacEwen C.J., Baines P. and Minassian D.C. (1996a). Epidemiology and implications of ocular trauma admitted to hospital in Scotland. *J Epidemiol Community Health*, **50(4)**, 436–441.

Desai P., MacEwen C.J., Baines P. and Minassian D.C. (1996b) Incidence of cases of ocular trauma admitted to hospital and incidence of blinding outcome. *Br J Ophthalmol*, **80**, 592–596.

Duma S.M., Kress T.A., Porta D.J., Woods C.D., Snider J.N., Fuller P.M. *et al.* (1996) Airbag-induced eye injuries: a report of 25 cases. *J Trauma Inj Inf Crit Care*, **41**, 114–119.

Easterbrook M. (1981) Eye injuries in racket sports: a continuous problem. *Physician Sportsman*, **9(1)**, 91–99.

Easterbrook M. (1988) Ocular injuries in racquet sports. *Int Ophthal Clin*, **28(3)**, 232–237.

Farmer D. (1982) Eye protection brought into perspective. *Health and Safety at Work*, **April**, 20–24.

Fong L.P. (1995) Eye injuries in Victoria, Australia. *Med J Aust*, **162**, 64–68.

Gervais G. (1989) Patient resistance to the wearing of safety spectacles. BSc final year project, Department of Optometry, UWCC, Cardiff.

Giovinazzo V.J., Yannuzzi L.A., Sorenson J.A., Delrowe D.J. and Cambell E.A. (1987) The ocular complications of boxing. *Ophthalmol (Rochester)*, **94**, 587–597.

Gregory P.T.S. (1986) Sussex Eye Hospital sports injuries. *Br J Ophthalmol*, **70**, 748–750.

Gross A. (1982) How the Norfolk and Western Railway drastically reduced the on the job injuries. *Sightsaving*, **51**, 14–17.

Grundy J.W. (1981) Eyes geared for the job. *Optical World*, **December**, 10–11.

Hall N.F., Denning A.M., Elkington A.R. and Cooper P.J. (1985) The eye and seat belt wear in Wessex. *Br J Ophthalmol*, **69**, 317–319.

Health and Safety Commission (1994) *Health and Safety Statistics. Statistical Supplement to the 1993/94 Annual Report*. HSE Books, UK.

Health and Safety Commission (1996) *Health and Safety (Safety Signs and Signals) Regulations*. HMSO, London.

John G., Witherspoon C.D., Feist R.M. and Morris R. (1988) Ocular lawn mower injuries. *Ophthalmology*, **95**, 1367–1370.

Johnson P.B. and Armstrong M.F.J. (1986) Eye injuries in Northern Ireland two years after seat belt legislation. *Br J Ophthalmol*, **70**, 460–462.

Jones N.P. (1988) One-year study of severe eye injuries in sport. *Eye*, **2**, 484–487.

Jones N.P. and Griffith G.A.P. (1992) Eye injuries at work – a prospective population-based survey within the chemical industry. *Eye*, **6**, 381–385.

Kelly S.P. (1987) Serious eye injuries in badminton players. *Br J Ophthalmol*, **71**, 746–747.

Lambah P. (1968) Adult injuries at Wolverhampton. *Trans Ophthal Soc (UK)*, **88**, 661.

La Roche G.R., McIntyre L. and Schertzer R.M. (1988) Epidemiology of severe eye injuries in childhood. *Ophthalmology*, **95**, 1603–1607.

Lathey M. (1973) Introduction of an eye protection programme. *Aust J Optom*, **56**, 321–326.

Leventhal H., Safer M. and Panagis D. (1983) Impact of communications on the self regulation of health beliefs, decisions and behaviour. *Health Ed Q*, **10**, 3–29.

MacEwen C.J. (1989) Eye injuries: a prospective survey of 5671 cases. *Br J Ophthalmol*, **73**, 888–894.

Manchee E.E., Goldberg R.A. and Mondino B.J. (1997) Airbag-related ocular injuries. *Ophthal Surg Lasers*, **28**, 246–250.

Moore M.C. and Worthly D.A. (1977) Ocular injuries in squash players. *Aust J Ophthalmol*, **5**, 46.

Moore A.T., McCartney A. and Cooling R.J. (1987) Ocular injuries associated with the use of air guns. *Eye*, **1**, 422–429.

Napier S.M., Baker R.S., Sanford D.G. and Easterbrook M. (1996) Eye injuries in athletics and recreation. *Surv Ophthalmol*, **41(3)**, 229–244.

Owen C.G., Margrain T.H. and Woodward E.G. (1995) Aetiology and prevalence of eye injuries within the United Kingdom fire service. *Ophthal Physiol Opt*, **9**, 54–58.

Pardham S., Shacklock P. and Weatherill J. (1995) Sport-related eye trauma: a survey of the presentation of eye injuries to a casualty clinic and the use of protective eyewear. *Eye*, **9**, 50–53.

Parver L.M. (1988) The national eye trauma system. *Int Ophthalmol*, **28**, 203–205.

Powell P., Hale M. and Simon M. (1971) *2000 Accidents: A Shop-floor Study based on 42 Months Continuous Observation*. National Institute of Industrial Psychology, London.

Randall K.A. (1985) First aid for home eye injuries. *Sightsaving*, **54(1)**, 10–14.

Rooke F.C.E., Rothwell P.J. and Woodhouse D.F. (1980) *Ophthalmic Nursing: Its Practice and Management*. Churchill Livingstone, London, pp. 75–77.

Rosenstock I., Derryberry M. and Carriger B.K. (1959) Why people fail to seek poliomyelitis vaccination. *Public Health Reports (UK)*, **74**, 98–103.

Taylor H.A. (1973) Maintenance of an eye protection programme. *Aust J Optom*, **56**, 86–90.

Van Nakagawara B. (1988) Functional model of an eye protection program: guide for the clinical optometrist. *J Am Optom Assoc*, **59**, 925–928.

Vinger P.F. (1980) Sports-related eye injury. A preventable problem. *Surv Ophthalmol*, **25(1)**, 47–51.

Vinger P.F. (1985) Setting performance standards for sports eye guards. *Sightsaving*, **54(1)**, 8–9.

Wigglesworth F.C. (1970) Motivation in eye protection programs. *Am J Optom AAAO*, **47(2)**, 891–898.

Wood K.H. (1973) Introduction of an eye protection programme. *Aust J Optom*, **56**, 63–69.

Woods T.A. (1988) The role of opticianry in preventing ocular injury. *Int Ophthal Clin*, **28(3)**, 251–254.

Wykes W.N. (1988) A 10-year survey of penetrating eye injuries in Gwent, 1976–85. *Br J Ophthalmol*, **72**, 607–611'

FURTHER READING

Gregg J.R. (1987) *Vision and Sports – An Introduction.* Butterworth-Heinemann, Stoneham, MA.

Loran D.F.C. and MacEwan C.J. (1995) *Sports Vision.* Butterworth-Heinemann, Oxford.

Nylman J.S. (ed.) (1989) *Problems in Optometry. Ocular Emergencies*, Vol. 1. J.B. Lippincott Company, Philadelphia.

4 Ocular injuries – mechanical

Chapter 3 outlined the causes and frequency of eye injuries, and this chapter will discuss the resultant effects upon the eye. Eye injuries, whatever their cause and however minor they appear to be, should always be treated seriously. All are potentially dangerous because of the possibility of infection or other secondary effects.

Ocular hazards can be divided into two main groups; mechanical and non-mechanical (Figure 4.1). The effects of these hazards upon the eye are numerous, and have been described in depth by several books. The main references used in compiling this chapter are Duke-Elder and MacFaul (1972), Fox (1973) and Shingleton et al. (1991).

Mechanical injuries may arise from a variety of causes, and their effects are generally divided into two main categories:

1. Contusion
2. Perforation.

CONTUSION INJURIES

Contusion injuries may result from a variety of causes, including flying blunt objects (such as a squash ball), falling objects, explosions or compressed air accidents, fluid under pressure escaping from burst pipes, and water jets from fire hoses (Acheson et al., 1987). More recently contusion injuries have been reported due to airbag inflation as a result of a car accident (Zabriskie; et al., 1997).

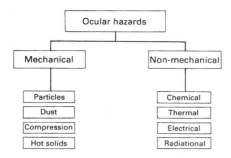

Fig. 4.1 *Classification of ocular hazards.*

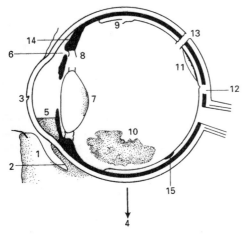

Fig. 4.2 *Composite diagram of the possible ocular effects of a contusion injury (modified from Coakes and Holmes Sellors, 1985, and courtesy of Butterworth Heinemann, Oxford. 1, black eye; 2, subconjunctival haemorrhage; 3, corneal abrasion; 4, blow-out fracture; 5, hyphaema; 6, iridodialysis; 7, cataract; 8, lens subluxation due to torn zonule; 9, retinal tear/detachment; 10, vitreous haemorrhage; 11, commotio retinae; 12, choroidal rupture; 13, scleral rupture; 14, angle recession; 15, retinal haemorrhage.*

The resultant ocular damage is due to a wave of pressure traversing the fluid content of the eye. As the fluid is incompressible, the blow will act as an explosive force in all directions from the centre outwards, resulting in the ocular contents being flung against their outer coat. The globe expands around the equator to take up a vertically oval shape. The effects of contusion on the various structures are numerous, and Figure 4.2 shows some of the possible ocular injuries that may occur.

The eyelids and orbit

Eye lids – black eye

Fortunately, the eyes have their own natural defence; they are deeply set in bony orbits and have a fast blink reflex. Hence the eye often escapes damage and the orbits and lids take the force of the blow, frequently resulting in the appearance of a black eye. Due to the vascularity and loose connective tissue structure of the lid, oedema and subcutaneous haemorrhages are common and usually occur rapidly after trauma. Haemorrhages may also spread under the conjunctiva, resulting in the lids being swollen and tightly shut. To examine the eye, the lids may need to be opened forcibly. A 'black eye' may spread to the other eye within 24 hours as a result of subcutaneous blood infiltration (Fox, 1973). The swelling and discolouration of the skin normally resolve within 2 weeks.

In more severe cases, the haemorrhages may be due to intracranial damage. Such haemorrhages become apparent after 12–24 hours, which is the time it takes for the blood to seep to the eyelids and forehead. This is a serious condition, and X-rays must be taken to see whether there are fractures of the orbital bones.

Ptosis

Trauma to the upper lid may cause it to droop, which narrows the palpebral aperture. This is known as ptosis, and may be caused by the lid being oedematous. In more severe cases there can be damage to the IIIrd nerve, which supplies the levator muscle, or detachment of the muscle itself; the latter case will require surgery. Occasionally a partial protective ptosis, or a tendency for the lid to close, will develop if there is an irritant causing discomfort and photophobia.

Ectropion

Damage to the lower lid may result in ectropion, a condition in which the lid margin turns away from the eye. This prevents the tears from draining properly through the puncta. Instead they flow down the cheek (epiphora) and can cause skin sores.

Fractures of the orbit

These can occur directly from a blow to the orbit, or indirectly from radiating skull fractures. These injuries may also be associated with other facial fractures, head injuries or severe lacerations.

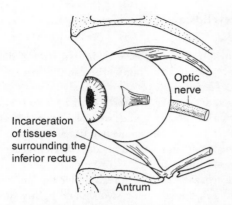

Fig. 4.3 *Orbital floor fracture (after Elkington, 1973a).*

Not surprisingly, the most common fracture affects the lateral wall of the orbit. The zygomatic bone and arch of the lateral wall may be fractured, resulting in depression of the lateral canthus and flattening of the cheekbone.

Fractures of the floor of the orbit may occur after a heavy blow, and are known as blow-out fractures. The blow increases the intraorbital pressure, which causes the very thin bone of the maxilla to collapse into the maxillary sinus; the orbital contents then prolapse into the antrum. Elevation of the eye will be defective because the tissues surrounding the inferior rectus and inferior oblique muscle become trapped in the fracture (Figure 4.3). Double vision will also be present in one or more directions of gaze. The herniation of the orbital contents results in a sinking or recession of the eye within the orbit (enophthalmos) with a narrowing of the palpebral fissure. There will also be loss of feeling on the same side of the face due to damage to the infraorbital nerve. Surgery, if required, should be carried out fairly promptly (within a week or two), before fibrous tissue has a chance to form. It will involve the insertion of a plate over the damaged orbital floor.

Damage to the nasal bone, ethmoidal sinuses and the medial wall is often apparent by the presence of air crepitus. Blowing the nose should be avoided, as air is forced under pressure into the soft tissue of the eyelids and surrounding skin, which results in swelling. As this can provide a route for the spread of infection, a course of systemic antibiotics is usually given (Sachsenweger, 1980).

Fractures of the superior orbital rim generally result in diplopia due to damage of the trochlear of the superior oblique muscle. This damage will be permanent unless there is early repair.

Inferior orbital rim damage is shown by ptosis or ectropion of the lower lid, and by anaesthesia of infraorbital nerve distribution. It is often associated with diplopia and hypotropia (Fox, 1973).

Whenever a fracture is suspected, X-rays should be taken.

Anterior segment damage

Damage to the anterior segment may result in corneal abrasions, hyphaema and associated damage to the ciliary body, iris, or lens. Secondary complications such as recurrent bleeding, uveitis, and abnormal intraocular pressure may also occur.

Subconjunctival haemorrhages

The conjunctiva, being the most superficial layer, often displays subconjunctival haemorrhages, but these reabsorb within several weeks and do not need treatment. However, subconjunctival haemorrhages caused by orbital bleeding can be so severe that the conjunctiva projects between the lids and, as mentioned above, this requires prompt attention.

Hyphaema

The anterior chamber may appear red as the result of the presence of blood. This is known as hyphaema, and is due to the rupture of a vessel in the iris or ciliary body. The chamber is generally only partially filled and the blood settles inferiorly. It will usually be reabsorbed without any serious consequences. However, in some cases the anterior chamber may completely fill with blood (total hyphaema). If the blood is not reabsorbed after a few days, its colour changes from red to purple to black. This occurs due to a lack of oxygen from the aqueous, and is sometimes referred to as an 'eight ball' hyphaema. This is a serious condition because the intraocular pressure is generally elevated, resulting in secondary glaucoma and possible blood staining of the cornea.

Re-bleeding may occur, resulting in secondary glaucoma, blood staining of the cornea, and permanent loss of vision. The source is uncertain, but it may arise from newly formed capillaries in the area of damage, or from the original leaking blood vessel. It usually occurs in the first 5 days after injury (Read and Goldberg, 1974). Surgery is frequently required in cases of re-bleeding, which should therefore be prevented if at all possible (Thomas *et al.*, 1986). Given the possible complications, hyphaema must always be referred, however small the amount of blood visible in the anterior chamber. The patient may be admitted to hospital and bed rest given for a couple of days.

Hyphaemas may also indicate the presence of scleral ruptures. The most common sites are in a circumferential arc parallel to the corneal limbus, opposite to the impact site at either the insertion of rectus muscles on the globe or at the equator of the globe. This type of injury commonly occurs as a result of a squash ball hitting the eye.

Iris

Damage to the iris may result in dilation or constriction of the pupil, which is known as traumatic mydriasis or traumatic miosis, respectively. Depending on the severity of the blow, the paralysis may be temporary, lasting only a few days or be permanent (Fox, 1973).

Ruptures may occur to the sphincter pupillae, leaving a permanently irregular, semi-dilated pupil that will not react to light or accommodation. The iris can be torn from its insertion to the ciliary body; this is known as iridodialysis. It is a permanent condition, usually accompanied by hyphaema, and results in a distortion of the pupil. Both conditions will cause symptoms of glare, especially in the case of iridodialysis, where a second pupil has formed, which will result in monocular diplopia.

Angle recession

Traumatic angle recession of the anterior chamber can lead to the development of unilateral glaucoma months or years later. It occurs when the ciliary body has been torn from the sclera. Extensive angles of recession have been found in subjects with prolonged primary hyphaemas. The site of the recession can be predicted from the presence of traumatic mydriasis. The affected area of the pupil is atonic, neither fully dilates nor constricts, and corresponds to the position of the angle recession (Eagling, 1974).

Lens

The zonular fibres that attach the lens to the ciliary body can be torn in a contusion injury. As a result, the lens may become totally dislocated from its attachment, or partially dislocated (subluxated). The dislocated lens may fall either posteriorly into the vitreous, where low-grade ophthalmitis may occur, or enter the anterior chamber, causing corneal endothelial damage. There will be a marked hyperopic shift in the refraction, and a tremulous iris (iridodonesis) may be seen due to the loss of support by the lens.

A subluxated lens produces a prismatic effect on vision, with the upward displacement of objects. This may cause symptoms such as diplopia, nausea and vomiting.

The sudden compression and expansion of the lens, with or without rupture of the capsule, can produce a cataract. In fact, trauma is the most common cause of unilateral cataract in the young (Kanski, 1984). There is a case report of a ruptured anterior lens capsule in a 10-year-old girl, caused by an airbag inflating after a minor car accident. She also presented with a corneal abrasion and a small hyphaema (Zabriskie *et al.*, 1997).

Various types of lens changes can occur, and these have been listed by Duke-Elder and MacFaul (1972) as follows:

1. *Vossius ring opacity.* A circle of iris pigment known as the vossius ring may be seen on the lens after impaction of the iris. This usually occurs only in the young, as older, more sclerosed lenses will not accept such an imprint. The pigment is usually absorbed and may be replaced by fine capsular dots, which gradually clear later in life.

2. *Sub-epithelial disseminated opacities.* The lens may appear to have small, discrete punctate or flake-like opacities, which lie beneath the anterior epithelium. These opacities may be transient, disappearing within a few days or weeks, or permanent. Occasionally, the development of these opacities is delayed, and they may not become apparent until several years after injury.

3. *Traumatic rosette-shaped cataract.* The rosette-shaped opacity may occur anteriorly or posteriorly and the onset may be delayed, in which case the opacities are usually found in the deeper cortical layers or the nucleus. This type of cataract may occur after perforating or contusion injuries.

4. *Diffuse cataract.* A diffuse concussion cataract is rare, and is usually associated with a tear of the lens capsule. If the tear is large, the lens fibres may spill into the anterior or posterior chamber.

This will result in secondary glaucoma or an inflammation of the iris and ciliary body (anterior uveitis).

5. *Zonular cataract.* Zonular (lamellar) cataracts are rare, and consist of a series of concentric, thin sheets of opacities surrounded by clear lens. They usually occur after extensive disseminated opacities or after rosette-shaped opacities.

Posterior segment damage

Damage to the posterior segment may initially be obscured from direct view by a hyphaema. The damage that may occur to the retina after contusion has been listed by Duke-Elder and MacFaul (1972) as:

1. Oedema, macular cysts and holes, necrosis, atrophic retinal changes
2. Vascular changes – haemorrhages (embolism, thrombosis, aneurysm)
3. Tears of the choroid and retina
4. Retinal detachment.

Oedema, cysts, holes, and necrosis

The retina may appear milky-white within a few hours of the trauma, and vision will be reduced. Commotio retinae is the term used to describe oedema of the retina; it is transient and reversible. The oedema usually subsides within 4 days, and vision returns to normal. (Some authorities believe that the white retinal appearance is not due to oedema but to derangement of the photoreceptors, whilst others believe it may be due to choroidal ischaemia; Deutsch and Feller, 1985.) In some cases vision may be permanently impaired due to the development of pigmentary changes at the macula, or to the formation of a macular cyst or hole. In severe injuries, intraretinal haemorrhages or haemorrhages into the anterior vitreous from the pars plana region may occur.

Vascular changes

Eyes with pathologically altered blood vessels (e.g. in patients with hypertension, arteriosclerosis or diabetes) are particularly vulnerable to haemorrhages. These haemorrhages may be retinal, subretinal, preretinal or vitreal. They may cause a sudden and profound loss of vision, and leave the site of retinal pathology obscured from view.

Tears of the choroid and retina

Although the choroid is firmly attached to the sclera, choroidal tears are common and generally occur between the disc and macula, or temporal to the macula. They are crescentic, vertical and of variable length; they may be single or multiple. Haemorrhages into the choroid, subretinal space or the retina itself may occur after such tears. These haemorrhages are usually absorbed, leaving yellowish-grey lesions in the choroid. The tears affect vision only if they are between the disc and macula. In one report, only 39 per cent of patients with choroidal and retinal lesions from contusion injuries regained a visual acuity of 6/12 or better (Archer and Canavan, 1983). A study by De Laey (1987) has noted that a late complication of choroidal ruptures may be choroidal neovascularization. This can usually be treated successfully by photocoagulation.

Choroidal detachment does not occur unless trauma is combined with decreased intraocular pressure. This allows fluid to pass into the suprachoroidal space, facilitating the detachment.

Retinal detachment

This is the separation of the retina from the pigment epithelium, which may occur gradually or suddenly. In cases of a gradual detachment the individual may be unaware of the condition, but symptoms such as floaters and photopsia (light flashes) due to vitreous traction on the retina may be experienced. Typically, if the retinal detachment occurs shortly after trauma, a peripheral retinal tear is found, frequently in the upper temporal region. The presence of tobacco dust (pigment cells) in the anterior vitreous is a strong indicator that there is a retinal tear present. People with predisposing factors, such as myopia, peripheral retinal degeneration and aphakia, where there are areas of retinal weakness, are more prone to retinal tears and hence detachments.

Scleral ruptures have been noted to occur after a severe blunt trauma, and are commonly seen in the superior and anterior portions of the globe (Russel *et al.*, 1988).

Nervous supply

The innervation to the eye may be affected after a contusion injury. Contusion of the infraorbital nerve will lead to decreased sensitivity or anaesthesia of the skin in the area of distribution of the nerve. The infra-orbital nerve is damaged most frequently after blunt trauma, whereas the supraorbital nerve is usually only affected after a sharp blow (Fox, 1973).

The innervation to the extraocular muscles, which are responsible for eye movements, may also be affected. Horizontal double vision may occur due to VIth cranial nerve damage, but fortunately recovery is complete in most cases. If the IVth trochlear nerve is involved, it gives rise to vertical double vision. Trauma to the IIIrd nerve may result in mydriasis, ptosis, double vision, lack of adduction and loss of accommodation. Traumatic hyperopia, due to the loss of accommodation, may be temporary or permanent. Myopic changes, which occur more commonly, are generally due to ciliary muscle spasm caused by irritation to the nerve or the muscle fibres. Myopic shifts in the order of 1–6 D may occur, but in most cases they are transient and the refraction returns to normal within about a month (Duke-Elder and MacFaul, 1972).

The optic nerve may be partially or completely ruptured, with partial or complete evulsion after blunt trauma (Williams *et al.*, 1987). Visual field defects will be found corresponding to the position of the damaged nerve fibres, so there will be permanent partial or total loss of vision, depending on the severity of the injury. Papillitis, swelling of the optic disc and optic atrophy may also occur following widespread retinal or choroidal damage (Duke-Elder and MacFaul, 1972).

PERFORATING INJURIES

Foreign bodies

The most common type of ocular trauma is due to foreign bodies (FBs), which account for about half of all eye injuries. They generally result from a person not realizing the hazard of the task – for instance, when using a hammer and chisel or grinding wheel, or cutting wire. The eye's natural defence mechanisms may be penetrated, and foreign bodies (FBs) may become embedded in the globe or pass through the cornea or sclera to become lodged within the globe. The symptoms can vary from little or no discomfort to severe pain. Figure 4.4 shows the common sites of foreign bodies.

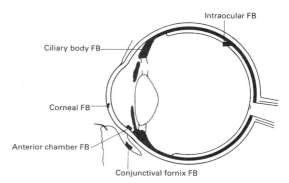

Fig. 4.4 *Sites of ocular foreign bodies.*

Subtarsal foreign bodies

Many small FBs will be washed out of the eye by the tears. Sometimes, however, the FB will become embedded in the subtarsal conjunctiva of the upper lid, which will cause pain on blinking and a vertical corneal abrasion. The area of abraded cornea, where the epithelium has been removed, will be seen as a disturbance of the corneal reflection. This can be viewed by instilling fluorescein and viewing the eye under ultraviolet light. The upper lid must be everted if these FBs are to be located and removed. The healing of the epithelium may sometimes be incomplete, resulting in recurrent corneal erosions.

Superficial foreign bodies

An eye with a corneal FB usually shows marked vascular injection closest to its position (Novak, 1970). Ocular pain will be experienced, but is difficult to localize. If the corneal FB has been present for a couple of days a grey ring of infiltration may occur around it, and on removal a small, pitted ulcer will remain. It may leave a permanent scar, although this will generally only affect the vision if it is over the centre of the cornea. A foreign body embedded in the conjunctiva or sclera is often surrounded by haemorrhages.

Many FBs are metallic, with iron particles being the most common, followed by copper and aluminium. The softer metals (e.g. magnesium) are less frequently a cause of FBs, as they tend to fragment less during drilling, sawing, grinding and cutting. Metallic FBs left embedded in the eye will rapidly oxidize under the influence of the enzymes of the cornea and tears, and this may set up a severe inflammation of the cornea or iris. The oxidation of steel is much faster than that of aluminium or magnesium, and a rust ring may be apparent within a couple of hours. A rust deposit left in the cornea will partially dissolve, and an iron stain will diffuse into stromal or subepithelial layers.

Intraocular foreign bodies

The possible presence of an intraocular foreign body (IOFB) should always be investigated, especially when the symptoms are a gush of fluid from the eye with blurring of vision. Small, hot FBs hitting the eye at great speed may penetrate the globe and actually seal their route of entry. Only a slight pain is experienced. It is essential not to miss an IOFB, as it may lead to loss of vision. Whenever the eye is perforated, an X-ray should be taken to exclude the presence of a metallic IOFB. The classic signs of a perforating injury are a shallow anterior chamber, eccentricity of the pupil, and prolapse of the iris. However, particular care must be taken with the following two presentations (Elkington, 1973a):

- Where a small conjunctival haemorrhage is the only clue; this may obscure deeper scleral laceration
- Where an eye appears normal, but there is a history suggestive of an IOFB.

The IOFB may have been stopped by the iris and then fallen down into the anterior chamber angle to be hidden from view. If an IOFB has penetrated through the vitreous, fibrous tissue will form along its path. The fibrous tissue may impair vision if it crosses over the visual axis, and a vitrectomy may then be required to restore vision and/or to prevent tractional retinal detachment.

There are various methods of localizing IOFBs, including X-ray techniques, ultrasonography, binocular indirect ophthalmoscopy, and the use of a Berman and Roper Hall localizer, which employs electric induction currents (Deutsch and Feller, 1985). Ultrasonography can locate non-metallic fragments, whereas X-rays show metallic FBs. Ultrasonography traces the rebound of high frequency pulsations, and by studying the resulting patterns the inside of the eye can be explored. Once the IOFB has been located it can be removed.

Retained intraocular foreign bodies

Vegetable FBs may cause infections so severe that a purulent panophthalmitis may occur in only a few hours. Other FBs, such as gold, silver, platinum, glass and many plastics, may be retained without noticeable reaction (Fox, 1973). Lead, zinc, nickel and aluminium particles are less well tolerated by the eye. These are often coated in an inert salt and later encapsulated by a fibrous tissue coating, rendering them less toxic.

The most dangerous IOFBs are iron and copper, which cause siderosis and chalcosis, respectively. In siderosis the iron oxidizes and causes a slow, insidious intraocular reaction as it permeates most of the ocular tissues (Elkington, 1973a); this can lead to complete blindness. It is a late-occurring syndrome, and the ferrous pigmentation causes a rusty coloration of the cornea, iris or lens. In addition, a series of chronic degenerative changes occur, which lead to pupil dilation because of atrophy of the sphincter pupillae, cataract, and then retinal detachment and open angle glaucoma. These complications usually occur between 2 months and 2 years after injury. Surgery is therefore urgently required after injury to remove the foreign body (Deutsch and Feller, 1985).

Pure copper will cause a rapid inflammation of the eye (chalcosis), and the eye may be lost if endophthalmitis occurs. Copper alloys (bronze and brass) may induce chronic degenerative processes by slow diffusion of the copper, which tends to be taken up by the limiting membranes of the eye (Elkington, 1973a). A green ring may develop in the peripheral cornea in Descemet's membrane (Kayser–Fleisher ring), and a sunflower cataract may form in the anterior capsule of the lens.

Another complication after IOFB trauma has been noted by Trimble and Schatz (1986), who reported cases where subretinal neovascularization occurred 6–8 months after a metallic IOFB. This was successfully treated by photocoagulation.

Lacerations

In cases where lacerations involve the cornea and sclera there may be a prolapse of the iris, ciliary body, lens and vitreous, resulting in complete disorganization of the globe. Posterior rupture of the globe is rare, and should be suspected when there is extreme conjunctival oedema and haemorrhage with marked hypotony. Unfortunately, useful vision is not often restored, even after prompt surgery. Lacerations may also occur after blunt trauma; for example, two cases of lacerations caused by jets of water from an agricultural sprinkler have been reported (Salminen and Ranta, 1983).

Infections of the eye

The main danger of IOFBs is that they may carry infections into the eye, resulting in uveitis, an inflammation of the entire uveal tract. Infections may be caused by brucellosis or toxoplasmosis (McWilliam, 1973). This is not as serious as a purulent infection, which usually results in the loss of the eye due to panophthalmitis or endophthalmitis.

A very rare and serious complication of perforating lacerations from an IOFB is sympathetic ophthalmitis, a type of uveitis affecting the non-injured eye, which can lead to blindness. The second eye usually becomes involved 2 weeks to 2 months after injury (Elkington, 1973b). Usually the initial treatment is topical and systemic steroids. But it has been suggested that the only effective therapy is preventive enucleation of the injured eye despite the use of immunosuppressive agents (Albert and Diaz-Rohena, 1989).

An individual who has received a perforating injury should be sent for immediate medical attention. The eye should never be padded, as this may cause the ocular contents to prolapse. A cardboard cone can be placed over the eye to protect it from dust, dirt etc. X-rays should be taken if the presence of an IOFB is suspected, to determine if it is metallic.

SUMMARY

Contusion and perforating injuries commonly occur after ocular trauma. The extent of the injuries can be minor or very severe, and any person with an eye injury should receive medical attention to assess the situation and the treatment needed.

REFERENCES

Acheson J.F., Wong D. and Chignell A.H. (1987) Eye injuries caused by direct jets of water from a fire hose. *Br Med J*, **292**, 481–482.
Albert D.M. and Diaz-Rohena R. (1989) A historical review of sympathetic ophthalmia and its epidemiology. *Sum Ophthalmol*, **34**, 1–14.
Archer D.B. and Canavan Y.M. (1983) Contusional eye injuries: retinal and choroidal lesions. *Aust J Ophthalmol*, **11**, 251–264.
Coakes R.L. and Holmes Sellors P.J. (1985) *An Outline of Ophthalmology*. Wright and Sons Ltd, Bristol.
De Laey J.J. (1987) Choroidal neovascularisation after traumatic choroidal rupture. *Bull Soc Belge Ophthalmol*, **220**, 53–59.
Deutsch T.A. and Feller D.B. (1985) *Paton and Goldberg's Management of Ocular Injuries*, 2nd edn. W.B. Saunders & Co., Philadelphia, PA.
Duke-Elder S. and MacFaul P.A. (eds) (1972) *System of Ophthalmology – Injuries*, Vol. XIV, Parts 1 and 2. Henry Kimpton, London.
Eagling E.M. (1974) Ocular damage after blunt trauma to the eye – its relationship to the nature and extent of the injury. *Br J Ophthalmol*, **58**, 126–139.
Elkington A.R. (1973a) Intraocular foreign bodies. *Nursing Times*, **December**, 1638–1639.
Elkington A.R. (1973b) Perforating wounds. *Nursing Times*, **November**, 1597–1598.
Fox S.L. (1973) *Industrial and Occupational Ophthalmology*. C.C. Thomas, IL.
Kanski J.J. (1984) *Clinical Ophthalmology*. Butterworths, London.
McWilliam R.J. (1973) Infection of the eye. *Nursing Times*, **February**, 145–146.
Novak J.F. (1970) Ocular trauma in industry. *J Occup Med*, **12**, 287–290.
Read J. and Goldberg M.F. (1974) Blunt ocular trauma and hyphema. *Int Ophthal Clin*, **14**, 57–59.
Russel S.R., Olsen K.R. and Folk J.C. (1988) Predictors of scleral rupture and the role of vitrectomy in severe blunt ocular trauma. *Am J Ophthalmol*, **105**, 253–257.
Sachsenweger R. (1980) *Illustrated Handbook of Ophthalmology*. Wright and Son Ltd, Bristol.
Salminen L. and Ranta A. (1983) Orbital laceration caused by a blast of water: report of two cases. *Br J Ophthalmol*, **67**, 840–841.
Shingleton B.J., Hersh P.S. and Kenyon K.R. (1991). *Eye Trauma*. Mosby Year Book, St Louis, MS.
Thomas M.A., Parrish R.K. II and Feuer W.J. (1986) Rebleeding after traumatic hyphema. *Arch Ophthalmol*, **104**, 206–210.
Trimble S.N. and Schatz H. (1986) Subretinal neovascularisation following metallic intraocular foreign body trauma. *Arch Ophthalmol*, **104**, 515–519.
Williams D.F., Williams G.A., Abrams G.W., Jesmanowicz A. and Hyde J.S. (1987) Evulsion of the retina associated with optic nerve evulsion. *Am J Ophthalmol*, **104**, 5–9.
Zabriskie N.A., Hwang I.P., Ramsey J.F. and Crandall A.S. (1997) Anterior lens capsule rupture caused by air bag trauma. *Am J Ophthalmol*, **123**, 832–833.

FURTHER READING

Catalano R.A and Belin M. (eds) (1992) *Ocular Emergencies.* W.B. Saunders & Co., London.

Deutsch T.A. and Feller B. (eds) (1985) *Paton and Goldberg's Management of Ocular Injuries.* W.B. Saunders & Co., Philadelphia, PA.

Duke-Elder S. and MacFaul P.A. (eds) (1972) *System of Ophthalmology – Injuries*, Vol. XIV, Parts 1 and 2. Henry Kimpton, London.

Fox S.L. (1973) *Industrial and Occupational Ophthalmology.* C.C. Thomas, IL.

Nyman J.S. (ed.) (1989) *Problems in Optometry. Ocular Emergencies*, Vol.1, No.1. J.B. Lippincott, Philadelphia, PA.

Roper-Hall M.J. (1987) *Eye Emergencies.* Churchill Livingstone, Edinburgh.

Shingleton B.J., Hersh P.S. and Kenyon K.R. (1991) *Eye Trauma.* Mosby Year Book, St Louis, MS.

5 Ocular injuries – non-mechanical

Non-mechanical ocular injuries fall into four main categories:

1. Chemical
2. Thermal
3. Electrical
4. Radiation.

CHEMICAL INJURIES

Most chemicals harm the eyes by direct contact with the external ocular tissues, and these are amongst the most urgent ocular emergencies. Concentrated sulphuric acid from exploding car batteries, household bleaches, detergents, disinfectants and lime are examples of chemicals that can cause burns to the eyes. However, it should not be forgotten that chemicals can also cause damage to the internal ocular structures (e.g. the retina and optic nerve) through systemic absorption.

Direct effect of chemicals

Chemicals may be in the form of gases, vapours, liquids or solids, and the main groups that produce damage are:

- Acids
- Alkalis
- Organic solvents
- Surfactants
- Irritants and allergens
- Aerosols.

Acids

The severity of the burn depends on the concentration of the chemical, the duration of the exposure and the pH of the solution. Inorganic acids include sulphuric acid, nitric acid and hydrochloric acid. When splashed, these acids may burn the eyelids and face, but fortunately the lid closure reflex is so fast that the eyeball is not generally affected. It may, however, suffer subsequently from exposure as a result of scar tissue formation and contraction of the lids. All solutions are irritating to the eye, but this is rarely serious if their pH is 2.5 or above (Fox, 1973). Diluted acids produce redness, oedema and small conjunctival haemorrhages, and prolonged exposure causes ulceration and opaqueness of the cornea and conjunctival epithelium. The epithelium normally regenerates to leave a clear cornea; however, if the acid is strong, then stromal opacification and corneal vascularization will occur. The tissues may even be charred by concentrated nitric or sulphuric acids, and in the severest cases complete destruction of the cornea and anterior structures will result.

The damage caused by acids depends upon the protein affinity of the acid anion and the concentration of the acid (Novak, 1970). The acids act by combining chemically with the protein of the more superficial tissues to form an insoluble acid proteinate. This acts as a buffer, which limits the penetration of the acid through the tissues, cornea etc.

Acid burns are generally less severe than alkali burns, and they tend to improve with treatment and time. They are common in artificial silk manufacturing, as the viscous process exposes the workers to a fine spray of sulphuric acid. Acid burns are also frequently associated with glass injuries resulting from flasks and bottles breaking, and there have been reports of exploding car batteries causing sulphuric acid burns to the eyes (Minatoya, 1978).

In general, organic acids have minimal penetration of the cornea and hence rarely cause dense corneal opacification. This group of acids includes formic, acetic and citric acids (Duke-Elder, 1972).

Alkalis

Alkalis penetrate tissues rapidly. They act by combining with the lipoid cells of the membranes, and produce total disruption of cells with softening of the tissues (Deutsch and Feller, 1985). Once the alkali has gained entry to the corneal stroma, it progresses to Descemet's membrane by the cations combining temporarily with the mucoproteins and

collagen. The mucoproteins are then denatured rapidly, and the released cations attach themselves to even deeper stromal proteins (Fox, 1973). The initial appearance of the eye after trauma may be deceptive, showing little apparent damage, but it may become worse with time, eventually resulting in a totally opaque cornea.

Salts of weak acids and strong bases (such as sodium carbonate) and organic amines have strong alkaline reactions; phenols also act similarly to alkalis.

The ocular effects of alkalis have been studied and noted to progress through three stages (Hughes, 1946; Brown et al., 1972):

1. The acute stage – ischaemic necrosis of the conjunctiva; sloughing of the corneal epithelium; oedema; and opacification of the subconjunctival tissue, the substantia propria, and acute iritis.
2. The reparation stage – the epithelium regenerates, vascularization appears and the iritis subsides.
3. Late complications – symblepharon; an opaque, vascularized cornea with recurrent ulcerations; uveitis; secondary glaucoma; and cataract.

There is a rapid increase in the intraocular pressure after severe chemical burns, especially with alkalis. The mechanisms responsible for the increase in intraocular pressure are a temporary shrinkage of the corneal collagen (Paterson and Pfister, 1974) and a breakdown of the blood aqueous barrier due to the lysis of the cells lining, and adjacent to, the anterior chamber. This causes intense exudation of cells etc. into the anterior chamber, which may lead to a severe fibrinous inflammatory reaction in the conjunctiva as well as in the anterior chamber of the eye. This leads to the later complication of symblepharon, an adhesion between the bulbar and palpebral conjunctiva, and a dry eye.

As the hydroxyl ion concentration increases, the severity of the effects increases; a pH above 11 is exceedingly dangerous. However, as alkalis have different fat solubilities, the penetration ability of the cornea varies. Ammonium hydroxide has the greatest ability to dissolve fats, and it penetrates the cornea rapidly to produce deep injury. Other chemicals frequently involved in burns are the sodium, potassium, ammonium and calcium hydroxides (Fox, 1973). Lime burns are very serious, and commonly occur in the building trades (Moon and Robertson, 1983).

Table 5.1 Classification of organic solvents and their uses (from Duke-Elder, 1972)

Type of organic solvent	Example	Industrial use
Hydrocarbons, aliphatic and aromatic	Benzene	In dyeing, leather, rubber, linoleum, paints, varnish and lacquer industries; motor fuels
Halogenated hydrocarbons	Trichloroethylene	Solvents for fats, waxes, gums, resins, oils. Used in rubber and cellulose industries and in manufacture of paints, lacquers and varnishes; insecticides; antiseptics
Alcohols	Ethanol	Solvents and used in lacquers and polishes
Ketones	Acetone	Solvent in plastics, rubber, dyes and paint industries
Aldehydes	Methyl aldehyde	Solvent for oils, resins, cellulose. Used in plastics and rubber industries
Ether	Ethylether	Solvent in plastics manufacture
Ester	Methyl formate	Solvent in many industries; it is the least toxic organic solvent

Calcium oxide is a major ingredient of substances such as cement, lime, mortar, whitewashes and numerous other compounds used in this industry. When water or tears are added to calcium oxide, heat is created, causing a thermal burn. In addition, calcium hydroxide is produced, which increases the damage to the eye. Lime in particular tends to adhere to the cornea and conjunctiva, causing excessive lacrimation.

Experiments on rabbits by Brown *et al.* (1969) have shown that corneal ulceration after an alkali burn is due to the collagenolytic enzyme produced by the cornea. This has led to the use of collagenase inhibitors, such as L-cysteine, in the treatment of alkali burns to reduce the corneal ulceration. Other types of treatment include the use of EDTA, ascorbic acid and citric acid (Pfister, 1983).

Organic solvents
Numerous substances of this type are used in various industries, but they rarely cause permanent damage. Exposure to their vapour causes irritation, and a more intense reaction occurs when liquids are splashed into the eye. Organic solvents cause superficial punctate keratitis of the cornea and conjunctiva. Some of the compounds are caustic, and may enter the stroma, denature the protein, and produce scarring. The subjective symptoms are pain, photophobia, lacrimation and stinging. Such complaints are reported by those working with lacquers when solvents such as alcohol, acetone, camphor, ether, toluene, benzol and acetates are used.

Table 5.1 lists the organic solvents, along with their uses in industry, as classified by Duke-Elder (1972). It

is important to note that, when absorbed, these solvents also have toxic effects that suppress the nervous system.

Surfactants
These compounds have a fat-soluble group at one end of the molecule and a water-soluble group at the other end. This structure allows the compound to lower the surface tension of water and to make fat-soluble materials miscible. They are used as industrial detergents and as emulsifying agents, and cause contact dermatitis and mucosal irritation. Surfactants are divided into three main groups; cationic, anionic and non-ionic (Duke-Elder, 1972; Fox, 1973; Grant, 1974). The cationic group of surfactants cause damage to the cornea and conjunctiva by precipitating the protein; if severe enough, this will lead to opacification of the corneal stroma, with subsequent vascularization. Quaternary ammonium compounds such as benzylkonium chloride belong to this group. Anionic surfactants, such as soap, cause slow saponification of intracellular lipoid substances and lysis of the cells. Healing occurs quite quickly, leaving no permanent damage (Fox, 1973). The non-ionic surfactants are usually esters of fatty acids with polyoxyethylene or sorbitol. These do not cause any permanent damage, as any corneal erosions produced heal with no scarring.

Irritants and allergens
Numerous substances may irritate the eyes without causing permanent damage. A true allergy requires sensitization of cells by prior exposure to an allergen,

and subsequent exposure to the allergen will then result in a typical allergic reaction. Common allergens are organic substances of animal or vegetable origin (e.g. wool, pollen and dairy products). They produce the characteristic redness and swelling of tissues of the lids and conjunctiva.

As new processes are introduced into industry the number of substances causing dermatitis and conjunctivitis increases, and many have not yet been isolated. Unfortunately, the appearance of the skin and conjunctiva often give no clue to the actual agent involved.

It is possible to desensitize people who are liable to attacks. In certain industries, allergic skin reactions are well known and are recognized as industrial diseases. Special trades may have easily identifiable irritants, but there is no explanation as yet for the fact that large numbers of people work for years with common irritants (such as soap) without any ill effects.

Industries with a high percentage of workers reporting dermatitis include baking, chemical manufacturing, engineering, metal working, painting, preserving and textile manufacturing. Adequate ventilation and protective goggles should be provided where necessary to prevent dust and fumes contacting the eyes, as these may cause serious secondary effects such as purulent conjunctivitis and corneal erosions.

Aerosols

Aerosols are commonly used in households as well as in industry. Their fine spray can cause a superficial corneal inflammation, known as superficial punctate keratitis. After staining with fluorescein, these show up quite clearly as small punctate dots when seen under ultraviolet (UV) light; they are temporary.

Indirect effects of chemicals

Chemicals come in various forms (solid, liquid, powder, dust, mist or vapour), and some can be toxic to the eye if they are accidentally ingested, absorbed or inhaled. Neurotoxic agents, such as organic solvents, heavy metals and their salts and alcohols, can cause optic neuritis or other ocular toxicities. Many industrial poisons affect the eyes, and Table 5.2 shows the effects of some commonly used chemicals upon the ocular tissues (for further details see Grant, 1974; Hunter, 1975).

Treatment of chemical trauma

Ideal treatment is to neutralize the chemical. As this is often not possible, and as speed is critical, immediate and prolonged irrigation of the eye with water or saline should be carried out. The faster the chemical is diluted, the better the prognosis. Water fountains, showers etc. must be available in areas where chemicals are being used so that accidental spills or splashes can be dowsed immediately with water. Irrigation should be continued for at least 20 minutes and the eye should not be padded, allowing the tears continue to wash out any residual chemical. Any chemical particles that remain should also be removed. Various solutions are recommended for lime, mortar and plaster, including 11 per cent disodium edetate, 10 per cent ammonium tartrate, and 10 per cent glucose solution (Porter, 1966). For other alkali injuries, 2 per cent boric acid or 2 per cent acetic acid solutions are advised (Porter, 1961). For acid burns, 3.5 per cent sodium bicarbonate solution is advised (O'Connor Davies, 1981).

The injured employee should be referred to the casualty department of the local hospital for further ocular irrigation. Treatment then depends on the severity of the burn. In mild cases, it may involve a short course of topical antibiotics to prevent secondary infection, topical steroids and a cycloplegic. However, the use of topical steroids is controversial. Whilst they have a beneficial effect in reducing the inflammatory reaction, they can retard the repair processes and hence lead to corneal melting and perforation (Pfister, 1983).

In cases of more severe burns, the treatment aims to reduce inflammation, promote epithelial healing and prevent sterile corneal ulceration. The treatment may include the use of topical steroids, topical citric acid, topical and systemic ascorbic acid, and topical and systemic tetracycline derivatives. Citric acid has been shown to reduce the incidence of corneal ulceration in experiments by inhibiting polymorphs (Pfister *et al.*, 1982). Collagenase inhibitors have also been reported to have a beneficial effect in preventing ulcers in alkali-burned corneas (Brown *et al.*, 1969). Tetracycline derivatives are effective collagen inhibitors, which reduce scar tissue formation.

The fitting of a scleral contact lens may help prevent adhesions of the bulbar and palpebral conjunctiva, i.e. symblepharon. A full-thickness corneal graft may be necessary if the cornea is opaque. Unfortu-

Table 5.2 Indirect effects of some commonly used chemicals

Structure	Effect	Chemical	Uses
Cornea and conjunctiva	Discoloration	Iron minerals, dinitrobenzene	Organic solvent
Cornea	Scarring	Hydroquinine	
	Deposits and opacities	Beryllium, gold, silver, mercury	
	Anaesthesia	Carbon disulphide	Rayon/viscose industry
	Inflammation	Ethylbenzene	
Lens	Opacities	Dinitrophenol, naphthalene	Dye industry, insecticides
	Deposits and discoloration	Copper, mercury	
Anterior uveal tract	Iris atrophy	Quinine	
	Dilated pupil	Carbon monoxide, nitrous fumes	
	Constricted pupil and ciliary body spasms	Parathion and lindane	Insecticides
Retina	Oedema	Cyanide, methanol	Solvent for shellacs
	Haemorrhages	Benzene, methyl bromide	Cleaning fluid, refrigerants and fire extinguishers
Optic nerve	Neuritis and atrophy	Lead, methanol, dinitrobenzol, trichloroethylene, carbon tetrachloride, carbon disulphide, benzene, methyl bromide, naphthalene	Heavy metals, organic solvents
	Papilloedema	Benzene, lead	
	Pigment degeneration	Copper, iron	
Visual pathways	Cortical blindness	Carbon monoxide	
	Homonymous hemianopia	Lead	

Compiled from Duke-Elder (1972), Grant (1974), Hunter (1975) and Teir (1984).

nately the prognosis is poor in many cases, due to raised intraocular pressure, dry eye and neovascularization of the cornea (Morgan, 1987).

Table 5.3 gives a summary of the prognosis for eyes affected by chemical burns, depending on the clarity of the cornea and severity of limbal ischaemia at the initial examination (Kanski, 1999). Limbal ischaemia is graded according to the patency of the deep and superficial limbal vessels, and is characterized by blanching and stasis of blood cells.

THERMAL INJURIES
Thermal burns
There are two types of thermal burns; flame and contact burns. These may be caused by hot bodies,

Table 5.3 Prognosis for eyes subjected to chemical burns (after J.J. Kanski, 1999)

Grade	Appearance	Prognosis
Grade I	Clear cornea and no limbal ischaemia	Excellent
Grade II	Hazy cornea but iris details visible and less than one-third of limbal ischaemia	
Grade III	No iris details visible and between one-third and one-half of limbal ischaemia	Guarded prognosis
Grade IV	Opaque cornea and more than one-half limbal ischaemia	Very poor

fluids or gases. Burns usually involve the eyelids and not the globe, which is often protected by the blink reflex. The characteristic picture is of marked oedema and tissue necrosis.

Flame burns

These occur frequently, and may result where high temperatures and inflammable liquids are being used. Gases, ovens, furnaces and petrol stores are liable to explode, and soaked overalls are also a potential fire hazard. The eye is rarely involved unless the heat is so intense and prolonged that the lids are destroyed. Generally the lashes and brow are scorched and the lids may be burnt with extensive damage to the face, but the globe is unaffected. The burnt lids may need plastic surgery and ectropion must be prevented. There may be continuous weeping due to damaged lacrimal puncta and canaliculi, which have become blocked by subsequent fibrosis.

Contact burns

These may be caused by molten substances such as metal or glass striking the cornea and entering the conjunctival sac. The molten substance solidifies as soon as it cools on hitting the eye and may fall into the lower fornix, where it continues to burn the surrounding tissue due to its latent heat. Prompt removal and irrigation reduces damage. The velocity of the hot particle may be such that it perforates the eye, causing intraocular damage.

According to Duke Elder (1972), two different reactions may occur, depending on the temperature of the particle, its capacity to retain heat, and whether it is in a solid or molten state. Glowing solid bodies that retain heat (e.g. slag, molten metal or glass at temperatures of, say, 1000°C) cause severe burns, scarring of the cornea and destruction of the conjunctiva, and this often leads to the loss of an eye. The intense reaction will lead to severe palpebral oedema, chemosis and a purulent discharge. While superficial lesions are accompanied by pain, photophobia and lacrimation, these corneal symptoms may be absent in severe cases because the nerves have been destroyed.

Molten metals of relatively low melting point, such as lead, tin or zinc, cause less damage if they are accidentally splashed onto the eye. Accidents generally occur when pouring metals into moulds or from solder splash/splatter. The metal forms a thin mould over the eye, which can be picked off. Generally the tissue remains undamaged, but occasionally the cornea may be dull. The conjunctiva may be oedematous in the contact area, and plaques of encrusted metal may cause superficial burns of the palpebral skin and lid margins where metal beads have adhered to the eyelashes. Vision is usually unimpaired, although small areas of symblepharon may result.

A burn to the cornea produces irregularity of its thickness and surface, and opacities, which cause distressing effects upon vision. Contact lenses may restore useful vision in mild cases, but corneal grafting may be needed if the burn is more severe.

Scalds

Burns by hot fluids frequently affect the lids and face, but the eyes are protected by the blink reflex. Scalds may be caused by the rupture of pipes containing steam, or by splashes of pitch, tar, molten sulphur or boiling oil, which usually result partial skin loss to the face and eyelids.

ELECTRICAL INJURIES

Lightning and high-tension electrical appliances are the two main causes of electrical injury. An electrical current may generate temperatures of up to 3000°C on a surface at the point of entry and exit. While tissues are generally bad conductors, nerve tissue conducts extremely well. If the current passes through the head, the hair, eyebrows and eyelashes will be singed, with superficial burns of the lids, usually associated with marked swelling and conjunctival chemosis. The cornea will become cloudy due to interstitial opacities and oedema. There may also be iritis, hyphaema, miosis, slow pupil reactions, retinal oedema, papilloedema, retinal detachment, choroidal rupture, chorioretinal atrophy, vitreous opacities or anterior cortical cataracts (Duke-Elder, 1972). The cataracts may have a delayed onset and are, in some cases, transient. A subcapsular cataract in the shape of a fern leaf was reported to have developed in the right eye of a 21-year-old man 6 days after being struck by lightning. The opacity resolved within a few weeks. Another case showed a permanent band-shaped subcapsular cataract and anterior uveitis (Novitskaya and Novitski, 1983).

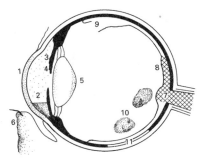

Fig. 5.1 *Some of the possible ocular effects of electrical injuries. 1, corneal oedema and interstitial opacities; 2, hyphaema; 3, iritis; 4, miosis; 5, subcapsular cataracts; 6, superficial burns; 7, papilloedema; 8, retinal oedema; 9, retinal detachment; 10, vitreous opacities; 11, chorioretinal atrophy.*

Van Johnson *et al.* (1987) reported cataract formation as a result of electrocution by a high-voltage power line, which fell on a worker. Diffuse anterior subcapsular cataracts were seen in both eyes 6 weeks after the accident. These progressed to complete subcapsular cataracts, and the left eye also developed a diffuse posterior subcapsular cataract. An extracapsular cataract extraction was performed on the left eye.

Figure 5.1 summarizes some of the ocular complications of electrical injuries.

RADIATION INJURIES

This section examines ocular injuries arising from different radiation sources, and is mainly summarized from Duke-Elder (1972), Lerman (1980a), Marshall (1985) and Waxler and Hitchins (1986).

The electromagnetic spectrum consists of radiant energy, both ionizing and non-ionizing. It comprises a large, continuous range of wavelengths, which extend from very short cosmic rays to the much longer Hertzian waves. The major natural source of electromagnetic radiation is the sun. Fortunately, the atmosphere acts as a filter, absorbing a significant amount of the harmful radiation. Ozone and oxygen absorb most of the ultra-violet (UV) radiation between 10 and 250 nm, and water and carbon dioxide absorbs some of the infra-red (IR) radiation. The highest intensity of radiation that penetrates the atmosphere is in the visible range 400–800 nm. Figure 5.2 shows the various wavelengths of the electromagnetic spectrum.

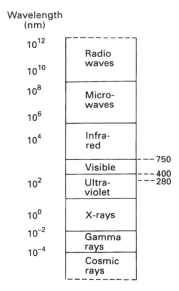

Fig. 5.2 *The electromagnetic spectrum.*

At present, the protection provided by the atmosphere and the ocular media against the harmful radiation appears to be adequate. However, there is currently great concern about the thinning of the ozone layer and the resultant health hazards, such as skin cancer.

Damage to the eyes occurs as a result of absorption of harmful radiation, and the effect upon the eye will depend upon the wavelength of the radiation and the photon energy (Lerman, 1980a):

- Long wavelength radiation has low photon energies. Infra-red radiation has photon energies that range from 0.01 to 1 eV. When it is absorbed, it will induce rotational and vibrational changes in the molecules. This increase in molecular agitation is generally referred to as a thermal effect.
- Visible and short wavelength radiation have higher photon energies. For visible and UV radiation, the photon energies range from 1 to 4 eV. Absorption results in changes to the electron energies within the molecule. This excitation of the electrons may be large enough to break some of the chemical bonds and even cause ionization (usually due to absorption of photon energies >6 eV).

Figure 5.3 illustrates the sites of absorption of the various wavelengths, and hence the potential sites of

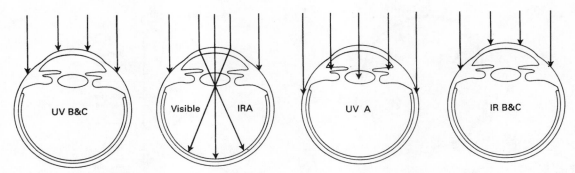

Fig. 5.3 *Sites of radiation absorption (reproduced by kind permission of J. Marshall and Butterworth-Heinemann (Oxford)).*

damage. The eye and the skin are particularly sensitive to the non-ionizing radiation normally present in the environment (280–1400 nm). Infra-red radiation does not cause any damage at normal ambient levels, whereas UV radiation can affect both the skin and the eye. Most ionizing radiation passes through the eye.

The effect of non-ionizing radiation depends upon the presence of absorbing molecules, known as chromophores. Cells that do not contain chromophores will transmit the wavelengths. Nucleic acids, for example (which are present in the cornea), absorb UV radiation (250–295 nm) but transmit visible light. Rhodopsin absorbs at 498 nm, and haemoglobin absorbs in the UV and visible region (275, 400 and 540–576 nm, respectively; Lerman, 1980a).

The ocular effects of radiation differ with the wavelengths, which can be grouped as follows:

1. Ionizing radiation
2. Non-ionizing radiation
   - ultraviolet radiation
   - visible light
   - infra-red radiation
   - microwave radiation.

Ionizing radiation

Source

Ionizing radiation has very short wavelengths (<0.01 nm) and is caused by the disintegration of atoms. It occurs naturally as cosmic radiation from radioactive isotopes (such as radium), or can be produced by artificial means. These artificial sources can produce X-ray and gamma radiation, as well as corpuscular radiation, which includes alpha and beta particles, electrons, positrons, protons and neutrons.

People employed in occupations such as radiology, nuclear physics, and uranium mining and engineering can be at risk from ionizing radiations.

Site of absorption

Most of the ionizing radiation passes through the eye, but a small amount is absorbed and, depending upon the exposure time and concentration, can cause damage to nearly all of the ocular tissues. In general, excessive and repeated exposure to low penetrating radiations, such as beta-particles, is required for damage (usually cataracts) to occur, whereas relatively small doses of high penetrating radiations, such as X-ray and gamma-radiation and neutrons, are required (Duke-Elder, 1972).

Ocular effects

Many changes may take place in ocular tissue when it is exposed to ionizing radiation. The sensitivity of the various ocular tissues will depend upon the miotic activity of the cells (i.e. division and growth) and the tissue's ability to repair radiation-induced damage; for example, the fetal eye is far more sensitive to radiation exposure than the adult eye. The conjunctiva, cornea and lens are the most susceptible ocular tissues, as they undergo constant replication and, in the case of the lens, growth throughout life. Merriam and Focht (1962) and Merriam *et al.* (1972) have listed the relative sensitivity of the ocular tissues in decreasing order: (i) lens; (ii) conjunctiva; (iii) cornea; (iv) vitreous; (v) iris and uveal tract; (vi) sclera; and (vii) retina.

The ionizing radiation may have a direct or an indirect effect upon the tissues. A direct action upon the cells can result in the development of

Table 5.4 Ultraviolet radiation and the eye (courtesy of J. Marshall and Butterworth-Heinemann, Oxford 1985)

Spectral domain		Wavelength (nm)	Sources	Site of ocular damage
Biological	Physical			
UV-C	Far UV	200–280	Sunlight, Lamps – arc, germicidal and mercury, excimer laser	Corneal epithelium resulting in photokeratitis, corneal opacity
UV-B	Far UV	280–315	Sunlight, sunlamps, welding arc, excimer laser	Corneal epithelium resulting in photokeratitis, corneal opacity
		295–315		Lens epithelium and nucleus, resulting in cataract
UV-A	Near UV	315–400	Sunlight, UV-A sunlamp, sunbeds, excimer laser	Lens epithelium and nucleus, resulting in cataract

abnormalities, or in cell death. Indirect damage can occur as a result of damage to the blood vessels, leading to a reduced blood supply to the tissues.

The most common effect of radiation exposure is the formation of cataracts, because the lens contains the ocular tissues that are most sensitive to this type of radiation. The lenticular changes are similar regardless of the type of radiation; fine dot-like subcapsular opacities in the anterior cortex, and granular and vacuolar subcapsular opacities at the posterior pole of the lens. These may progress to involve the peripheral portions of the posterior cortex (Palva and Palkama, 1978; Hayes and Fisher, 1979). It may take several years for the cataracts to develop after exposure to the radiation. The latent period and the severity of lens damage depends on:

- The radiation dose – duration and concentration, single or multiple exposure. A single dose of 250 rad appears to be the threshold level above which radiation is capable of inducing cataracts in humans. (1 rad is defined as the absorbed dose of radiation when 1 g of material absorbs 100 ergs of energy; $1\,\text{rad} = 10^{-2}\,\text{Jkg}^{-1}$. However, dose-splitting can increase the threshold to 550 rad if the doses are spread over 3 months (Merriam and Focht, 1957).
- The type of radiation – low or high penetration.
- The age of the person – the younger the

person, the shorter the latent period and the greater the lens damage.

When a patient is undergoing radiation treatment for ocular tumours such as retinoblastoma, there is the risk of unwanted side effects such as cataract formation. If the eyelids are being irradiated because of the presence of a basal cell carcinoma, the eye should be protected by a lead contact lens. Unfortunately, the loss of lashes, pigmentary changes to the skin and 'dry eye' due to atrophy of the accessory lacrimal glands are not easy to prevent.

Non-ionizing radiation

Ultra-violet radiation
Source
Table 5.4 shows the range of wavelengths in the UV region and their sources. Ultra-violet radiation ranges from 200 to 400 nm, and can be subdivided into three groups: UV-A, 315–400 nm; UV-B, 280–315 nm; and UV-C, 200–280 nm. The most common sources of UV radiation, apart from sunlight, are germicidal lamps, high-pressure mercury arc lamps, special fluorescent lamps and welding arcs. Of particular concern is the increasing use of sunlamps and sunbeds, which are sources of UV-A and UV-B radiation.

Site of absorption
The corneal epithelium and conjunctiva absorb the wavelengths between 200 and 315 nm (UV-C and UV-B), and the lens nucleus and epithelium absorb the wavelengths between 295 and 400 nm (i.e. UV-A

and part UV-B; see Figure 5.3). With age, the filtering effect of the crystalline lens increases as a result of the increase in concentration of chromophores, which absorb the radiation. Therefore most of the UV radiation is absorbed by the cornea and some by the crystalline lens, which results in photochemical damage.

Ocular effects

1. Direct – radiation is absorbed by chromophores within the tissue. Direct effects of UV radiation include cornea-photokeratitis, pingeculae, pterygia and band-shaped keratopathies, cataracts and in aphakic eyes, vitreous shrinkage and retinal damage.
2. Indirect – radiation is absorbed by photosensitizing drugs or other compounds, causing damage to the crystalline lens and retina.

Cornea-photokeratitis occurs when UV-B and UV-C are absorbed by the corneal epithelium. This results in a reduction of the cell division in mild cases, or in complete death of the epithelial cells and corneal ulceration in extreme cases (English, 1973). The accumulation of damaged and exfoliated cells on the surface of the cornea can act as an effective filter to limit the total exposure dose and filter specific wavelengths of UV radiation.

Unfortunately, unlike the skin, the eye cannot build up resistance to UV radiation; exposure has a cumulative effect over a 24-hour period. Therefore, while a single exposure may not be harmful, if it is repeated the cumulative effect may rise above the threshold and result in epithelial damage (English, 1973; Cullen, 1980).

The maximum efficiency for experimental photokeratitis is seen to occur at 288–290 nm, with a small peak at 254–260 nm (Bachem, 1956; Pitts and Tredici, 1971). These peaks correspond to the presence of the absorbing chromophores in the cornea (nucleic acids at 260 nm and tyrosine and tryptophan at 275–290 nm).

Following exposure to UV radiation, there is a latent period of 6–12 hours before any symptoms are noticed. This period varies inversely with the dose of UV radiation exposure. The symptoms experienced are:

● A sensation of sand in the eyes, due to congestion of the conjunctival and episcleral blood vessels

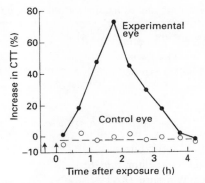

Fig. 5.4 *Corneal sensitivity after absorption of UV radiation. The arrows indicate UV exposure; CTT, corneal touch threshold (reproduced by kind permission of Millodot, M., R.A. Earlam and publishers S. Karger AG 1984).*

● Lacrimation
● Photophobia
● Chemosis
● Blepharospasm
● Erythema (redness) of the lids.

The condition is generally self-limiting, and almost all the discomfort disappears within 48 hours due to the repair mechanisms of the corneal epithelium. Photokeratitis is common amongst welders, when the condition is referred to as 'arc eye' or 'welder's flash'.

The latent period appears to be due to a marked decrease in corneal sensitivity. A study by Millodot and Earlam (1984) found that after exposure to UV radiation from an electric arc welder the corneal sensitivity decreased. The sensation of sand and pain in the eyes is experienced as the corneal sensitivity is restored (Figure 5.4).

Therapy consists of instillation of lubricating ointment and decongestant drops. A local/topical anaesthetic can be given, and the eye can be patched if pain is severe and blepharospasm is present.

Although the primary short-term effect of acute exposure of the cornea to UV radiation is photokeratitis, damage to the corneal endothelium may also occur (Cullen *et al.*, 1984). It appears that chronic UV radiation exposure also contributes to the increased endothelial polymegethism seen with age (Good and Schoessler, 1988).

Pingeculae, pterygia and band-shaped keratopathies

are thought to be caused partially by long-term chronic exposure to UV radiation. A significantly high incidence of pingeculae and pterygia is found amongst outdoor workers, such as fishermen and welders, who are exposed to UV radiation (Klintworth, 1972; Norm, 1982, Karai and Horiguchi, 1984; Moran and Hollows, 1984; Mackenzie *et al.*, 1992).

A nodular band-shaped keratopathy has been noted in people who live in areas of the world with high levels of UV. White or cream opacities occur between the epithelium and Bowman's membrane in the palpebral fissure (Rodger, 1973). Anderson and Fuglsang (1976) also reported similar degenerative changes of the cornea associated with UV exposure.

Cataracts are thought to be caused by absorption of UV radiation. The crystalline lens epithelium and nucleus absorb wavelengths between 295 and 400 nm (i.e. part UV-B and UV-A). As only the shorter wavelengths are filtered out by the cornea, the lens is constantly exposed to the longer wavelengths (295–400 nm) throughout life. It has been shown that these wavelengths are responsible for generating fluorescent compounds, and for the protein cross-linking associated with lens ageing and cataract formation. A young lens will transmit approximately 90 per cent of incident light > 400 nm, but with age the amount of short-wave radiation transmitted is reduced, particularly in the region of 300–400 nm (Lerman, 1980a; Lerman, 1983).

Chronic cumulative photochemical damage results in increased absorption of UV radiation and some visible light due to photochemically generated chromophores. The chromophores increase in concentration and number with age and are responsible for the increased yellow colour of the lens nucleus, which enables the lens to act as an effective filter, protecting the retina from cumulative photochemical damage by the second to third decade (Weale, 1983; Zigman, 1983). Lerman (1980b) reported that 'senile' cataracts have occurred at an earlier age (40–50 years) in workers exposed to industrial sources of UVA – e.g. printing works, dentistry and medicine.

So is there any evidence to suggest that exposure to UV radiation is responsible for cataract formation? Many papers now suggest that UV radiation is a causative factor in cataract formation. Animal studies have shown that cataracts can be induced by UV radiation. One study found that high doses were required in the region of 295–320 nm to produce

cataracts (Bachem, 1956), whilst another found that long-term exposure can also produce cataracts, usually anterior subcapsular cataracts (Zigman and Vaughn, 1974). Other studies have established threshold levels of exposure for near-UV radiation. However, permanent lens changes were not induced until the radiant exposure levels reached twice the threshold value (Pitts, 1978). Epidemiological studies are also inconclusive; some have shown that in areas of high levels of sunlight and UV radiation there is a higher incidence of cataracts (Hiller *et al.*, 1977; Hollows and Moran, 1981; Zigman, 1983, Delcourt *et al.*, 2000), whilst one reported a lower incidence (Crabbe, 1983). The different results in these studies may well be due to such factors as general health and diet, which were not taken into account (Minassian *et al.*, 1984).

It has also been suggested that the brown (brunescent) cataract that occurs in the nucleus of the older lens results from exposure to sunlight. However, this has not yet been proven, and there are arguments against the hypothesis (Harding and Dilley, 1976; Dolin, 1994).

To summarize, although the evidence is not entirely conclusive as to the relationship between UV radiation and cataracts, it would seem sensible to assume from all the research so far that a causal relationship is possible (Pitts, 1981).

A summary of the possible anterior segment complications of UV radiation are shown in Figure 5.5.

Vitreous shrinkage occurs when the eye is aphakic and has no protection against certain wavelengths. The vitreous is normally protected from damage by the cornea and lens, which filter wavelengths up to 400 nm; however, if the eye is aphakic the vitreous has no protection against wavelengths > 295 nm. The vitreous gel possesses UV-absorbing chromophores,

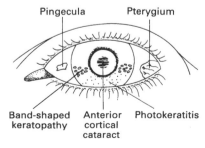

Fig. 5.5 *Some of the possible effects of UV radiation on the anterior segment of the eye.*

Work and the Eye

Table 5.5 Visible radiation and the eye (courtesy of J. Marshall and Butterworth-Heinemann, Oxford 1985)

Visible wavelength (nm)	Sources	Site of ocular damage
400–780	Sunlight; incandescent, fluorescent and arc lamps Lasers – argon, krypton	Retinal pigment epithelium, haemoglobin, macular pigment photoreceptors, resulting in visual loss, colour vision problems, accelerated ageing

and there is experimental evidence that damage, such as vitreous shrinkage and denaturation of the collagen network, can occur (Balazs *et al.*, 1959).

Retinal damage can also occur in aphakes. The retina is generally protected from UV radiation by the cornea and lens, but damage can occur to aphakes who lack the filtering effect of the lens. Aphakes are prone to cystoid macular oedema, and this is now thought to be due to absorption of wavelengths > 295 nm. A study by Kraff *et al.* (1985) reported that patients who had been given UV-absorbing intraocular lenses after cataract extraction had a lower incidence of cystoid macular oedema than those who did not receive absorbing implants. However, this report did not describe the absorption characteristics of the eye, intraocular lenses and spectacles. Wittenberg (1986) makes the point that, until the study by Kraff *et al.*, there were no reports of apparent retinal damage in people who had been aphakic from an early age. Therefore, the association between retinal damage and UV radiation due to sunlight is uncertain.

The aphakic eye is also at risk from retinal detachments due to vitreous shrinkage and denaturation of the collagen network. Ageing is known to cause a loss of rod and cone cells, and it has been suggested that this is due to a potential cumulative action of light (i.e. a phototoxic effect), during the normal ageing process. As studies suggest that UV and short-wave visible radiation (320–450 nm) are significant factors in retinal photochemical damage, it is advisable to provide protection, especially for aphakics, by giving UV-absorbing spectacle lenses or intraocular lenses.

Indirect effects of UV radiation have been reported by Lerman *et al.* (1980), Boukes *et al.* (1985) and Woo (1985), who reported that UV radiation can be indirectly absorbed by photosensitizing drugs and cause damage to the crystalline lens and retina. A treatment for psoriasis, known as PUVA therapy, consists of the ingestion of a psoralen compound (e.g. 8-methoxypsoralen (8-MOP) or methoxsalen) followed by exposure to UV-A radiation. Ocular protection must be provided, as the UV-A radiation causes binding of the psoralen compound to lens and retinal proteins in aphakic individuals. This protection must be provided for at least 12–24 hours after ingestion – i.e. until there is no psoralen compound remaining in the lens (Boukes *et al.*, 1985). The opacities occur in the anterior and posterior cortical layers; some are punctate and others are wedge-shaped. It is believed that the opacification is mainly due to binding of tryptophan and lens proteins, which remain in the lens (Lerman *et al.*, 1980).

Visible light
Sources and site of absorption
Table 5.5 shows the sources and site of absorption of visible light. The range of visible radiation is from 400–780 nm, most of which reaches the retina.

Ocular effects
Visible light may cause damage by thermal photocoagulation. Retinal burns may occur when high intensities of light are focused on the retina. The severity of the damage will depend upon the intensity of the source. Non-thermal damage can occur with long-term exposure to ambient light levels with intensities well below that required for thermal damage.

Experimental animal studies have shown that

Table 5.6 Infra-red radiation and the eye (courtesy of J. Marshall and Butterworth-Heinemann Ltd, 1985)

Spectral domain		Wavelength (nm)	Sources	Site of ocular damage
Biological	Physical			
IR-A	Near IR	780–1400	Sunlight, furnaces, arc lamp, electric fires, neodymium-YAG laser	Pigment epithelium of retina, iris, lens, resulting in visual loss and cataract
IR-B	Far IR	1400–3000	Sunlight, furnaces, erbium laser	Corneal and lens epithelium, resulting in corneal opacity, aqueous flare and cataract
IR-C	Far IR	3000–10 000	Furnaces, carbon dioxide laser	Corneal epithelium, resulting in corneal opacity

retinal damage can occur at relatively low levels of visible radiation energy, and hence there is concern that such exposure may be responsible for retinal degeneration in humans (Noell *et al.*, 1966; Kuwabara and Gorn, 1968; O'Steen *et al.*, 1972; Lanum, 1978; Ham *et al.*, 1982). Long-term exposure to low levels of visible and UV radiation has been shown to cause damage to the photoreceptors, especially the cones, and to the retinal pigment epithelium (Heriot, 1985; Marshall, 1985; Mainster, 1987; Young, 1988). It appears that the overloading of the photopigments results in a chain of metabolic events that can lead to reversible or irreversible damage to the photoreceptors. Whether the damage to the retinal pigment epithelium occurs before or at the same time as the damage to the photoreceptors remains an open question.

The following degenerative changes are believed to occur to the rods and cones (Kuwabara and Gorn, 1968):

1. There is vacuole formation of the outer tip of the photoreceptor
2. The outer segment loses its lamellar structure and becomes tortuous and swollen
3. The outer segment breaks off from the inner segment
4. The outer segments are phagocytosed by retinal pigment epithelium
5. The photoreceptors disappear but the remaining layers are intact.

The cones appear to be more sensitive to photopic damage than the rods (Marshall *et al.*, 1972; Sykes *et al.*, 1981), and are especially sensitive to the blue region of visible light and UV (Harwerth and Sperling, 1971). Marshall (1985) has suggested that the difference in sensitivity between the rods and cones is not due to a difference in threshold for damage, but rather to different capacities for repair. There has been concern about the output of various light sources and their potential hazards (Sliney and Wolbarsht, 1980). Artificial illumination levels generally vary between 200 and 500 lm/m^2, and these levels are below the levels of irradiance that produce retinal photopathology in primates and man. However, the trend for higher lighting levels should be approached with caution in view of the photic damage that may be incurred at these high levels (Lerman, 1987).

Infra-red radiation

Sources and site of absorption

The range of infra-red wavelengths lies between 780 and 10 000 nm (Table 5.6), and can be sub-divided into three groups: IR-A, 780–1400 nm; IR-B, 1400–3000 nm; IR-C, 3000–10 000 nm. Wavelengths of 3000 nm and longer do not usually reach our environment because they are absorbed by the atmosphere. The most common sources of IR radiation are sunlight, arc lamps, electric fires, and steel and glass furnaces.

Infra-red radiation, when absorbed, leads to rotational and vibrational changes, which result in a thermal effect on the tissue. The major sites of absorption are shown in Figure 5.3. The cornea absorbs wavelengths >3000 nm (i.e. IR-C), the crystalline lens absorbs wavelengths <3000 nm (i.e. IR-A and IR-B), and the retina absorbs wavelengths <1400 nm (i.e. IR-A). There is some absorption in all the ocular tissues, but the absorption by the crystalline lens and retina are of greatest concern.

Ocular effects

The damage that occurs to the eye after absorption of IR radiation is due to thermal effects, and affects the cornea, the crystalline lens and the retina.

The cornea Absorption of IR-C results in opacification, especially of the stroma, due to thermal photocoagulation of the corneal proteins.

The crystalline lens Cataracts generally occur in workers who are exposed to intense heat for many years, such as steelworkers and glass blowers. The opacification occurs in the cortex of the crystalline lens, and is often associated with lamellar splitting and exfoliation of the anterior lens capsule. This damage results from both direct and indirect absorption of IR radiation. Indirect absorption by the pigment epithelium of the iris results in heat transfer to the underlying lens, which may in turn lead to anterior subcapsular opacities (Langely *et al.*, 1960; Pitts and Cullen, 1981). Direct absorption at the posterior pole of the lens, where radiation from a large source is focused, may induce posterior cortical or subcapsular cataracts (Goldman, 1935; Edbrooke and Edwards, 1967).

Retinal burns have been reported after exposure to IR radiation (750–1400 nm) under a variety of conditions, such as solar retinopathy (Agarwal and Malik, 1959; Tso and La Piana, 1975), eclipse blindness (Penner and McNair, 1966), exposure to high-intensity light sources such as xenon lamps, MIG (metal-arc inert gas) welders (Brittain, 1988), and exposure to IR lasers. The IR radiation is focused on the retina and will be absorbed by the melanin pigment granules in the pigment epithelium and underlying choroid. This results in a thermal reaction and inflammatory response involving the neural retina.

Microwave radiation

Sources

Microwave radiation consists of wavelengths ranging from 0.001 m to 0.3 m. Man-made sources of

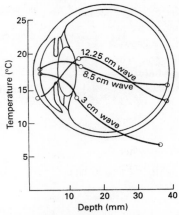

Fig. 5.6 *Temperature gradients in the exposed eye to 12.25, 8.5, and 3 cm pulsed microwaves (from Richardson* et al. *copyright 1951, American Medical Association).*

microwave radiation are used in microwave ovens, FM radio, television and radar.

Site of absorption

The direct effect of microwave radiation is due to an increase in temperature of the tissue. The absorption depends on:

1. *The type of tissue.* Water-based tissue absorbs much more energy than fat or bone, which microwaves can penetrate with little loss of energy. Tissues with higher amounts of water and greater conductivity, such as muscle tissue, will absorb the microwave energy, which results in a temperature rise. Conduction and convection of the heat will diminish the temperature differences induced by the absorption of the microwave radiation. The relative avascularity of the intraocular cavity will result in a temperature increase within the eye. This is markedly higher than in other well-vascularized tissues absorbing an equivalent amount of radiation. The crystalline lens is avascular and, being unable to dissipate heat, is particularly prone to thermal damage from microwave radiation. From experimental animal studies, the dose required to produce a cataract is believed to be 100–150 mW/cm^2 (Richardson *et al.*, 1951; Daily *et al.*, 1952; Williams *et al.*, 1955).

2. *Wavelength.* The degree of penetration of microwave radiation is directly related to the

wavelength. The thermal effects of the longer wavelengths are more penetrating. For example, a 12-cm microwave will penetrate about 1 cm into the eye, whereas a 3-cm microwave will penetrate only 1 mm. The temperature gradients created by different wavelengths are shown in Figure 5.6 (Richardson *et al.*, 1951). The maximum temperature rise in the posterior cortex of the lens occurs when it is exposed to 12-cm microwaves, whereas the maximum temperature rise in the cornea occurs with exposure to 3-cm microwaves.

3. *Frequency.* There is a relationship between the microwave frequency and the amount of absorption. The amount absorbed at the surface of exposed tissues increases with increasing microwave frequency (Schwan and Piersal, 1954).

Ocular effects

The ocular effects of microwaves can only be assessed by experimental or clinical means. The experimental production of anterior and posterior subcapsular cataracts in animals at relatively high intensities (> 100 mW/cm^2) has been documented by several researchers (Daily *et al.*, 1952; Van Ummerson and Cogan, 1965; Stewart-DeHann *et al.*, 1985). However, it is believed by some that lower levels of microwave exposure can also induce cataracts due to cell membrane damage if there is repeated exposure to subthreshold doses (Lipman *et al.*, 1988).

The only available human data are from retrospective population surveys comparing microwave workers with controls matched for age and sex. So far, all population surveys have failed to show a correlation between occupational exposure and cataract formation. One of the largest surveys was carried out by Appleton *et al.* in 1975, of 2343 military personnel. They concluded that there was no difference in the incidence of lens opacities between the control group and experimental subjects, and that lens damage due to microwave radiation from military equipment had not occurred. These findings suggested that the existing safety level of 10 mW/cm^2 is adequate. (For a review of the studies, see Lipman *et al.*, 1988.)

Instruments using specific man-made sources of radiation

These include lasers (an acronym for Light Amplifica-

tion by Stimulated Emission of Radiation) and ophthalmic instruments.

Lasers

Sources

The use of laser technology has increased greatly in recent years, and lasers have many applications in engineering, science, medicine and the defence industry. A laser beam is a monochromatic, highly coherent, parallel, very high-energy beam. It is produced by the excitation of atoms to a higher than usual energy state by the input of radiant energy, which causes the emission of light as the atoms return to their original energy state. Many substances can be used as a laser source, e.g. ruby, argon, carbon dioxide and YAG (yttrium–aluminium–garnet). Lasers have been produced to emit at many monochromatic wavelengths, ranging from far UV (< 300 nm) to far IR (> 1400 nm).

Different types of exposure can be produced from a laser depending upon the mode of operation (Lerman, 1980a; Mainster *et al.*, 1983a):

- In the continuous wave mode, the exposure time can vary from a few milliseconds to minutes
- In the long pulsed mode, the exposure time ranges from 100 µs to 2 ms
- In the Q-switched mode, the exposure time is less than 100 ns (1 ns $= 10^{-9}$ s)
- When mode-locked, the exposure may vary from 20–40 ps pulses (1 ps $= 10^{-12}$ s).

The Q-switched mode and mode-locked methods of operation allow high peaked power to be produced by compressing the laser output in time.

There are four important radiometric terms in medical laser applications:

1. Energy, measured in joules (J) (1 J $= 1$ W $\times 1$ s)
2. Power, measured in watts (W)
3. Radiant energy density, measured in joules per cm^2 (J/cm^2)
4. Irradiance, measured in watts per cm^2 (W/cm^2)

The laser output is quantified in joules or watts, and its effect upon the tissue is determined by the spot size, which will determine the energy density or irradiance. The power of a continuous beam laser, such as an argon laser, is measured in watts, while pulsed lasers, e.g. neodymium (Nd):YAG, provide a reading of energy per pulse in joules.

Continuous wave laser systems, such as argon and krypton lasers, focus light energy on an area of tissue to cause a temperature rise, which in turn causes coagulation of the tissue. The temperature rise depends on the spot size, amount of energy and wavelength. The wavelength determines the efficiency with which the light source is absorbed and converted into heat by the pigment of the tissues (Mainster *et al.*, 1970, 1983b). An excessive temperature rise can cause an explosion and haemorrhage in the tissue; a temperature rise of only 10°C is required for retinal photocoagulation. Short pulse lasers, such as Nd:YAG, will disrupt transparent tissue, and hence are known as photodisruptors. They are generally used for the relatively transparent anterior portion of the eye.

There are various mechanisms whereby the short pulse laser systems disrupt the transparent membranes (Mainster *et al.*, 1983a):

- The high irradiance (power/area) disintegrates tissues by removing electrons from atoms (i.e. ionizing them) and creating a 'plasma', which is a gaseous state consisting of electrons and ions
- The rapid outwards expansion of the plasma

creates shock and acoustic waves, which mechanically disrupt adjacent tissue
- Latent stress in the membrane causes further disruption
- A specific photochemical reaction has been reported with UV lasers, which results in the ablation of corneal tissues without thermal damage to the adjacent structures (Trokel *et al.*, 1983).

Figure 5.7 shows the pulse energy required to produce retinal damage for laser exposures of different durations (Mainster *et al.*, 1983a). It can be seen that mode-locked exposures are potentially more hazardous than Q-switched, and that short pulses can produce retinal damage with less energy (or irradiance) than the longer pulses. The margin between retinal damage and explosion is also much lower for short pulse than for continuous wave.

Site of absorption
The site of absorption depends upon the wavelength being emitted by the laser. Radiation from lasers emitting in the UV region will be absorbed by the cornea and crystalline lens. Visible and IR lasers will cause problems, not necessarily because of their power but due to the fact that the collimated beam will be focused onto the retina.

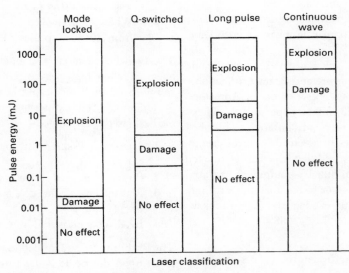

Fig. 5.7 *Pulse energy required to produce retinal damage or haemorrhage for laser exposures of different durations (after Mainster et al., 1983a; published courtesy of* Ophthalmology*).*

Table 5.7 Classification of lasers according to BS EN 60852 (1992)

Class of laser	Description	Upper limit of radiant emission
Class 1	Safe	0.4 µW
Class 2	Low power	1 mW
Class 3A	Low-medium power lasers (visible)	5 mW, and irradiance should not be > 25 W/m^2 *
Class 3B	Medium power	500 mW
Class 4	High power	> 500 mW

* The beam must be sufficiently divergent so that the amount of radiant emission of the laser passing through a 7-mm pupil does not exceed an irradiance of 25 W/m^2.

Ocular effects

Ultra-violet lasers emitting radiation <300 nm can be absorbed by the cornea and, as described, will cause damage to the corneal epithelium. Lasers emitting UV from 300–400 nm can cause cataracts because the radiation is absorbed by the crystalline lens. UV-emitting lasers can therefore cause damage to the cornea and crystalline lens, if they are exposed for a sufficient time and at power densities above threshold level. As a result of this, the excimer laser is now being used, particularly for corneal surgery, as the depth of incision can be accurately controlled by the photons that break the molecular bonds when absorbed. This has the advantage that the adjacent tissue does not suffer from thermal damage. Marshall *et al.* (1986) found that the wavelength of 193 nm was optimal for corneal surgery. The excimer laser was initially used in the printing and electronics industries, where its properties allowed submicron patterns to be etched into the surface of materials without damaging the adjacent non-irradiated areas. A study by Trokel *et al.* (1983) shows that 1 J/cm^2 ablates corneal tissue to a depth of 1 µm.

Radiation from visible and IR lasers are focused on to the retina and can cause:

- Thermal injury following absorption by the melanin, the pigment epithelium and choroid
- Photochemical damage, especially in the blue region of the visible spectrum, which is absorbed by the inner retinal layers
- Shock waves, which are produced by the Q-switched high-intensity beams and cause disruption of the internal cellular structure.

The type and degree of retinal damage caused by a laser will depend upon (Ham *et al.*, 1970):

- The power density of the laser (W/cm^2)
- The time of exposure
- The wavelength and transmission through the ocular media
- The size of image upon the retina
- The blink reflex
- The degree of retinal and choroidal pigmentation.

Industrial ocular laser burns have been reported by Boldrey *et al.* (1981). The damage ranged from minor retinal burns to extensive areas of damage with retinal oedema and vitreous haemorrhages. A variety of lasers were involved, including Nd : YAG, argon, krypton, and rhodamine dye. The haemorrhages and oedema subsided during the weeks following the injury and, with the exception of one case, the final visual acuity was 6/6, although a paracentral scotoma was usually present. In all but one case eye protection was not being worn; in the case where eye protection was being worn, it was not fitted correctly and the spectacles slipped as the worker bent over the laser, the beam being reflected from a piece of test paper into his left eye. There are other reports of ocular injury from lasers where the visual outcome was not as good. Many of the cases resulted in a markedly reduced vision, one case being due to a macular hole (Jacobson and McLean, 1965; Rathkey, 1965; Zweng, 1967; Curtin and Boyden, 1968; Armstrong, 1970; Henkes and Zuidema, 1975).

Lasers can be grouped into four main classes, 1, 2, 3A and 3B, and 4 (BS EN 60825) as shown in Table 5.7. Classes 1, 2 and 3A are believed to be safe due to the blink reflex and to the aversion response, which means that the head is turned away before sufficient energy has entered the eye to cause irreversible damage. Classes 3B and 4 can cause irreversible

Table 5.8 Safe viewing time for various ophthalmic instruments (reprinted with permission of *Vision Research*, vol.20, Calkins *et al.*, Potential hazards from specific ophthalmic devices. 1980. Copyright, 1980, Pergamon Press).

Instrument	Average retinal irradiance (mW/cm^2)	Safe time (s)*
Direct ophthalmoscope (A.O. Giantscope: Welch Allyn)	29.0	–
Indirect ophthalmoscopes (Binocular-AO and Frigi-Xonix)	68.6 (6.5 V)	42
	125.0 (7.8–8.4 V)	23
Slit lamp (Haag Streit)	140.0 (5 V)	21
	217.0 (6 V)	13
	358.0 (7.5 V)	8
Operating microscope		
emmetrope and myopes	100.0–970	29–1.8
aphakic	59.0–590	49–3.7

* Safe time is defined as the time required to reach an integrated retinal irradiance of 2.92 J/cm^2.

damage to the eye, and all ophthalmic surgical lasers are Class 4 (for full details refer to BS EN 60825). There has been concern about the use of laser pointers causing eye injuries. Laser pointers should be Class 1 or 2 according to the European Codes of Practice, and in a review article by Marshall (1998) he concluded that laser pointers are not an eye hazard if used appropriately, and even if used inappropriately they will not cause permanent eye damage. However, Kar (1998) reported that many laser pointers manufactured overseas are incorrectly classified for sale in the UK, so care needs to be taken and it is advisable to check the power of the pointer.

Ophthalmic instruments

There is concern that radiation from ophthalmic instruments may cause damage to the eye being examined, especially to the retina. The proceedings of a symposium on intense light hazards in ophthalmic diagnosis and treatment (Calkins *et al.*, 1980) have shown that various ophthalmic instruments are capable of causing damage to the retina. Estimates were made of the critical exposure time for the retina when using the indirect ophthalmoscope, slit lamp, operating microscope and overhead surgical lamp. The retinal irradiance of the instruments was calculated for a person with clear ocular media and a dilated pupil. This was correlated with the recommended maximum permissible exposure (MPE) time based on the ANSI Z-136 guidelines for laser safety to provide a safe viewing time for the various instruments (Table 5.8). The 'safe time' indicates how long

exposure at the particular level of retinal irradiance must be maintained before the ANSI laser safety guidelines are exceeded (2.92 J/cm^2). However, these studies did not take into account the spectral power distribution of the light sources.

Ophthalmoscopes

Indirect ophthalmoscopes can produce levels of retinal irradiance up to five times greater than that produced by a direct ophthalmoscope. There are obviously differences between the types of ophthalmoscopes; for example, the Keeler Indirect produces nearly 3.6 times more irradiance than the American Optical at maximum voltage setting (Kossel *et al.*, 1983). The power of the condensing lens also affects the retinal irradiance, which increases as the power of the condensing lens decreases – a 14-D lens can give 81 per cent more retinal irradiance than a 20-D lens (Calkins *et al.*, 1980). Therefore, an indirect ophthalmoscope is considered to be unsafe, when compared with the laser safety standard, after 23 s of exposure in a normal patient with clear media and dilated pupils. The time taken for fundus examination should not, therefore, be prolonged unnecessarily.

The light sources in ophthalmoscopes are usually an incandescent bulb (tungsten halogen) and are composed of one-third visible and UV radiation, and two-thirds IR radiation. It has therefore been suggested that an IR filter should be incorporated in all ophthalmoscopes to avoid thermal damage from extensive viewing (Lerman, 1985). The higher the voltage at which the bulbs are operated, the greater the amount of UV radiation emitted. As UV-A and blue light can cause damage to the retina, especially in aphakes whose natural filter has been removed, it has been suggested that a cut-off filter at 450 nm should also be incorporated (Kossol *et al.*, 1983; Cullen and Chou, 1984).

A survey by James *et al.* (1988) has investigated the light hazard of hand-held direct ophthalmoscopes. Studying the spectral irradiance of ophthalmoscopes at maximum output, they found that the levels of UV and IR radiation are not hazardous, although they may be potentially harmful to certain groups of patients, such as aphakes. They therefore recommended the use of UV- and IR-blocking filters. For most ophthalmoscopes, the safe time was found to be in excess of 1 hour.

Slit lamps
Slit lamp examination of the retina produces up to three times more irradiance than indirect ophthalmoscopy. The level of irradiance obviously depends upon the lamp voltage, and can range from 140 mW/cm^2 for a 5 V lamp to 358 mW/cm^2 for a 7.5-V lamp (Calkins *et al.*, 1980). The safe durations for retinal examination are also shorter than for indirect ophthalmoscopy, being as little as 8 s. It has therefore been suggested that medium voltage settings should be used and short examination times of 10 s employed. This applies particularly to the examination of patients with macular or retinal degeneration.

Operating microscopes
These can produce up to 10 times more retinal irradiance than indirect ophthalmoscopes (i.e. up to 970 mW/cm^2). The retinal irradiance, and hence safe time, is seen to vary with the patient's refractive error. The safe time varies from 1.8 to 49 s, which is still relatively short when considering the time taken during operation procedures (Calkins *et al.*, 1980). It has therefore been suggested that corneal occluders should be used during prolonged procedures with operating microscopes. Although microscopes do not produce much UV radiation, it is still advisable to incorporate a pale yellow filter to absorb blue light and UV-A. Care should be taken with certain conditions, such as retinitis pigmentosa, when light exposure may accelerate the disease.

Light sources such as the surgical illuminating lid speculum provide a safe retinal irradiance (Calkins *et al.*, 1980), as they provide 900 times less retinal irradiance than conventional operating microscopes.

Recommendations
To summarize, the following recommendations have been given regarding ophthalmic instruments:

1. Use IR filters to absorb wavelengths longer than 700 nm
2. Absorb wavelengths below 450 nm to eliminate blue light and UVA; this will improve image quality by reducing the light scattering and chromatic aberration
3. Use the minimum amount of light and time necessary for examination
4. In some cases, use corneal occluders to prevent unnecessary exposure from operating microscopes.

It is interesting to note that scanning laser ophthalmoscopes have been designed in which the light intensities required for illumination of the retina are considerably less than in conventional instruments (Mainster *et al.*, 1982; Plesch *et al.*, 1987). In the system described by Mainster *et al.* (1982), the light level was less than 70 μW/cm^2 compared with 100 000 μW/cm^2 for direct ophthalmoscopes. This means that it is possible to view the retina through an undilated pupil, and the examination will be more comfortable for the patient compared with indirect ophthalmoscopy. A laser that emits IR light can also be used to view the retina, and this provides a very comfortable method of examination for the patient, who is unaware of the light (Webb *et al.*, 1987).

In 1994, Sliney and Campbell reported on the efforts being made to develop an International and European Standard on ophthalmic diagnostic instruments. The following limits were tentatively made for irradiance at the cornea:

- Ultra-violet irradiance limit – 50 μW/cm^2 (305–400 nm)
- Infra-red irradiance limit – 100 mW/cm^2 (700–1100 nm).

No agreement was made regarding limits on visible light, but it was recommended that manufacturers should provide the spectral radiance of the instrument and give a maximal value for the phakic and aphakic eye.

SUMMARY

Chapters 4 and 5 have discussed the various ocular injuries that may occur due to mechanical and non-mechanical hazards. The most urgent condition is that of a chemical burn, which requires immediate action; the eye should be irrigated as soon as possible. Other ocular injuries requiring urgent attention include penetrating injuries of the globe, a corneal ulcer or abrasion, hyphaema, acute vitreous haemorrhage, retinal tear or detachment, corneal foreign body, and thermal and radiant burns (Fox, 1973).

REFERENCES

Agarwal L.P. and Malik S.R.K. (1959) Solar retinitis. *Br J Ophthalmol*, 53, 366–370.

Anderson J. and Fuglsang H. (1976) Droplet degeneration of the cornea in the North Cameroons. Prevalence and clinical appearances. *Br J Ophthalmol*, 60, 256–262.

Appleton B., Hirsch S., Kinion R.O., Soles, M., McCrossan G.C. and Neidlinger R.M. (1975) Microwave lens effect in humans. 1 – Results of 5-year survey. *Arch Ophthalmol*, 93, 257–258.

Armstrong C.E. (1970) Eye injuries in the modern radiation environment. *J Am Optom Assoc*, 41, 55–62.

Bachem A. (1956) Ophthalmic ultra-violet action spectra. *Am J Ophthalmol*, 41, 969–974.

Balazs E.A., Laurent T.C., Howe F.C. and Varga L. (1959) Irradiation of mucopolysaccharides with ultraviolet light and electrons. *Radiant Res*, 11, 149–164.

Boldrey E.E., Little H.L., Flocks M. and Vassiliadis A. (1981) Retinal injury due to industrial laser burns. *Ophthalmology*, 88, 101–107.

Boukes R.J., Van Balen A.Th.M. and Bruynzeel D.P. (1985) A retrospective study of ocular findings in patients treated with PUVA. *Doc Ophthalmol*, 59, 11–19.

Brittain, G.P.H. (1988) Retinal burns caused by exposure to MIG welding arcs: report of two cases. *Br J Ophthalmol*, 72, 570–575.

Brown S.I., Akiya S. and Weller C.A. (1969) Prevention of ulcers of the cornea: preliminary studies with collagenase inhibitors. *Arch Ophthalmol*, 82, 95–97.

Brown S.I., Tragakis M.P. and Pearce D.B. (1972) Treatment of alkali burned cornea. *Am J Ophthalmol*, 74, 316–320.

BS EN 60825 (1992) Radiation safety of laser products, equipment classification, requirements and user's guide. British Standards Institute, London.

Calkins J.L., Hochheimer B.F. and D'Anna S.A. (1980) Potential hazards from specific ophthalmic devices. *Vis Res*, 20, 1039–1053.

Crabbe M.J.C. (1983) Low incidence of cataract in Hawaii despite high exposure to sunlight. *Lancet*, 1, 649.

Cullen A.P. (1980) Additive effects of ultraviolet radiation. *Am J Optom Physiol Opt*, 57, 808–814.

Cullen A.P. and Chou B.R. (1984) Blue free fundus examination. *Can J Optom*, 46, 153–156.

Cullen A.P., Chou B.R., Hall M.G. and Jang S.E. (1984) Ultraviolet B damages corneal endothelium. *Am J Optom Physiol Opt*, 61, 473–478.

Curtin T.L. and Boyden D.G. (1968) Reflected laser beam causing accidental burn of the retina. *Am J Ophthalmol*, 65, 188–189.

Daily L., Wakim K.G., Herrick J.F. *et al.* (1952). The effects of microwave diathermy on the eye of the rabbit. *Am J Ophthalmol*, 35, 1001–1017.

Delcourt C., Carriere I., PontonSanchez A., Lacroux A., Covacho M.J. and Papoz M.J. (2000) Light exposure and the risk of cortical, nuclear and posterior subcapsular cataract. *Arch Ophthalmol*, 118, 385–392.

Deutsch T.A. and Feller D.B. (1985) *Paton and Goldberg's Management of Ocular Injuries*, 2nd edn. W.B. Saunders Co., London.

Dolin P.J. (1994) Assessment of the epidemiological evidence that exposure to solar ultraviolet radiation causes cataract. *Doc Ophthalmol*, 88, 327–337.

Duke-Elder S. (ed.) (1972) *System of Ophthalmology – Injuries*, Vol. XIV, Parts 1 and 2. Henry Kimpton, London.

Edbrooke C.M. and Edwards C. (1967) Industrial radiation cataract: the hazards and the protective measures. *Ann Occup Hyg*, 10, 293.

English W.P. (1973) Eye protection for welders. *J Am Soc Saf Eng*, July, 39–43.

Fox S.L. (1973) *Industrial and Occupational Ophthalmology*. C.C. Thomas, Illinois.

Goldman H. (1935) The genesis of the cataract of the glass blower. *Am J Ophthalmol*, 18, 590.

Good G.W. and Schoessler J.P. (1988) Chronic solar radiation exposure and endothelial polymegethism. *Curr Eye Res*, 7, 157–162.

Grant W.M. (ed.) (1974) *Toxicology of the Eye*, 2nd edn. C.C. Thomas, Illinois.

Ham W.T. Jr., Clarke A.M., Geeraets WJ., Cleary S.F., Mueller H.A. and Williams R.C. (1970) The eye problems in laser safety. *Arch Environ Health*, 20, 156–160.

Ham W.T., Mueller H.A., Ruffolo J.J., Guerry D. and Guerry R.K. (1982) Action spectrum for retinal injury from near ultraviolet radiation in the aphakic monkey. *Am J Ophthalmol*, 93, 299–306.

Harding J.J. and Dilley K.J. (1976) Structural protein of the mammalian lens: a review with emphasis on changes in development, aging and cataract. *Exp Eye Res*, 22, 1–73.

Harwerth R.S. and Sperling H.G. (1971) Prolonged colour blindness induced by intense spectral lights in Rhesus monkeys. *Science (NY)*, **174**, 520–523.

Hayes B.P. and Fisher R.F. (1979) Influence of prolonged period of low dosage X-rays on the optic and ultrastructural appearance of cataract of the human lens. *Br J Ophthalmol*, **63**, 457–464.

Henkes H.E. and Zuidema H. (1975) Accidental laser coagulation of the central fovea. *Ophthalmologica*, **171**, 15–25.

Heriot W.J. (1985) Light and the retinal pigment epithelium: the link in senile macular degeneration? In *Hazards of Light, Myths and Realities* (eds Cronly-Dillan J., Rosen E.S. and Marshall J.). Pergamon Press, Oxford, pp. 187–196.

Hiller R., Giacometti L. and Yuen K. (1977) Sunlight and cataract: an epidemiological investigation. *Am J Epidemiol*, **105**, 450–459.

Hollows F. and Moran D. (1981) Cataract – the ultra-violet risk factor. *Lancet*, **2**, 1249–1250.

Hughes W.F. Jr (1946) Alkali burns of the eye II. Clinical and pathological course. *Arch Ophthalmol*, **36**, 189–214.

Hunter D. (1975) *The Diseases of Occupations*, 5th edn. Hodder and Stoughton, London.

Jacobson J.H. and McLean J.M. (1965) Accidental laser retinal burns. *Arch Ophthalmol*, **74**, 882.

James R.H., Bostrom R.G., Remark D. and Sliney D.H. (1988) Handheld ophthalmoscopes for hazards analysis: an evaluation. *Appl Opt*, **27**, 5072–5076.

Kanski J.J. (1999) *Clinical Ophthalmology*, 4th edn. Butterworth-Heinemann, Oxford, pp. 646–662.

Kar A.K. (1998) The optical safety of laser pointers. *Optician*, **215(5643)**, 27–32.

Karai I. and Horiguchi S. (1984). Pterygium in welders. *Br J Ophthalmol*, **68**, 347–349.

KIintworth G.K. (1972) Chronic actinic keratopathy – a condition associated with conjunctival elastosis (pingeculae) and typified by characteristic extracellular concretions. *Am J Pathol*, **67**, 327–348.

Kossol J., Cole C. and Dayhaw-Barker P. (1983) Spectral irradiances of and maximal permissible exposures to two indirect ophthalmoscopes. *Am J Optom Physiol Opt*, **60**, 616–621.

Kraff M.C., Saunders D.R., Jampol L.M. and Lieberman H.L. (1985) Effect of ultraviolet filtering intraocular lens on cystoid macular edema. *Ophthalmology*, **92**, 366–369.

Kuwabara T. and Gorn R.A. (1968) Retinal damage by visible light: an electron microscopic study. *Arch Ophthalmol*, **79**, 69–78.

Langely R.K., Mortimer C.B. and McCullough C. (1960) The experimental production of cataracts by exposure to heat and light. *Arch Ophthalmol*, **63**, 473.

Lanum J. (1978) The damaging effect of the light on the retina. Empirical findings, theoretical and practical implications. *Surv Ophthalmol*, **22**, 221–249.

Lerman S. (1980a) *Radiant Energy and the Eye*. Macmillan Publishing Co. Inc., New York.

Lerman S. (1980b). Human ultraviolet radiation cataracts. *Ophthalmic Res*, **12**, 303–314.

Lerman S. (1983) An experimental and clinical evaluation of lens transparency and aging. *J Gerontol*, **38**, 293–301.

Lerman S. (1985) Ocular photoxicity. In *Recent Advances in Ophthalmology* (eds Davidson S.I. and Fraunfelder F.T.). Churchill Livingstone, London, pp. 109–136.

Lerman S. (1987) Light induced changes in ocular tissues. In *Clinical Light Damage to the Eye* (ed. Miller D.). Springer Verlag, New York, pp. 183–215.

Lerman S., Megaw J. and Willis I. (1980) Potential ocular complications of PUVA therapy and their prevention. *J Invest Dermatol*, **74**, 197–199.

Lipman R.M., Tripathi H.J. and Tripathi R.C. (1988) Cataract induced by microwave and ionizing radiation. *Surv Ophthalmol*, **33**, 200–210.

Mackenzie F., Hirst L., Battistutta D. and Green A. (1992) Risk analysis in the development of pterygia. *Ophthalmology*, **99**, 644–650.

Mainster M.A. (1987) Light and macular degeneration: a biophysical and clinical perspective. *Eye*, **1**, 304–310.

Mainster M.A., White T.J. and Allen R.G. (1970) Spectral dependence of retinal damage produced by intense light sources. *J Optom Soc Am*, **60**, 848–855.

Mainster M.A., Timberlake G.T., Webb R.H. and Hughes G.W. (1982) Scanning laser ophthalmoscopy. *Ophthalmology*, **89**, 852–857.

Mainster M.A., Sliney D.H., Beleher C.D. III and Buzney S.M. (1983a) Laser photodisruptors. Damage mechanisms, instrument design safety. *Ophthalmology*, **90**, 973–991.

Mainster M.A., Ham W.T. Jr. and Delori F.C. (1983b) Potential retinal hazards – instrument and environmental light sources. *Ophthalmology*, **90**, 927–932.

Marshall J. (1985) Radiation and the ageing eye. *Ophthal Physiol Opt*, **5**, 241–263.

Marshall J. (1998) The safety of laser pointers: myths and realities. *Br J Ophthalmol*, **82**, 1335–1338.

Marshall J., Mellerio J. and Palmer D.A. (1972) Damage to pigeon retinae by moderate illumination from fluorescent lamps. *Exp Eye Res*, **14**, 164–169.

Marshall J., Trokel S., Rothery S. and Krueger R.R. (1986) A comparative study of corneal incisions induced by diamond and steel knives and two ultra-violet radiations from an excimer laser. *Br J Ophthalmol*, **70**, 482–501.

Merriam G.R. Jr and Focht E.F. (1957) A clinical study of radiational cataracts and the relationship to dose. *Am J Roentgenol*, **77**, 759–785.

Merriam G.R. Jr and Focht E.F. (1962) A clinical and experimental study of the effect of single and divided doses of radiation on cataract production. *Trans Am Ophthalmol Soc*, **60**, 35–52.

Merriam G.R. Jr, Szechter A. and Focht E.F. (1972) The effects of ionizing radiation on the eye. *Radiat Ther Oncol*, **6**, 346–362.

Millodot M. and Earlam R.A. (1984) Sensitivity of the cornea after exposure to ultra-violet light. *Ophthalmic Res*, **16**, 325–328.

Minassian D.C., Mehra V. and Jones B.R. (1984) Dehydrational crises from severe diarrhoea or heat stroke and risk of cataract. *Lancet*, **1**, 751–753.

Minatoya H.K. (1978) Eye injuries from exploding car batteries. *Arch Ophthalmol*, **96**, 477–481.

Moon M.E.L. and Robertson I.F. (1983) Retrospective study of alkali burns of the eye. *Aust J Ophthalmol*, **11**, 281–286.

Moran D.J. and Hollows F.C. (1984) Pterygium and ultraviolet light: a positive correlation. *Br J Ophthalmol*, **68**, 343–346.

Morgan S.J. (1987) Chemical burns of the eye: causes and management. *Br J Ophthalmol*, **71**, 854–857.

Noell W.K., Walker V.S., Kang B.S. and Bergman S. (1966) Retinal damage by light in rats. *Invest Ophthalmol Vis Sci*, **5**, 450–473.

Norm M.S. (1982) Spheroid degeneration, pingecula, and pterygium among Arabs in the Red Sea territory, Jordan. *Acta Ophthalmol*, **60**, 949–954.

Novak J.F. (1970) Ocular trauma in industry. *J Occup Med*, **12**, 287–290.

Novitskaya V.V. and Novitski I.Y. (1983) Two cases of ocular damage from lightning. *Vestn Oftalmol*, **100**, 71–72.

O'Connor Davies P.H. (1981) *The Actions and Uses of Ophthalmic Drugs*, 2nd edn. Butterworth-Heinemann, London.

O'Steen W.K., Shear C.R. and Anderson K.V. (1972) Retinal damage after exposure to visible light: a light and electron microscopic study. *Am J Anat*, **134**, 5–21.

Palva M. and Palkama A. (1978) Ultrastructural lens damage in X-ray induced cataract of the rat. *Acta Ophthalmol*, **56**, 587–598.

Paterson C.A. and Pfister R.R. (1974) Intraocular pressure changes after alkali burns. *Arch Ophthalmol*, **91**, 211–218.

Penner R. and McNair J.N. (1966) Eclipse blindness: a report of an epidemic in the military population in Hawaii. *Am J Ophthalmol*, **61**, 1452–1457.

Pfister R.R. (1983) Chemical injuries to the eye. *Ophthalmology*, **90**, 124–153.

Pfister R.R., Haddox J.L. and Patterson C.A. (1982) The efficacy of sodium citrate in the treatment of severe alkali burns of the eye is influenced by the route of administration. *Cornea*, **1**, 205–211.

Pitts D.G. (1978) The ocular effects of ultraviolet light. *Am J Optom Physiol Opt*, **55**, 19–35.

Pitts D.G. (1981) Threat of ultraviolet radiation to the eye – how to protect against it. *J Am Optom Assoc*, **52**, 949–957.

Pitts D.G. and Cullen A.P. (1981) Determination of infra red radiation levels for acute ocular cataractogenesis. *Graefes Arch Klin Exp Ophthalmol*, **217**, 285.

Pitts D. and Tredici T. (1971) The effects of ultra-violet light radiation on the eye. *Am Ind Hyg Assoc J*, **32**, 231–246.

Plesch A., Klingbeil U. and Bille J. (1987) Digital laser scanning fundus camera. *Appl Optics*, **26**, 1480–1486.

Porter W.J. (1961) Emergency treatment. *Ophthalmic Opt*, **1**, 483–485 *et seq.*

Porter W.J. (1966) Drugs in everyday practice. *Ophthalmic Opt*, **6**, 491–8, 507.

Rathkey A.S. (1965) Accidental laser burn of the macula. *Arch Ophthalmol*, **74**, 346–348.

Richardson A.W., Duane T.D. and Hies H.M. (1951) Experimental cataract produced by 3-centimetre pulsed microwave irradiations. *Arch Ophthalmol*, **45**, 382–386.

Rodger F.C. (1973) Clinical findings, course and progress of Bietti's corneal degeneration in the Dahlak Islands. *Br J Ophthalmol*, **57**, 657–664.

Sachsenweger R. (1980) *Illustrated Handbook of Ophthalmology*. Wright and Sons Ltd, Bristol.

Schwan H.P. and Piersol G.M. (1954) The absorption of electromagnetic energy in body tissues. *Am J Phys Med*, **33**, 371–404.

Sliney D.H. and Campbell C.E. (1994) Ophthalmic instrument safety standards. *Lasers Light Ophthalmol*, **6**, 207–215.

Sliney D.H. and Wolbarsht M.L. (1980) Safety standards and measurement techniques for high intensity light sources. *Vision Res*, **20**, 1133–1141.

Stewart-DeHaan P.J., Creighton M.O., Larsen L.E. *et al.* (1985) In vitro studies of microwave-induced cataract: reciprocity between exposure duration and dose rate for pulsed microwaves. *Exp Eye Res*, **40**, 1–13.

Sykes S.M., Robinson W.G., Waxler M. and Kuwabara T. (1981) Damage to the monkey retina by broad spectrum fluorescent light. *Invest Ophthalmol Vis Sci*, **20**, 425–434.

Teir H. (1984) Toxicological effects on the eyes at work. *Acta Ophthalmol*, *Suppl.* **161**, 60–65.

Trokel S.L., Srinivasan R. and Braren B. (1983) Excimer laser surgery of the cornea. *Am J Ophthalmol*, **96**, 710–715.

Tso M.O. and La Piana F.G. (1975) The human fovea after sun gazing. *Trans Am Acad Ophthalmol Otolaryngol*, **79**, 788–795.

Van Johnson E., Kline L.B. and Skalka H.W. (1987) Electrical cataracts: a case report and review of the literature. *Ophthalmic Surg*, **18**, 283–285.

Van Ummerson C.A. and Cogan F.C. (1965) Experimental microwave cataracts: age as a factor in induction of cataracts in the rabbit. *Arch Environ Health*, **11**, 177–178.

Waxler M. and Hitchings V.M. (1986) *Optical Radiation and Visual Health*. CRC Press Inc., Florida.

Weale R.A. (1983) Senile cataract: the case against light. *Ophthalmology*, **90**, 420–423.

Webb R.H., Hughes G.W. and Delori F.C. (1987) Confocal scanning laser ophthalmoscope. *Appl Optics*, **26**, 1492–1499.

Williams D.B., Monahan J.P., Nicholson W.J. and Aldrich J.J. (1955) Biological effects and studies on microwave radiation; time and power thresholds for production of lens opacities by 12.3-cm microwaves. *Arch Ophthalmol*, **54**, 863–874.

Wittenberg S. (1986) Solar radiation and the eye: a review of knowledge relevant to eyecare. *Am J Optom Physiol Opt*, **63**, 676–689.

Woo T.Y. (1985) Lenticular psoralen photoproducts in cataracts of PUVA treated psoriatic patients. *Acta Dermatol*, **121**, 1307–1308.

Young R.W. (1988) Solar radiation and age-related macular degeneration. *Surv Ophthalmol*, **32**, 252–269.

Zigman S. (1983) The role of sunlight in human cataract formation. *Surv Ophthalmol*, **27**, 317–325.

Zigman S. and Vaughn R. (1974) Effects of near UV light on the lens and retinas of mice. *Invest Ophthalmol Vis Sci*, **13**, 462–465.

Zweng H.C. (1967) Accidental Q-switched laser lesion of the human macula. *Arch Ophthalmol*, **78**, 596–569.

FURTHER READING

Deutsch T.A. and Feller B. (1985) *Paton and Goldberg's Management of Ocular Injuries*. W.H. Saunders, Philadelphia PA.

Miller D. (ed.) (1987) *Clinical Light Damage to the Eye*. Springer-Verlag, New York.

Roper-Hall M.J. (1987) *Eye Emergencies*. Churchill Livingstone, Edinburgh.

Sliney D. and Wolbarsht M. (1980) *Safety with Lasers and other Optical Sources. A Comprehensive Handbook*. Plenum Press, London.

Waxler M. and Hitchings V.M. (1986) *Optical Radiation and Visual Health*. CRC Press Inc., Florida.

6 Construction of eye-protectors*

Potential ocular hazards, such as flying particles and chemical splashes, should be eliminated or controlled at source. However, if this is not possible, the appropriate type of eye protection must be provided and worn. Screens or fixed shields can be used alone or in addition to eye-protectors to guard against potential hazards. People are now becoming more aware of the need to protect their eyes, and eye-protectors should not only be provided to fulfil legal obligations at work but also for the many other leisure activities, such as DIY, skiing, squash and ice hockey.

Ideally, an eye-protector should be:

- Constructed to provide the necessary protection against the hazard for which it is designed, e.g. flying particles or radiation
- Comfortable during wear and not liable to condensation
- Lightweight, and not interfere with movements
- Easily cleaned
- Readily replaced at reasonable cost
- Constructed so that it does not impair visual function
- Durable, non-flammable and non-irritant to the skin
- Of suitable optical quality
- Cosmetically acceptable
- Compatible with other protective devices, such as ear and respiratory protective equipment.

*This chapter is a revised version of North and Earlam (1988).

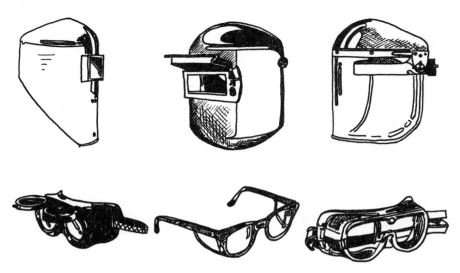

Fig. 6.1 *Different types of eye-protectors.*

Eye-protectors may be in the form of spectacles, goggles (cup or box), screens or visors supported by a headband, or a helmet (Figure 6.1).

LENS MATERIALS
The lenses for these eye-protectors may be made of:

- Glass–heat and special heat-toughened, chemically-toughened, and laminated
- Plastics–polymethylmethacrylate (PMMA), allyl diglycol carbonate (CR39), polycarbonate or cellulose acetate
- Wire gauze.

Glass

Heat-toughened glass
Glass is a fragile and brittle material, which breaks into very sharp splinters. It is therefore unsuitable for an impact-resistant eye-protector, unless it is heat or chemically toughened.

Heat-toughened glass lenses are usually made from spectacle crown glass. The toughening process begins when the edged lens is placed in a furnace and heated to 637°C for 50–300 s (Collins, 1983). The time spent in the oven depends on the weight, size and average thickness of the lens. After heating, the lens is withdrawn and cooled rapidly, usually by a jet of cold air. The sudden cooling creates a state of compression at the lens surface and a state of tension in the lens mass. This produces a compression tension coat, often referred to as the compression envelope. As glass is stronger in compression than in tension, the compression envelope improves the impact resistance. After the lenses have been manufactured, they are fitted into the frame or housing.

Advantages:

1. Heat-toughening is a comparatively quick process.
2. It does not need skilled labour.
3. The equipment needed is inexpensive and requires little bench space.
4. It is a relatively cheap process.

Disadvantages:

1. Prescription lenses over +5.00 D are not ideal for toughening, as the bulk of glass requires prolonged heating. This can cause warping, which degrades the optical qualities. Warping can be seen easily when viewing the focimeter image produced through the reading portion of fused bifocals. Lenses of over −5.00 D have poor impact resistance due to the relatively small centre substance (Collins, 1983).
2. A heat-toughened lens will always be thicker than an untoughened lens of equivalent power.

3. Impact resistance is markedly reduced by scratches and other surface abrasions, and lenses that conformed to BS EN 166 (1996) when first received from the factory will not retain the same level of impact resistance throughout life. As the lens surface will naturally become scratched with use, lenses should be inspected regularly and replaced when distinct scratches are present (Silberstein, 1964).

4. The heat-toughening process has an adverse effect on the photochromic salts present in photochromic lenses. It reduces the range of activity, and the lens does not lighten to the original transmission. To restore most of this activity it is necessary to apply a secondary annealing process.

5. When heat-toughened glass lenses are viewed through a polariscope or strain tester, a shadow or strain pattern can be seen (the Maltese Cross shape is typical). This pattern is induced during the heat-toughening process when the lens is cooled. The method of thin lens toughening does not give the characteristic Maltese Cross stress pattern, but shows a shadow pattern that varies from lens to lens.

Chemically-toughened glass

This is a method of toughening glass, which is more popular in the USA. As with heat toughening, the impact resistance is formed by the creation of a compression–tension coat, but in this case it is produced by a chemical process. The lenses are first preheated and then lowered into a potassium nitrate solution at 470°C for 16 hours (Jalie, 1984). The compression coat is produced by exchanging the larger potassium ions present in the solution for the smaller sodium ions present in the glass. As this treatment occurs on the surface of the glass only, it produces a very thin (100 μm) but very tough compression coat. For photochromic lens toughening, the solution normally used is 40 per cent potassium nitrate and 60 per cent sodium nitrate at a reduced temperature of 400°C. This process does not generally affect the photochromic activity of lenses.

Advantages:

1. Although chemically-toughened lenses are thin-

ner than heat-toughened lenses, they have been shown to possess a greater impact resistance.

2. Chemically-toughened glass has a greater impact resistance to large particles/missiles than conventionally heat-toughened glass (Woodward and Melling, 1977).

3. Chemical toughening is suitable for many lenses of stock thickness; specially surfaced lenses are therefore required only infrequently.

4. The toughening process takes the same time for all types of lenses.

5. The temperature required for chemical toughening is lower than that used for the heat treatment of lenses, and warping is therefore not a problem.

Disadvantages:

1. Chemical toughening is an expensive process, as it requires equipment that must withstand the chemicals and the temperatures involved.

2. It is not ideally suited for crown glass, and a special type of glass is needed for the best results. This glass is more expensive.

3. Scratches on the lens surface reduce the impact resistance because of damage to the very thin compression coat (Woodward and Melling, 1977).

4. It is difficult to determine whether the lens has been toughened, as there is neither a stress pattern nor a conventional method that will provide this information.

When chemically- or heat-toughened glass lenses fracture they usually show a radial fracture pattern, although concentric cracks can also occur (Figure 6.2). Therefore, only a few splinters of glass are produced and the fragments tend to stay in the spectacle frame.

Laminated glass

Laminated glass lenses are made by the adhesion of two layers of crown glass to an inner layer of plastic material. This type of lens has an impact resistance only slightly higher than crown glass. If it shatters, the glass is supposed to stick to the plastics interlayer; however, large, low velocity missiles may result in

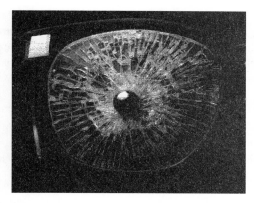

Fig. 6.2 *Fracture pattern of a heat-toughened lens. The lens was impacted with a steel ball bearing, which did not penetrate it (copyright B. Tarr).*

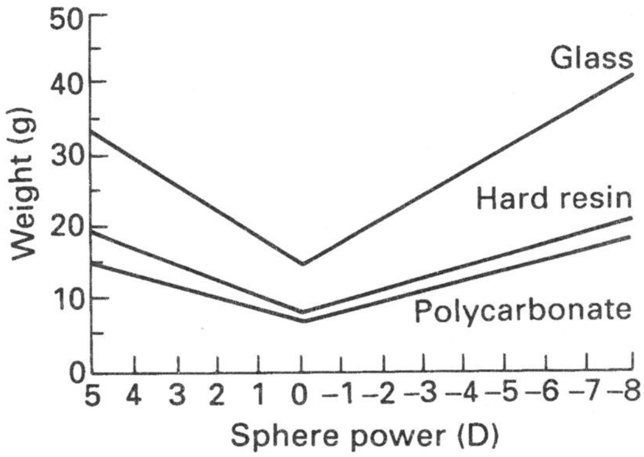

Fig. 6.3 *The weight of different lens materials (after Herbert, 1984, Courtesy of Gentex Corporation ITD and Optical World).*

slivers of glass from the back glass surface injuring the eye.

Plastics

Plastic lenses have many advantages over glass and are widely used as eye-protectors, especially where impact resistance is required.

Advantages (Jalie, 1984):

1. They offer greater impact resistance, particularly against high velocity particles.
2. Scratches on the lens surface do not obviously affect the impact resistance.
3. If the lens is fractured, the fragments tend to be larger and relatively blunt.
4. The weight is about 50 per cent of that of a glass lens of equivalent power (Figure 6.3).
5. A plastics lens can be thinner than a glass lens of equivalent power, as it may not be necessary to thicken the lens as much to maintain the impact resistance.
6. Plastics generally withstand molten metal splashes and hot sparks better than glass, as the metal does not fuse with the lens surface.
7. Plastic lenses are less susceptible to condensation, which is due to the lower thermal conductivity.
8. Plastics offer greater protection against UV radiation.

Disadvantages:

1. The lens surface is easily abraded because the material is soft; it needs an abrasion-resistant coating. Unfortunately, this has been shown to reduce the impact resistance of some lenses.
2. The refractive indices for plastic lenses range from 1.49 to 1.60. The higher index is usually accompanied by a lower V-value (Abbe number), which is the reciprocal of the dispersive power for the material. In general, the greater the V-value the better the material optically, as the chromatic aberrations produced decrease as V increases (Jalie, 1984).

Polymethyl methacrylate (PMMA) and Columbia Resin 39 (CR39)

PMMA (ICI perspex) was the first plastic material used in the UK for prescription lenses (Igard/Igard Z). These lenses have to a large extent been replaced by the thermosetting plastic CR39 (allyl diglycol carbonate). CR39 offers a greater impact resistance than PMMA, but when the lens breaks it produces sharper fragments. However, both these materials are suitable for eye-protectors. Lenses can be made up as a combination of PMMA and CR39. Prescription lenses for eye-protectors are commonly made from CR39, which can easily be tinted if required, using a dying technique. This method of tinting cannot be applied to PMMA lenses, as it causes deformation of the lens.

Polycarbonate

This has the highest impact resistance of all lens materials, but unfortunately it has a very soft and easily abraded surface. To avoid abrasion, a quartz coating is often used. Polycarbonate is commonly used for plano eye-protectors, where lenses and front are made in one piece by injection moulding. Its popularity for use as a prescription lens material in eye-protectors is increasing.

Advantages:

1. Polycarbonate has a much greater impact resistance than heat-toughened glass. If the lens does fracture upon impact, it cracks; it does not break into particles.
2. Silica-coating lenses makes them more abrasion-resistant than uncoated lenses.
3. There is no age-related warping, chipping, or discoloration.
4. Polycarbonate is the lightest lens material available (specific gravity 1.2).
5. Polycarbonate has a fairly high refractive index (1.586).
6. The material absorbs UV radiation.

Disadvantages:

1. Compared with glass or CR39, the surface quality of polycarbonate is poor.
2. Polycarbonate lenses can be tinted only by a vacuum coating process.
3. The V-value is poor (30) and causes colour fringes. This is most marked when viewing through the periphery of the lens, especially with high power prescriptions.
4. Abrasion-resistant coatings can decrease the impact resistance from 244 m/s to 152 m/s (Greenberg *et al.*, 1985).

Cellulose acetate

This has a relatively poor impact resistance compared with polycarbonate, and it is therefore used only for basic eye-protectors. However, it does have good resistance to chemicals, and is more often used for chemical visors and box goggles.

Wire gauze

Goggles made from wire gauze have a very good impact resistance, but are generally not accepted because they degrade the visual function and give no protection against splashes of molten metal, etc.

Testing procedures for protective lenses

The lenses used in eye-protectors must be tested to establish whether they are suitable for the specific hazard for which they were designed. The following factors may be assessed:

- Impact resistance
- Surface hardness
- Chemical resistance
- Thermostability
- Flammability
- Resistance to hot particles
- Radiosensitivity.

Impact resistance

The impact resistance of a lens can be influenced by:

- Abrasions/scratches on the lens surface
- The size and speed of the missile/particle
- The lens thickness
- The type of material.

The impact resistance of all types of lenses may be reduced when the surface has been abraded. There are two modes of failure, which partly depend upon the size of the missile. Large particles (> 16 mm) hitting a lens cause it to bend, and so the failure is initiated on the back surface. Therefore, any scratches that occur on the front surface due to wear and tear will not have a significant effect on the impact resistance. Smaller particles do not cause the lens to bend upon impact, so the fracture is generally initiated on the front surface. In this case, the impact resistance to smaller particles will be reduced for all types of lenses when the front surface has been abraded (Welsh *et al.*, 1974). The impact resistance was reduced by 20 per cent for heat-toughened lenses, and by more than 30 per cent for chemically toughened lenses (Woodward and Melling, 1977).

In general, as the missile size decreases, the impact resistance of the lens (measured as the fracture velocity) increases (Wigglesworth, 1971a). Table 6.1

Table 6.1 Mean fracture velocities of lens materials (m/s) (after Wigglesworth, E.C. (1972). A comparative assessment of eye-protective devices and proposed system of acceptance testing and grading. *Am. J. Optom. A.A.A.O.*, **49**, 287–304. Copyright The Am. Acad. of Optom; amd Greenberg *et al.* 1985)

Lens material	Thickness of lens (mm)	Missile diameter (mm)		
		25.4	6.5	3.2
CR39	3	6.6	49	88
CR39	2	5.0	39	63
Polymethyl methacrylate	3	4.5	34	58
Toughened glass	3	7.6	18	29
Toughened glass	2	3.7	12	23
Untoughened glass	3	3.1	12	23
Laminated glass	3	2.2	12	25
Polycarbonate coated*	3		152	
uncoated *	3		244	

Data from Wigglesworth (1972) and * Greenberg *et al.* 1985.

shows the mean fracture velocities of lens materials for different sizes of missile. When a 3-mm heat-toughened glass lens is hit by a large missile (19.1–28.6 mm), it demonstrates more impact resistance than a CR39 lens of similar thickness. However, when the missile is small (3.2–6.3 mm), the CR39 lens performs best. It has also been shown that for small missiles (< 6.4 mm), chemically-toughened lenses are not as resistant as heat-toughened lenses, whilst for larger missiles (> 6.4 mm) they have a slightly superior performance (Woodward and Melling, 1977).

As the lens thickness increases, the impact resistance also increases; impact resistance also increases slightly as the lens is curved. The strength increases with increasing base curve (6.00–10.00 D) with both heat-toughened and CR39 lenses (Wiggleworth, 1971b).

The type of material used for an eye-protector gives an indication of the mean fracture velocity that can be tolerated. Figure 6.4 shows the fracture velocity for some of the materials available. The samples were all of the same thickness and were struck by a 6.5-mm steel ball. Polycarbonate offers the greatest fracture resistance of all lens materials (Welsh *et al.*, 1974; Greenberg *et al.*, 1985).

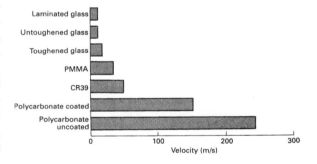

Fig. 6.4 *Fracture velocity of a 3-mm thick sample of different lens materials when struck by a 6.5-mm diameter steel ball (data from Table 6.1).*

Surface hardness

There have been many efforts to study the problems associated with surface abrasion, not all of which fully represent natural wear and tear. There are distinct advantages in coating plastic lenses, particularly polycarbonate, which is a soft thermoplastic. A thinly coated (5 µm) polycarbonate lens is superior to an uncoated CR39 lens.

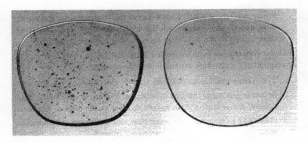

Fig. 6.5 *Resistance to hot particles by a glass lens (left) and a CR39 plastic lens (right). After equal exposure to spatter from an arc welder the glass lens is considerably more pitted than the CR39 plastic lens (copyright B. Tarr).*

Chemical resistance

Glass lenses are resistant to most chemicals. Plastics, however, may show crazing and surface clouding with some strong chemical solutions. CR39 has quite good chemical resistance, and is frequently used for chemical visors and box goggle windows.

Thermostability

Polycarbonate and polymethyl methacrylate are prone to distort more readily than glass.

Flammability

All the plastic materials are flammable. However, as their ignition temperatures are high, they are considered safe for use.

Resistance to hot particles

Eye-protectors must be able to withstand hot particles impinging upon them, as can occur in such processes as grinding or welding. A glass surface is very easily pitted by these particles, as they fuse with the surface. Plastics, on the other hand, do not pit easily (Figure 6.5). This is possibly due to the elasticity of the surface when heated by the particle.

Radiosensitivity

This should be considered in cases where a lens has broken and particles have penetrated the eye. A series of X-rays taken from different angles may locate the particle(s). Glass fragments can be observed by X-ray techniques when they are not too small (> 0.5 mm),

but plastic particles are very difficult to find (Collins, 1983).

A summary of the properties of the various materials used for lenses in eye-protectors is given in Table 6.2.

Materials for lens housing

The frames or lens housing may be made of metal (e.g a nickel alloy) or plastics (e.g. polycarbonate, polyamide, cellulose acetate or cellulose acetate butyrate). These materials may be used in the manufacture of:

1. Spectacle frames
2. Goggles – both cup and box type
3. Face shields
4. Helmets.

Spectacle frames

Protective spectacle frames may be manufactured by three methods (Fatt, 1977):

1. The front may be cut from a flat sheet of plastic material. Frames manufactured by this process are generally used for prescription eye-protectors and are made from cellulose acetate.
2. The frame may be formed by injection moulding from plastics granules. This technique again uses cellulose acetate for frames, which are generally glazed with prescription lenses. Polyamide (e.g. nylon) or polycarbonate is often used for plano eye-protectors.
3. The frames may be made from wire (e.g. nickel type). These frames have been shown to cause more damage upon impact than a plastic frame, as injury may occur when a blow forces the frame against the upper brow and cheek. Frames with adjustable toggle pads can cause more injury to the nose than those with a plastic bridge.

Particular concern has been expressed about the use of metal frames for prescription eye-protectors for the following reasons:

- The screws quickly work loose (notably the rim-securing screws).
- Accurate glazing of the lens is critical; if the lens is too small it may fall out, and if too

Table 6.2 A comparison of the major properties of glazing materials for eye-protectors (modified from Grundy 1987, courtesy of J. Grundy and *Optometry Today*)

Material	Impact resistance		Hardness	Chemical resistance	Thermostability	Fracture pattern	Resistance to hot particles	Weight
	Large missile	Small missile						
Glass								
Heat- toughened	Good	Good	Good	Very good	Very good	Fair	Poor	Heaviest
Chemically toughened	Good	Poor	Good	Very good	Very good	Fair	Poor	Heavy
Laminated	Fair	Fair	Good	Good	Fair	Poor	Poor	Heavy
Plastics								
PMMA	Fair	Fair	Poor	Good	Fair	Good	Very good	Light
CR39	Good	Good	Fair	Good	Good	Fair	Good	Light
Cellusose acetate	Good	Good	Poor	Good	Fair	Good	Fair	Light
Polycarbonate (coated)	Very good	Very good	Poor	Fair	Good	Very good	Good	Light

large it may induce stresses at the edge of the lens.

- Metal frames have narrower rims than plastic frames, which makes the glazing of high power lenses more difficult.

Recommendations relating to the use of metal frames (Grundy, 1982) are as follows:

- Rim screws should be secured by a lock nut, peening, or adhesives that bond the thread.
- Plastic lenses should be used instead of glass.
- Separate rim-securing screws and side-hinge screws should be used.

Side shields for spectacle frames

Side shields must not restrict the wearer's field of vision, and they should therefore be made of a transparent material that does not discolour with age. Injection-moulded side shields are best, as their shape does not alter (unlike those made from a flat sheet, which tend to warp). Any warping of the side shield will produce gaps between the shield and the front, allowing particles direct access to the eye. Ideally, side shields should be made of injection-moulded polycarbonate material. They may also be made from wire gauze or perforated plastics, to allow a better airflow and so prevent condensation.

The main advantage of spectacle eye-protectors is that they can be made to fit well, as there is a range of sizes available. Spectacles are not suitable for protection against such hazards as medium- or high-energy impact, dusts, gases, molten metal, hot solids, or liquid droplets or splashes (BS EN 166).

Afocal one-piece eye-protector

An afocal one-piece eye-protector is usually moulded in a single piece from polycarbonate. This type of protector has the advantage that the lenses cannot be dislodged, as may occur with a spectacle frame. They are suitable for emmetropes, but are usually manufactured in only one size and, as the fit required is different for each person, they do not always fit well. If not fitted correctly, eye-protectors will not provide the necessary protection and eye injury may still occur. Prescription eye-protectors are normally fitted by an optometric practitioner or dispensing optician, and should be adjusted carefully on collection. It is unfortunate that afocal eye-protectors are often handed out by safety officers, who do not have the necessary training or the facilities to fit them.

Afocal eye-protectors are often disliked by employees who do not normally wear spectacles, and are therefore worn very reluctantly. The employees' complaints include (Garner, 1973):

- A restricted field of view due to the frame
- The magnification effect – afocal lenses can give a small magnification, caused by the shape of the lenses (base curve)
- Reflections from the lens surfaces, which give rise to unwanted ghost images

● Peripheral displacement effects of afocal lenses increase with centre thickness, base curve and angle of ocular rotation, but the vertical displacement effect induced on ocular rotation is only a problem if the lenses of a pair have different base curves.

Goggles

The uses, advantages and disadvantages of the two different types of goggles can be summarized as follows (Rousell, 1979; Grundy, 1987).

Cup-type goggles

These may be used to provide protection against molten metal, flying particles, dust, etc. A good tight fit to the face is required. The housing is generally made of polyvinyl chloride (PVC).

Advantages:

1. They have an adjustable nasal fitting, i.e. distance between the rims.
2. Screw rim types allow the lenses to be replaced or exchanged for another type of lens, e.g. tinted or impact resistant.
3. Large bridge aprons are often available to protect the nose.

Disadvantages:

1. They cannot normally be worn over prescription spectacles.
2. Ventilation is often poor, which causes the lenses to mist. If present, the ventilation holes must be screened to prevent penetration and blocking by dust or chemicals, etc.
3. They are sometimes uncomfortable, as the cup is hard. The separation of the lenses is often too large, causing an obstruction of central vision.
4. Peripheral vision is restricted.

Box-type goggles

Box-type goggles are normally made of PVC, which gives a good fit around the brows and cheeks. The one-piece lens may be of cellulose acetate, polycarbonate or possibly toughened glass.

Advantages:

1. They can normally be worn over prescription spectacles.

2. They usually have good ventilation.
3. They are lightweight.
4. There is no central obstruction of vision.
5. There is a wide field of view.

Disadvantages:

1. The nasal fitting is not adjustable.
2. The one-piece lenses are not always easy to replace, and hence the whole eye-protector may have to be discarded.
3. Prescription wearers may sometimes have difficulty in achieving comfort or a proper fit of the goggles over their prescription spectacles.

Face shields

These are usually headband-supported visors that cover the face and neck. They are used to provide protection from flying particles, molten metal and chemical splashes, and can easily be worn over prescription spectacles or other types of eye-protection, if required. They provide an excellent field of view. Face shields are generally made from either polycarbonate or cellulose acetate. They can also be made so that they can be hand-held, e.g. the arc welding screens, which have a filter as the ocular (i.e. a tinted window). Face shields are also used to provide protection in occupations such as motorcycling, cricket and the security industry.

Helmets

Helmets are commonly worn during welding. They provide protection of the face and neck from intense radiation and spatter, and an ocular containing a filter prevents harmful radiation from reaching the eyes. The filter may be designed so that it can be flipped up to expose a clear, impact-resistant lens, which can be used during grinding and chipping operations. There are some superior variations of this appliance where the window is fitted with a polarizing cell, which darkens to welding density as soon as the arc is struck. These appliances usually have their own air supply, as the gases from welding rods are toxic.

Table 6.3 summarizes the different types of eye-protection required for specific ocular hazards according to BS EN 166.

Table 6.3 Type of eye-protectors available for ocular hazards according to BS EN 166

	Spectacles	Goggles	Face shields
Mechanical strength:			
Increased robustness	Yes	Yes	Yes
Low energy impact	Yes	Yes	Yes
Medium energy impact		Yes	Yes
High energy impact			Yes
Liquid droplets/ splashes		Yes	Yes
Large dust particles		Yes	
Gas, fine dust particles		Yes	
Short circuit electric arc			Yes
Molten metals/hot solids		Yes	Yes

Table 6.4 Eye wear for sports players (source: Eyecare Information Service, London)

Sport	Spectacles	Contact lenses
Abseiling*	Yes, or goggles	Scleral
Badminton	Yes, goggles better	All, soft CLs best
Basketball*	Yes, or goggles	All
Cricket*	Yes, or goggles	All
Hang gliding and parachuting*	Yes, under goggles	Soft CLs, under goggles
Hockey*	Goggles best	All
Scuba diving	Diving mask	Soft CLs, with mask goggles
Squash	Squash goggles	All types under goggles
Tennis*	Yes, or goggles	All, soft best
Water sports*	Ventilated goggles	Scleral best
Wrestling/judo	No	Soft or scleral
Yachting/sailing*	Yes, consider polarized	Soft

*Ultraviolet absorbers in the contact lens would be useful, or in some cases tinted spectacles lenses.
NB CLs provide very little eye protection and eye-protectors should be worn over CLs when necessary and appropriate.

EYE-PROTECTORS FOR SPORTS

As stated in Chapter 3, an increasing number of serious eye injuries are resulting from sports. Table 6.4 outlines the type of eye wear advised for some of the sports. For further information, refer to Loran and MacEwan (1995) and the *AOP Members Handbook*.

The following recommendations have been made regarding eye-protectors for sports.

Guidelines for frames:

- Frames should be lightweight but resistant to strong impact
- Frames should be fitted with curl sides
- Frames should be fitted with an elasticated sports band
- If made from metal, frames should fitted with a padded bridge.

Lenses guidelines:

- Lenses should be made of impact-resistant plastics, preferably polycarbonate
- Glass lenses should be avoided
- For indoor use, lenses should not be tinted and should have an anti-reflection coat.

SUMMARY

Various types of eye-protectors have been described, which can offer protection against different types of ocular hazards. However, it is essential that the hazards are correctly identified in order for the appropriate eye-protector to be supplied.

REFERENCES

BS EN 166 (1996) Personal eye protection – specifications. British Standards Institution, London.

Collins M. (1983) *Occupational Public Health Optometry*. Queensland Institute of Technology, Brisbane, pp. 25-41.

Fatt I. (1977) Is the frame safe? *Mfg Opt Int*, **March**, 109-110.

Garner L.F. (1973) Optical requirements for personal eye-protectors. *In Vision and its Protection. A Symposium on Visual Efficiency and Eye Protection at Work* (ed. Wigglesworth E.G. and Cole B.L.). Australian Optometrical Publishing Company, Sydney, pp. 77-93.

Greenberg I., Chase G. and Lamarre D. (1985) Statistical protocol for impact testing prescription polycarbonate safety lenses. *Optical World*, **March/April**, 7-8.

Grundy J.W. (1982) Eye protectors constructed with metal spectacle frames. *Ophthal Optician*, **July 31**, 550-552.

Grundy J.W. (1987) A diagrammatic approach to occupational optometry and illumination. Part 3. Industrial hazards and eye protection. *Optom Today*, **September 12,** 562-574.

Herbert S. (1984) The polycarb story could have a happy ending. *Optical World*, **April/May**, 4-8.

Jalie M. (1984) *The Principles of Ophthalmic Lenses*, 4th edn. Association of Dispensing Opticians, London.

Loran D.F.C. and MacEwan C.J. (1995) *Sports Vision*. Butterworth–Heinemann, Oxford.

North R.V. and Earlam R.A. (1988) Eye protection. In *Optometry* (eds Edwards K. and Llewellyn R.). Butterworth-Heinemann, Oxford, pp. 523–534.

Rousell D. (1979) *Eye Protection*. Publication No. 1S126, obtainable from: the Royal Society for the Prevention of Accidents, Cannon House, The Priory, Queensway, Birmingham, UK.

Silberstein I.W. (1964) The fracture resistance of industrially damaged safety glass lenses. Plano and prescription – an expanded study. *Am J Optom AAAO*, **41**, 199-220.

Tunnacliffe A.H. (1989) *Ophthalmic Lens Data. The Complete Reference*. J.R. Stallwood & Assoc., West Sussex.

Welsh K.W., Miller J.W., Kislin B., Tredici T.J. and Rahe A.J. (1974) Ballistic impact testing of scratched and unscratched ophthalmic lenses. *Am J Optom Physiol Opt*, **51**, 304-311.

Wigglesworth E.G. (1971a) A ballistic assessment of eye protector lens material. *Invest Ophthal Vis Sci*, **10**, 985-991.

Wigglesworth E.G. (1971b) The impact resistance of eye protector lens material. *Am J Optom AAAO*, **48**, 245-261.

Wigglesworth E.G. (1972) A comparative assessment of eye protective devices and proposed system of acceptance testing and grading. *Am J Optom AAAO*, **49**, 287-304.

Woodward A. and Melling R. (1977) Glass, the basic material. *Ophthal Optician*, **March 19**, 231-233.

7 Regulations and standards relating to eye protection

Under the Health and Safety at Work Act 1974, six new regulations were introduced:

- The Management of Health and Safety at Work Regulations 1992
- The Personal Protective Equipment at Work Regulations 1992
- The Workplace (Health, Safety and Welfare) Regulations 1992
- The Provision and use of Work Equipment Regulations 1992
- The Health and Safety Display Screen Equipment Regulations 1992
- The Manual Handling Operations Regulations 1992.

The Management of Health and Safety at Work Regulations 1992 requires employers to identify and assess the risks to health and safety present in the workplace, so that the most appropriate method of reducing the risks to an acceptable level can then be decided. The regulations state that the provision of personal protective equipment (PPE) should be viewed as a last resort. Risks should be controlled by other means wherever possible. For example, a fixed shield placed in front of a grinding wheel could provide protection against flying particles, instead of eye-protectors.

PERSONAL PROTECTIVE EQUIPMENT REGULATIONS

The Personal Protective Equipment Regulations 1992 came into force on 1 January 1993. The Regulations cover protective clothing (e.g. gloves and footwear) and equipment (e.g. lifejackets and eye-protectors). The PPE Regulations are divided into two parts;

Work and the Eye

Table 7.1 Personal Protective Equipment Regulations 1992

Part 1:	
Regulation 1	Citation and commencement – 1 January 1993
Regulation 2	Interpretation
Regulation 3	Disapplication of these regulations
Regulation 4	Provision of personal protective equipment
Regulation 5	Compatibility of personal protective equipment
Regulation 6	Assessment of personal protective equipment
Regulation 7	Maintenance and replacement of personal protective equipment
Regulation 8	Accommodation for personal protective equipment
Regulation 9	Information, instruction and training
Regulation 10	Use of personal protective equipment
Regulation 11	Reporting loss or defect
Regulation 12	Exemption certificates
Regulation 13	Extension outside Great Britain
Part 2: Selection, use and maintenance	Head protection
of personal protective equipment	Eye protection
	Foot protection
	Hand and arm protection
	Protective clothing for the body
Appendices	

Part 1 includes 13 regulations about PPE, and Part 2 aims to assist employers with their responsibilities for selection, use and maintenance of PPE (Table 7.1).

It is the responsibility of employers to make sure that any PPE supplied to their employees is appropriate for the risks concerned.

The employer must:

- Identify the hazard(s) present, such as chemicals, flying particles or radiation sources
- Assess the degree of risk, for example the probable size and velocity of any flying particles
- Select a suitable type of PPE from the range of 'CE' marked equipment (indicating that the equipment has a certificate of conformity)
- Ensure that PPE fits correctly, after adjustment if necessary
- Ensure that, where more than one type of PPE is necessary, they should be compatible and still effective against the risks.

The PPE should be maintained so that it continues to provide the protection required. This may include cleaning, examination, replacement, repair and testing. A stock of spare parts, when appropriate,

should be made available to the wearers. The regulations also require employers to provide suitable information, instruction and training so that effective use of PPE will be made by the employees. They must be trained in the correct use, fitting, wearing and storage of the equipment.

The employees also have a responsibility to wear the PPE provided, and to report any loss or defect to the employer as soon as possible.

Any PPE supplied for use at work must comply with the UK legislation implementing the European Community directives concerning design or manufacture with regard to health and safety. These are listed in Schedule 1 of the Regulations. The PPE Regulations require that most PPE supplied for use at work must be certified by an independent inspection body. If the PPE conforms to the basic safety requirements, a certificate of conformity will be issued and the manufacturer is then able to mark the product with 'CE'. It is illegal for suppliers to sell PPE unless it is 'CE' marked.

Part 2, regarding the selection and use of PPE, lists the various types of ocular hazards as:

- Impact
- Splashes from chemicals or molten metal

- Liquid droplets
- Dusts
- Gases
- Welding arcs
- Non-ionizing radiation
- Lasers.

The types of eye protection listed include:

- Safety spectacles
- Eyeshields (one-piece)
- Safety goggles
- Face shields.

Maintenance of PPE includes:

- Wet and dry cleaning. Dry cleaning involves the removal of grit with a brush and use of a silicone-treated non-woven cloth to wipe the lenses. NB: polycarbonate and other plastic lenses should not be dry cleaned
- The use of antistatic and anti-fog lens solutions as required
- Replacement of scratched or pitted lenses
- The provision and use of suitable storage cases for eye-protectors.

The Health and Safety Executive has compiled a document to provide guidance on the PPE Regulations. It states each Regulation and then gives a section on guidance. This document is very useful and should be consulted, as the above is only an outline. The actual Regulations should be consulted by employers.

EUROPEAN STANDARDS FOR EYE-PROTECTORS

The Regulations refer to relevant British and European Standards for eye-protectors, and include:

- BS EN 165 Personal eye protection – vocabulary
- BS EN 166 Personal eye protection – specifications
- BSEN 167 Personal eye protection – optical test methods
- BS EN 168 Personal eye protection – non-optical test methods
- BS EN 169 Personal eye protection – filters for welding and similar operations

- BS EN 170 Personal eye protection – ultra-violet filters
- BS EN 171 Personal eye protection – infra-red filters
- BS EN 172 Personal eye protection – sunglare filters
- BS EN 175 Personal eye protection – equipment for eye and face protection during welding and allied processes
- BS EN 207 Personal eye protection – filters and eye-protectors against laser radiation
- BS EN 379 Personal eye protection – welding filters with switchable luminous transmittance and with dual luminous transmittance.

BS EN 166 Personal eye protection – specifications

The standard that is the most important to an optometrist is BS EN 166 (which replaced BS 2092).

Ocular markings

The order of the ocular markings is shown in Table 7.2.

Filters

The first number refers to the type of filter that may be present in the eye-protector (Table 7.3).

Optical class

The optical class indicates the measure of optical tolerance to which the lenses have been manufactured (Table 7.4).

Properties of oculars

The different types of protection provided are shown in Table 7.5.

The following are examples of the ocular markings (Ⓡ represents the manufacturers' mark).

12 Ⓡ 1	Welding filter, optical class 1
3–1.7 Ⓡ 1	Ultra-violet filter, optical class 1
Ⓡ 3 B N	Optical class 3, medium energy impact and non-fogging properties
Ⓡ S K	Increased robustness and resistance to damage by fine particles

Table 7.2 BS EN 166 – order of ocular marking

Order of ocular marking	Marking/symbol
Scale number (where appropriate)	Combination of code (2-6) and shade number (see Table 7.3)
Manufacturers' identification mark	
Optical class	1, 2, 3 (see Table 7.4)
Symbol for mechanical strength	S, F, B, A, (see Table 7.5)
Symbol for non-adherence of molten metal and hot solids	9
Symbol for resistance to surface damage by fine particles	K
Symbol for resistance to fogging	N

Table 7.3 BS EN166 – code numbers for filters

Filter code number	Filter property
(no code number)	Welding filters
2	UV filters where colour recognition may be affected
3	UV filters with good colour recognition
4	IR filter
5	Sunglare filter without IR specification
6	Sunglare filter with IR specification

Table 7.4 BS EN 166 - optical class - tolerances

Number	Sphere & cylinder	Horizontal prism	Vertical prism
1	±0.06 D	0.75 Δ out 0.25 Δ in	0.25 Δ up & down
2	±0.12 D	1.00 Δ out 0.25 Δ in	0.25 Δ up & down
3	+0.12 D −0.25 D	1.0 Δ out 0.25 Δ in	0.25 Δ up & down

Table 7.5 BS EN 166 – types of protection provided by the oculars

Symbol	Oculars - property
S	Increased robustness
F	Low energy impact
B	Medium energy impact
A	High energy impact
9	Non-adherence of molten metal and resistance to penetration of hot solids
K	Resistance to damage by fine particles
N	Non-fogging properties

Table 7.6 BS EN 166 – order of housing markings

Manufacturers' identification mark
The EN standard (EN 166)
The field of intended use (See Table 7.7)
Symbol of resistance of high-speed particles

Marking of the housing

The housing must be marked as well as the oculars to indicate the protection that it provides. The markings must be given in the order shown in Table 7.6.

The symbols to indicate the field of intended use and the resistance to high-speed particles are shown in Tables 7.7 and 7.8, respectively.

There are two tests for increased robustness:

1. The oculars have to withstand the impact of a 22-mm diameter steel ball weighing 43 g travelling at 5.1 m/s.
2. The eye-protector must withstand the impact of a 6-mm diameter steel ball weighing 0.86 g travelling at 12 m/s.

The following are examples of frame/housing markings (® represents the manufacturers' mark):

® BS EN 166 3 9 - B	Protection against liquids (droplets or splashes), molten metals and hot solids, medium energy impacts
® BS EN 166 4	Protection against large dust particles
® BS EN 166 - F	Protection against low energy impact particles.

Table 7.7 BS EN 166 – symbols to indicate field of use

Symbol	Designation	Field of use
No symbol	Basic use	
3	Liquids	Liquid droplets or splashes
4	Large dust particles	> 5 μm
5	Gas & fine dust particles	Gases, vapours, sprays, smoke and dust particles < 5 μm
8	Short circuit electric arc	Electric arc due to short circuit in electrical equipment
9	Molten metals and hot solids	Splashes of molten metals and penetration of hot solids

Table 7.8 BS EN 166 – grades of impact resistance

Symbol	Level of impact resistance*		Types of eye-protector
−F	Low energy	45 m/s	All types
−B	Medium energy	120 m/s	Goggles and face shields
−A	High energy	190 m/s	Face shields

* The eye protector must withstand the impact of a 6-mm diameter steel ball of mass 0.86 g.

Filters
Ultra-violet and infra-red radiation
BS EN 170 and BS EN 171 deal with filters for protection against ultra-violet and infra-red radiation respectively. Filters are marked with two numbers; the code number and shade number (the combination of these two numbers is known as the scale number). Code numbers 2 and 3 are for filters to protect against ultra-violet radiation, and code number 4 is for protection against infra-red radiation.

Table 7.9 shows some of the typical applications of filters to protect against ultra-violet radiation (according to BS EN 170).

The selection of filters for protection against infra-red radiation is made according to the mean temperature of the source in degrees Celsius (Table 7.10).

Sunglare
Filters for protection against sunglare listed in BS EN 172 have code numbers 5 and 6 for without and with infra-red specification respectively. The shade numbers range from 1.1 to 4.1.

Welding
Filters recommended for various welding processes are listed in BS EN 169. The filters need to provide protection against ultra-violet, intense visible and infra-red radiation. Tables 7.11 and 7.12 and Figure 7.1 indicate the scale numbers required for the different types of welding processes. (Welding filters do not have a code number).

BS EN 167 and BS EN 168 – optical and non-optical tests for eye-protectors
These standards provide details of the various test procedures that the eye-protectors must undergo to ensure that they are suitable for the purpose intended. The tests are varied, and precise details of each test are given for the manufacturers.

The non-optical tests in BS EN 168 include:

- Increased robustness
- Minimum robustness
- Stability at elevated temperature
- Resistance to ultra-violet radiation
- Resistance to ignition
- Resistance to corrosion
- Resistance to high speed particles (see Table 7.8)
- Protection against molten metal
- Resistance to penetration by hot solids
- Protection against droplets and liquid splashes
- Protection against large dust particles
- Protection against gases and fine particles
- Resistance to surface damage by fine particles
- Resistance of the oculars to fogging.

Table 7.9 BS EN 170 - filters to protect against ultra-violet radiation

Scale number	Colour perception	Typical applications	Typical sources*
2-1.2	May be impaired	For use with sources which emit predominantly ultra-violet radiation and when glare is not an important factor	Low pressure mercury lamps such as lamps used to stimulate fluorescence or 'black lights'
2-1.4	May be impaired	For use with sources which emit predominantly ultra-violet radiation and when some definite absorption of visible radiation is required	Low pressure mercury lamps such as actinic lamps
3-1.2 3-1.4 3-1.7	No significant degradation	For use with sources which emit predominantly ultra-violet radiation at wavelengths shorter than 313 nm and when glare is not an important factor. This covers the UVC and most of the UVB bands†	Low pressure mercury lamps such as germicidal lamps
3-2.0 3-2.5	No significant degradation	For use with sources which emit intense radiation in both the UV and visible spectral regions and therefore require the attenuation of visible radiation	Medium pressure mercury lamps such as photochemical lamps
3-3 3-4			High pressure mercury lamps and metal halide lamps such as sun lamps for solaria
3-5			High and very high pressure mercury and xenon lamps such as sun lamps, solaria, pulsed lamp systems

* The examples given are for general guidance.
† The wavelengths of these bands are as recommended by CE (that is, 280 nm to 315 nm for UVB and 100 nm to 280 nm for UVC).

BS 7930 – eye-protectors for racket sports

In 1998 a British Standard was published relating to eye-protectors for racket players, BS 7930. At present only Part 1 is available, and this covers eye-protectors for squash players. The standard only applies to eye-protectors with polycarbonate oculars, and it includes prescription lenses. However, it does not cover eye-protectors designed for use over spectacles.

The test for resistance to impact is similar to that of BS EN 166, except that a yellow dot squash ball is used as the projectile. The protector is tested at four points using a squash ball with an impact velocity of 40 m/s. It should be noted that impact testing is performed only on plano protectors. Prescription eye-protectors are acceptable if the central lens thickness is no less than that subjected to impact testing. This information should be available from the manufacturers.

SUMMARY

It is important that eye-protectors are correctly selected and marked appropriately. Table 7.13 summarizes the markings of the oculars and housing and

Table 7.10 BS EN 171 – filters for protection against infra-red radiation

Scale number	Typical application in terms of mean temperature sources,°C
4-1.2	Up to 1050
4-1.4	1070
4-1.7	1090
4-2	1110
4-2.5	1140
4-3	1210
4-4	1290
4-5	1390
4-6	1500
4-7	1650
4-8	1800
4-9	2000
4-10	2150

When the level of radiation is very high, filters with reflective surface treatment are recommended for IR protection because the reflection of radiation results in a smaller rise in filter temperature.

the form of eye-protector available according to BS EN 166.

REFERENCES

The BS EN 169 (1992), BS EN 170 (1992) and BS EN 171 (1992) are reproduced with permission of BSI under licence number 2000SK/0064. British Standards can be obtained by post from BSI Customer Services, 389 Chiswick High Road, London W4 4AL, UK (Tel 020 8996 9000 or Fax 020 8996 7400).

BS EN 165 Personal eye protection - vocabulary

BS EN 166 Personal eye protection - specifications

BS EN 167 Personal eye protection - optical test methods

BS EN 168 Personal eye protection – non-optical test methods

BS EN 169 Personal eye protection - filters for welding and similar operations

BS EN 170 Personal eye protection - ultra-violet filters

BS EN 171 Personal eye protection - infra-red filters

BS EN 172 Personal eye protection - sunglare filters used in personal eye-protectors for industrial use

BS EN 175 Personal eye protection - equipment for eye and face protection during welding and allied processes

BS EN 207 Personal eye protection – filters and eye-protectors against laser radiation

BS EN 379 Personal eye protection – welding filters with switchable luminous transmittance and with dual luminous transmittance

BS 7930 Part 1 (1998) Specifications for eye-protectors for racket sports - squash

Personal Protective Equipment Regulations 1992. Guidance on Regulations L25 is available from HMSO, mail order telephone 071 873 9090 or telefax 071 873 0011.

Table 7.11 BS EN 169 – scale numbers of filters to be used during gas welding and braze welding[*]

Work	$q =$ flow rate of acetylene (l/h)			
	$q \leq 70$	$70 < q\ 200$	$200 < q \leq 800$	$q > 800$
Welding and braze welding of heavy metals[**]	4	5	6	7
Welding with emittive fluxes (notably light alloys)	4a	5a	6a	7a

[*]According to the conditions of use, the next greater or the next smaller scale number can be used. [**]The term heavy metals applies to steels, alloy steels, copper and its alloys, etc.

Table 7.12 BS EN 169 – scale numbers of filters to be used during oxygen cutting[*]

Work	$q =$ flow rate of oxygen (l/h)		
	$900 \leq q \leq 2000$	$2000 < q \leq 4000$	$4000 < q \leq 8000$
Oxygen cutting	5	6	7

[*]According to the conditions of use, the next greater or the next smaller scale number can be used.

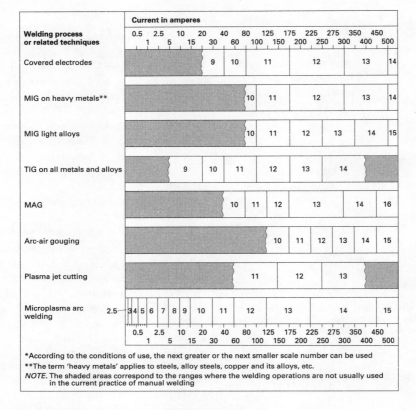

Fig. 7.1 *BS EN 169 Scale numbers* of filters recommended for use during arc welding.*

Table 7.13 Types of eye-protectors and their markings according to BS EN 166

	BS EN 166		Type of eye-protector		
	Housing	Oculars	Spectacles	Goggles	Face shields
Optical class	–	1	Yes	Yes	Yes
	–	2	Yes	Yes	Yes
	–	3	Yes	Yes	
Mechanical strength					
Increased robustness	–	S	Yes	Yes	Yes
Low energy impact	– F	F	Yes	Yes	Yes
Medium energy impact	– B	B		Yes	Yes
High energy impact	– A	A		Yes	
Field of use					
Liquid droplets/splashes	3	–		Yes	Yes
Large dust particles	4	–		Yes	
Gas, fine dust particles	5	–			Yes
Short circuit electric arc	8	–		Yes	
Molten metals/hot solids	9	9		Yes	Yes
Resistance to fogging	–	N	Yes	Yes	Yes
Resistance to surface damage	–	K	Yes	Yes	Yes

8 Lamps and lighting

This chapter aims to outline the units of light, summarize the different types of light sources and luminaires, and describe lighting design procedures.

CONCEPTS AND UNITS OF LIGHTING

Light is a form of radiant energy that induces a luminous sensation in the eye. The eye, as mentioned in Chapter 1, is more sensitive to some wavelengths than others, and this sensitivity is different for photopic and scotopic vision (Figure 8.1). For photopic vision, the eye has a peak sensitivity at a wavelength of 555 nm, a yellow-green colour. For scotopic vision, the peak sensitivity shifts to 505 nm, a blue-green colour. There are, however, individual variations, and not everyone has the same sensitivity. To overcome this problem the CIE (Commission Internationale de l'Eclairage), an international lighting body, has adopted an agreed standard response called the CIE standard observer. This is also known as the v (λ) curve, which has maximum sensitivity under photopic conditions at 555 nm. At 400 nm the sensitivity is poor, being about one-thousandth of the maximum level. Therefore, 1 W of radiation of yellow-green colour will be 1000 times more effective than 1W of radiation of a deep blue-colour (Thorn Lighting, 1991).

Photometric units

There are four important photometric units, which represent luminous flux, illuminance, luminous intensity and luminance.

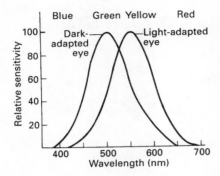

Fig. 8.1   *The relative spectral sensitivity of the human eye.*

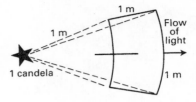

Fig. 8.2   *Luminous intensity. One lumen is the flow of light through an area of one square metre on a surface of a sphere of one metre radius with a point source of one candela at its centre (courtesy of EASL and LIF 1986).*

Luminous flux

The quantity of light emitted from a light source or received by a surface is expressed in units of lumens (lm). This is a measurement of the rate of flow of luminous energy, which is more commonly called the luminous flux (**F**). It is not practical to use the watt as a measure of light because of the variation in sensitivity of the eye with wavelength.

Illuminance

When a ray of light reaches a surface, it is referred to as illumination. The quantity of illumination or illuminance (**E**) is defined as the luminous flux (**F**) that is incident on a given surface area (**A**), i.e. the luminous flux per unit area. This is expressed in SI units of lumens per square metre, or lux, where $E = F/A$. For example, if an area of 0.1 square metres receives a luminous flux of 40 lumens, the illuminance, **E**, will equal 40/0.1, i.e. 400 lux.

One of the basic laws to enable the calculation of illuminance is the inverse square law, which states that the illuminance (**E**) equals the intensity of the light source (I) divided by the square of the distance (**d**); $E = I/d^2$. In principle this applies only to a single point source of light in a completely dark room. However, for most practical applications a luminaire can be considered to be a point source if its largest dimension is less than one-fifth of the distance from itself to the point of illumination. Therefore, the inverse square law can be applied to a 1-m fluorescent tube at a distance greater than 5 m. For example, light from a small point source with a luminous flux of 1 lm strikes a surface 1 m away, illuminating an area of 1 m². Hence, the illuminance ($E = F/A$) is 1 lux. If the

surface is moved to 2 m from the light source, the luminous flux will remain the same but the illuminated area will increase in size to 4 m², i.e. the area has increased in proportion to the square of the distance of the light source. The illuminance will be reduced to 0.25 lux, i.e. the illuminance has changed inversely with the square of the distance.

Luminous intensity

This is a measure of the capacity of a source or illuminated surface to emit light in a given direction. It is the luminous flux emitted in a very narrow cone containing the given direction divided by the solid angle of the cone. Luminous intensity (**I**) is expressed in candelas (cd). One candela is equal to one lumen per steradian; $I = lm/sr$ (Figure 8.2).

If a source emits the same luminous flux in all directions, its luminous intensity is uniform in all directions. However, for most sources the flux is not the same in all directions. A spotlight, for example, may have a luminous intensity of 2000 cd at the centre of the beam, but if it were angled, the intensity directed downwards may be reduced to only 200 cd. Applying the inverse square law to the spotlight when directed downwards on to a surface 2 m below, the illuminance will be:

$$E = I/d^2$$

$$E = 2000/2^2 = 500 \text{ lux}$$

where I = intensity in candelas and d = distance in metres. This law applies to light striking a surface at right angles. However, if the surface is tilted or turned so that the rays hit it at an angle, the illuminated

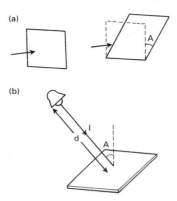

(a)

(b)

Fig. 8.3 *(a) The effect upon the illuminance of tilting a surface. (b) Inverse square law and the Cosine Law (from the Thorn Lighting Technical Handbook, courtesy of Thorn Lighting Ltd).*

surface will increase in size and the illuminance will decrease. The ratio of the originally illuminated area to the new area is equal to the cosine of the angle through which the surface has been tilted. The illuminance will decrease by the factor of the cosine of the angle. This is known as the cosine law of illuminance. For example, if a surface originally illuminated to 200 lux is tilted through an angle of 60°, the illuminance will be reduced by half, to 100 lux, because the cosine of 60° is 0.5 (Figure 8.3a).

The cosine law can be combined with the inverse square law (Figure 8.3b) thus:

$$E = (I \cos A)/d^2$$

This equation can be used for one or more light sources provided the total illuminance at a point is the sum of the illuminance by the individual sources; this is known as the point-by-point method.

Luminance

Luminance is the intensity of light emitted or reflected in a given direction per projected area of a luminous or reflecting surface. Luminance is expressed in candelas per square metre. For a matt surface, the relationship is:

$$\text{Luminance} = \frac{\text{Illuminance} \times \text{reflectance}}{\pi}$$

It should be noted that the terms 'luminance' and 'brightness' have similar meanings. However, the objectively measured photometric quantity should be referred to as luminance.

For physiological purposes, the following approximate luminance ranges are recognized:

- Scotopic conditions, 10^{-6} to 10^{-3} cd/m^2
- Mesopic conditions, 10^{-3} to 3 cd/m^2
- Photopic conditions, > 3 cd/m^2.

Contrast

Contrast is a term that is used subjectively and objectively. It expresses the luminance differences of two parts of the visual field. It may be expressed as:

$$\text{Contrast} = \frac{L_t - L_b}{L_b}$$

where L_t is the task luminance and L_b is the background luminance.

LIGHT SOURCES

There are two basic sources of light; natural daylight and electric (artificial) light.

Daylight

Although daylight appears to have a great advantage over electric light in being free of charge, it does have a major disadvantage in that it is a continually varying source. An electric light source is constant and, provided there is a supply of electricity, it is always available. Daylight, unfortunately, varies in quantity, colour and direction, depending upon the time of day, the season, and weather conditions. For example, the range of illuminances can vary from 100 000 lux on a bright, sunny day to 5000 lux on an overcast day, and 0.5 lux from moonlight. Cricket followers will have heard the expression 'bad light stops play'. This means that the light level is about 1000 lux.

To utilize the available daylight efficiently, large windows are required. These have several disadvantages; they are poor thermal and noise barriers, and require regular cleaning.

The spectral composition of daylight varies, as do the correlated colour temperatures (CCT), which can vary from 4000 K on an overcast day to 40 000 K on a clear, bright day; the most common value is about 6000 K. Five phases of CCT have therefore been agreed, which represent the typical spectral

Table 8.1 Colour rendering classification (CIBSE 1994) (courtesy of The Chartered Institution of Building Services Engineers)

Colour rendering group	CIE colour rendering index (R_a)	Typical application	Examples of lamps
1 A	$R_a \geq 90$	Accurate colour matching required, e.g. colour printing inspection	Artificial daylight
1 B	$80 \leq R_a < 90$	Accurate colour judgements are necessary or good colour rendering is required for reasons of appearance, e.g. shops	Kolor-Rite 38
2	$60 \leq R_a < 80$	Moderate colour rendering is required	Warm white
3	$40 \leq R_a < 60$	Colour rendering is of little significance, but marked distortion is unacceptable	Colour 35
4	$20 \leq R_a < 40$	Colour rendering of no importance	

distribution of irradiances produced by the sun. As the CCT increases, i.e. with clear sky conditions, the blue end of the spectrum becomes more dominant. Correlated colour temperature is the temperature of a full radiator that emits radiation having a chromaticity nearest to that of the light source being considered, and is measured in degrees Kelvin.

Electric light

To enable a comparison to be made between the different light sources, the following factors can be assessed.

Luminous efficacy

This is the amount of light given by a lamp for each watt of power consumed, and is measured in (lumens/watt).

It is important to note that a discharge lamp cannot normally be operated directly from mains electricity supply unless it has control gear to stabilize the lamp current. This control gear also consumes energy, and therefore the efficiency of the discharge lamp circuit depends on the power taken by both lamp and control gear.

Colour properties

These are related to the spectral composition of the emission, and include colour rendering and colour appearance.

Colour rendering

This expression describes the appearance of colours under a given light source compared with their appearance under a reference source. Good colour rendering implies similarity of appearance under an acceptable light source, such as daylight. However, the colour appearance of light from a source is not a guide to its colour properties, as it is possible for the light from two lamps to be apparently identical in appearance but to have different colour rendering properties.

The CIE has developed a method of indicating the colour rendering properties of a light source. The colour rendering index ranges from 0 to 100, where 100 represents no colour distortion (Table 8.1). The Chartered Institution of Building Service Engineers (CIBSE) Code 1994 also provides a classification of colour rendering for light sources. It defines five groups ranging from 1A to 4, where 4 represents very poor colour rendering.

Accurate colour matching requires good colour rendering. Hence, light sources from Group 1A should be used. These have a high CIE general colour rendering index, being greater than or equal to 90.

Colour appearance

The colour appearance is the colour the light source, or a white surface seen by its light, appears to be. It is generally described as being warm, intermediate or cold. Cold colours have a bluish tinge, while warm

Table 8.2 Classification of colour appearance (CIBSE 1994) (courtesy of The Chartered Institution of Building Services Engineers)

Correlated colour temperature	CCT Class	Examples of fluorescent lamps
Less than 3300 K	Warm	Colour 93, Warm white
3300–5300 K	Intermediate	Polylux, Natural 25
>5300 K	Cold	Artificial daylight, Northlight 55

Table 8.3 Classification of light sources

Lamp group	Lamp type	Old code*	New code*
Incandescent	Filament – tungsten, – tungsten halogen	GLS/TH	I/HS
Discharge – Low pressure	Fluorescent (tubular and compact)	MCF	FD/FS
	Low pressure sodium	SOX	LS
Discharge – High pressure	High pressure sodium	SON	S–
	High pressure mercury	MBF	QE
	High pressure metal halide	MBI	M–

*International Lamp Coding System

colours are at the red end of the spectrum. Filament lamps have a warm appearance, whilst high-pressure mercury lamps have a cool appearance.

The colour appearance of a light source is classified according to the correlated colour temperature range (CCT). The colour temperature of a radiator is the absolute temperature (K) of a full radiator (black body) which emits radiation of the same chromaticity as the radiator under consideration. (A full radiator (black body) is a theoretical perfect absorber of all incident radiation and if it is heated to sufficient temperatures it will emit visible radiation, the wavelength depending on the temperature.) For filament lamps the colour temperature approximates to the temperature of the filament itself.

The correlated colour temperature is the term given to the temperature of a full radiator (black body) having the chromaticity nearest to that of the light source being considered. For example, the colour of a full radiator at 3500 K is the nearest match to that of a white tubular fluorescent lamp. Each lamp has its own specific CCT, but for practical purposes these have been divided into three classes as previously mentioned; warm, intermediate and cold. It can be seen from Table 8.2 that light sources that have a cold appearance have a high CCT, and those that have a warm appearance have a low CCT. (This is

contrary to what might be assumed. As red is a warm colour we would expect the CCT to be high, and as blue is cold we would expect the CCT to be low, but in fact the opposite is true.)

Lamp life

The term 'life' of an electric lamp can have two different meanings:

1. The time after which the lamp ceases to operate, e.g. filament lamps fail due to filament breakage
2. The time after which the light output is so reduced that it is more economical to replace the lamp, e.g. discharge lamps.

It is convenient to divide lamps into two main categories; incandescent and discharge lamps (Table 8.3). These will be considered below. Most of the information was gathered from CIBSE (1994), Pritchard (1999), Thorn Lighting (1991) and EASL and LIF (1986).

Incandescent lamps

Tungsten

Tungsten lamps operate by heating a tungsten filament to incandescence in a glass envelope filled with an inert gas, usually argon or krypton (Figure 8.4). The

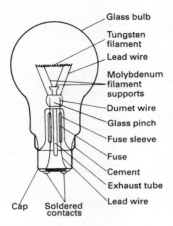

Glass bulb
Tungsten filament
Lead wire
Molybdenum filament supports
Dumet wire
Glass pinch
Fuse sleeve
Fuse
Cement
Exhaust tube
Lead wire
Cap
Soldered contacts

Fig. 8.4 *A tungsten filament lamp (from the Thorn Lighting Technical Handbook, courtesy of Thorn Lighting Ltd).*

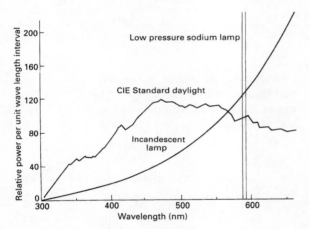

Fig. 8.5 *Types of radiant energy as produced by different light sources.*

passage of electricity through the filament raises the temperature of the tungsten molecules to the point where they emit light, or incandesce. The resulting spectral emission is a function of the temperature of the filament. The main characteristic of the incandescent lamp is that the spectral emission forms a continuum (Figure 8.5). As the temperature of the filament increases, the peak of its emission moves from the red to the blue end of the spectrum. Although the melting point of tungsten is 3600 K, the rate of evaporation increases markedly above 2800 K. This can be reduced by raising the vapour pressure in the lamp with an inert gas such as argon.

Advantages:

1. There is generally immediate full light output
2. The lamp operates in all positions
3. It is easy to control the lamp output by varying the applied voltage.

Disadvantages:

1. Tungsten lamps have a short life (1000–2000 h) and frequent replacement is necessary
2. The running costs are high due to poor luminous efficiency (11–19 lm/W)
3. The lamp emphasizes red strongly, and yellows and greens to a lesser extent; blue is strongly subdued
4. Tungsten lamps should not be used for colour matching
5. The light output and life are sensitive to small voltage variations
6. These lamps are sensitive to vibration
7. At too high a temperature the tungsten evaporates from the filament, leaving black deposits on the inside of the bulb, which reduce the light output.

Tungsten halogen

These are filament lamps. The filament is contained in a tube of fused silica or quartz, which is filled with a halogen compound gas. Whereas conventional tungsten filament lamps must not be run at too high a temperature, a tungsten halide lamp can be run at much higher temperatures because although the tungsten is evaporated off the filament, it combines with the halogen (e.g. iodine vapour) to form a reusable compound – a halide. This compound is carried on the convection currents within the bulb, and when it passes the filament it dissociates into tungsten, which is deposited on the filament, and the halogen, which is released to repeat the cycle (Figure 8.6). This increases lamp efficacy and life.

Advantages:

1. These lamps have a higher luminous efficacy than tungsten (17–25 lm/W)
2. The life of the lamp is longer (2000–4000 h)
3. There is no decline in light output with time (there is no blackening of the inner surface of the glass)

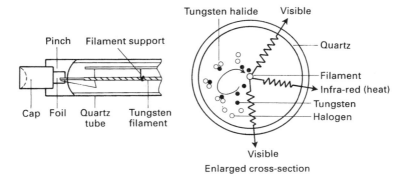

Fig. 8.6 *Simplified mechanism of the tungsten halogen lamp (from the Thorn Lighting Technical Handbook, courtesy of Thorn Lighting Ltd).*

4. The colour temperature is higher
5. The lamps can be made small and compact, and are therefore ideal for optometric instruments.

Disadvantage:

1. The surface of the bulb is liable to deteriorate if touched with the fingers (the fats from the skin migrate into the quartz envelope, causing it to blister).

Extra low voltage lamps are used for projectors and car headlamps. The low voltage dichroic reflector lamps frequently used for display lighting are designed to reflect light forward and transmit the heat (infra-red radiation) through the back of the lamp.

Gas discharge lamps

These lamps utilize the ionization of a gas to produce light. As electrons pass through the gas between the electrodes, they accelerate and collide with the atoms of the gas (usually sodium or mercury). The collisions may cause ionization of the atoms (i.e. release an increasing number of free electrons, which themselves cause collisions, resulting in a cumulative ionization) or absorption by the gas atoms of most of the energy of the electrons, which raises the energy state of the electrons to higher levels. Subsequently, when the electron falls back to a lower energy level it emits radiation.

The spectral emissions from discharge lamps tend to be discontinuous (line spectra), unlike those of incandescent lamps. At low gas pressure the emission is concentrated in narrow spectral lines, but these broaden as the pressure is raised. The envelope of the lamp is filled with a mixture of gases and vapours. The main gas is the one responsible for the emission of light, i.e. mercury or sodium, and other gases are included to aid the starting of the electron discharge, such as argon, neon, xenon, or argon mixed with nitrogen.

Control gear is necessary, first to be able to provide a high voltage for starting the lamp and secondly to be a current limiter/controller once the arc has been established. This is achieved by either a large resistor or an inductive resistor, which is known as a choke or ballast. Virtually all discharge lamps require control gear of some sort, and it will vary in size and weight in proportion to the lamp wattage and lamp complexity.

Discharge lamps can be grouped according to:

- Pressure – high or low
- Gas – sodium or mercury.

Fluorescent (low-pressure mercury) lamps

These lamps are often known as tubular fluorescent lamps, or strip lights. This type of lamp produces radiation in the visible and UV regions, the latter being absorbed by a phosphor coating on the inside of the glass tube, which re-emits the radiation in the visible region (Figure 8.7a). Any UV radiation that is not absorbed by the phosphor is absorbed by the glass tube. The spectral emission can be altered by varying the composition of the phosphors, and by introducing an additional compound into the discharge tube.

There is a wide range of phosphors available, which can produce almost any colour of light and different

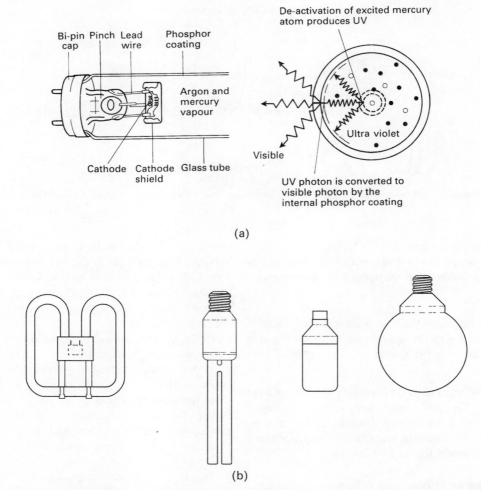

Fig. 8.7 *(a) Simplified mechanism of a low pressure mercury vapour fluorescent lamp (from the Thorn Lighting Technical Handbook, courtesy of Thorn Lighting Ltd). (b) Examples of compact fluorescent lamps.*

colour rendering properties. Phosphors commonly used are halophosphates (artificial phosphors), which produce 'white' light from a single phosphor. Triphosphors, which use three phosphors (red, green, and blue) in various combinations, give different shades of white (e.g. polylux and pluslux). The spectrum is a continuum (which varies with the phosphors used) on which the visible lines from the mercury discharge are superimposed.

Introducing an additional compound into the discharge tube, such as sodium, thallium or other metal halides, improves both the colour properties and the light output.

Compact fluorescent lamps

These are smaller versions of the long discharge tube, in that they have been folded into a more compact form – for example, a D or L shape (Figure 8.7b). They use approximately one-quarter the power of tungsten filament lamps and last, on average, five to ten times longer. They fall into two categories; energy-saving plug-in replacements for general lighting systems (GLS), or light sources for new luminaires.

It is possible to dim some of the tubular and compact fluorescent lamps by using high frequency technology. A disadvantage of the fluorescent lamps

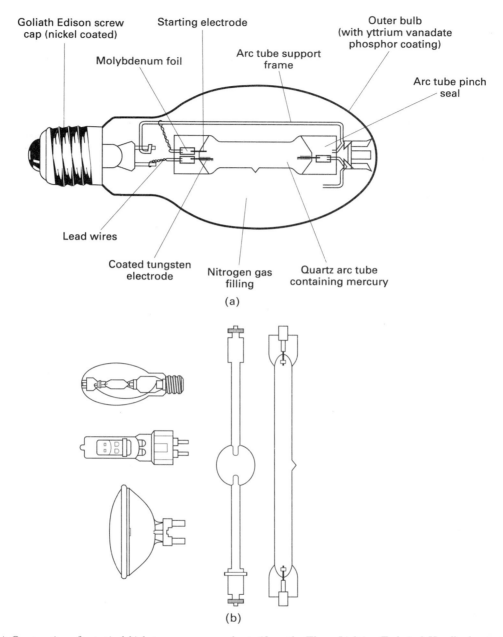

Goliath Edison screw cap (nickel coated)

Starting electrode

Outer bulb (with yttrium vanadate phosphor coating)

Molybdenum foil

Arc tube support frame

Arc tube pinch seal

Lead wires

Coated tungsten electrode

Nitrogen gas filling

Quartz arc tube containing mercury

(a)

(b)

Fig. 8.8 *(a) Construction of a typical high-pressure mercury lamp (from the Thorn Lighting Technical Handbook, courtesy of Thorn Lighting Ltd). (b) Examples of metal halide lamps.*

is that the light output is markedly affected by the atmospheric temperature - the lower the temperature, the lower the light output. This is a point worth remembering when, for example, choosing a light for the garage or outside porch.

High pressure mercury and metal halide lamps
Figure 8.8a shows the construction of a typical high-pressure mercury lamp (MBF). It consists of a quartz arc tube, containing a small amount of mercury and an inert gas, enclosed in a glass tube envelope with

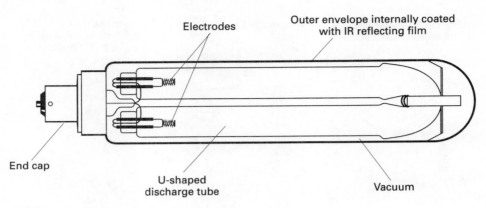

Fig. 8.9 *Construction of a low-pressure sodium lamp.*

phosphor coating, such as magnesium fluorogerminate or yttrium. The outer glass envelope is filled with nitrogen or a nitrogen/argon mix. The phosphor coating converts the ultra-violet light to visible light, and also improves the colour rendering. These lamps are mainly used for industrial and road lighting. Reflector versions of these lamps are also available.

Mercury blended lamps (MBT) have a tungsten filament and mercury arc tube in the same envelope. The filament is in series with the arc discharge, and it acts as a ballast as well as adding a warm colour to the light emitted. These lamps do not need control gear for operation, and due to the tungsten filament there is immediate light output. They are not dimmable and have a low luminous efficacy (10–26 lm/W), but they can usually be operated in any position.

Metal halide lamps (MBI) have the same construction as mercury discharge lamps except that the quartz arc tube also contains metal halides, which increases the luminous efficacy of the lamp to 45–80 lm/W and improves the colour appearance and colour rendering of the lamp. The metal halides are used in powder form, and may include indium, thallium or tin, which produce blue, green and orange-red radiation respectively. Additional colour correction and efficacy can be achieved by adding a fluorescent coating to the outer envelope. Figure 8.8b shows examples of the various metal halide lamps.

These lamps are not dimmable and have limited operational positions. They are commonly used in commercial interiors, industry, floodlighting and for colour TV lighting in studios.

High-pressure mercury lamps are available in a large range of wattages and colours. They are smaller than low-pressure mercury (fluorescent) lamps and have approximately the same life and range of luminous efficacy.

High intensity discharge lamps (HID) are a type of metal halide lamp that operate at higher pressures to provide a high intensity light source. Due to their small size and good colour rendering properties, they are often used for projection systems.

Low-pressure sodium lamps

Radiation emitted from these lamps is monochromatic and has a characteristic yellow colour. Figure 8.9 shows the typical construction of a low-pressure sodium lamp. The spectral emission is concentrated at 589 and 589.6 nm, which lie close to the peak of the photopic curve, i.e. maximum luminous efficiency of the eye (see Figure 8.5). These lamps have the highest luminous efficacy of all types (70–135 lm/W). It should be noted that during the start-up period the lamp is seen to have a red appearance, which is due to the neon/argon filling in the discharge tube.

These lamps are commonly used for street lighting due to their high luminous efficacy, but they also have the advantage that in foggy or misty conditions the monochromatic yellow light is not dispersed by the water droplets. Full light emission is not available instantly; the run-up time to 90 per cent output takes from 6–12 minutes. The light emitted is virtually monochromatic (yellow) and can therefore be used only where colour distortions are not important, as in street lighting. The lamps are not dimmable, and can be only be operated in limited positions.

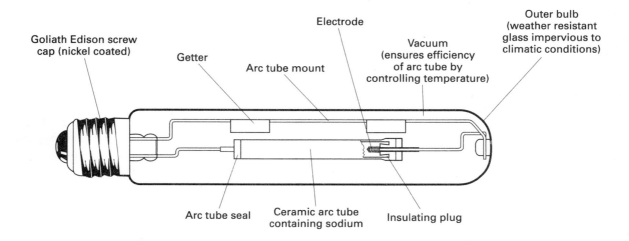

Fig. 8.10   *Construction of a high-pressure sodium lamp (from the Thorn Lighting Technical Handbook, courtesy of Thorn Lighting Ltd).*

High-pressure sodium lamps

Figure 8.10 shows the typical construction of a high-pressure sodium lamp. These lamps emit a more continuous spectrum than the low-pressure sodium lamps, and therefore have better colour properties. They have a luminous efficacy of 65–100 lm/W and, although this is not as high as the low-pressure lamp, it is being used increasingly in industry, for road lighting in cities, and for floodlighting etc. where the better colour properties are considered worthwhile despite the lower luminous efficacy. It is also a smaller lamp and easier to handle. Full light emission is not available instantly, as the lamp takes about 5 minutes to warm up. If switched off, there is an interval of about 10 minutes before the lamp will re-ignite, although special circuits can reduce this time to about 1 minute.

There are new high-pressure sodium deluxe lamps, which have good colour rendering properties and are designed primarily for interior lighting as an energy-saving alternative to other sources, e.g. SONDL-T and SONDL-E (Thorn Lighting, 1991). These lamps operate at higher pressure and temperature, which results in improved colour rendering properties. The main applications are for leisure centres, social areas, swimming pools, sports halls, and as uplighters in office areas where there are visual display units.

Induction lamps

This is a relatively new type of lamp, also known as an

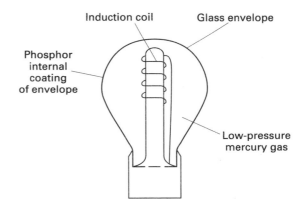

Fig. 8.11   *Construction of an induction lamp.*

electrodeless lamp. Figure 8.11 shows the construction and operating principle of an induction lamp. The lamp has a glass envelope filled with low-pressure mercury. There is a primary coil and a ferrite core, which together are known as the antenna.

The primary coil is supplied with an alternating current with a frequency of, usually, 2.65 MHz. The induced current causes an emission of UV as it circulates through the low-pressure mercury vapour, and these UV photons activate the phosphor coating on the glass envelope, thus producing visible radiation (as in fluorescent lamps).

Induction lamps have a very long lamp life (60 000 hours), and the light output is free from stroboscopic effects.

Advantages of discharge lamps

In general, discharge lamps have a higher luminous efficacy, have a longer lamp life and can have excellent colour rendering properties.

Disadvantages of discharge lamps

Two particular problems are associated with electric lights, and especially with fluorescent lights:

1. *Flicker.* Most lamps are supplied by alternating current (AC) at a frequency of 50 or 60 Hz. A 50 Hz supply has 50 cycles or reversals of direction of the current each second, giving 100 pulses of current per second. The light output does not generally follow the curve of the current, and the output from each half cycle is overtaken by the output from the next half cycle before it has decayed significantly. The effect of a succession of half cycles gives a 'ripple' in the output, and hence the flicker is not significant. The absence of flicker in most light sources is due to their construction - for example, in high-pressure mercury lamps the contribution to the light output from the phosphors is marked and, as the phosphors have a long after-glow, this tends to smooth the light output. However, as the lamp ages the flicker may be reduced to 50 Hz or less; this is usually most noticeable as a flicker at the end of the tube. It is usually best to replace the tube if flickering occurs, but sometimes it can be alleviated by shielding the ends of the tube.

2. *Stroboscopic effects.* The oscillation of the light output from a lamp can produce a stroboscopic effect even when the oscillation flicker is not detectable. This can cause moving machinery etc. to appear stationary or seem to move more slowly than it actually is doing, or can appear to reverse the actual direction of rotation (CIBSE, 1994). These effects occur particularly when all the lamps contributing to the illuminance are supplied by the same phase of the same supply. The stroboscopic effects may be reduced by the following methods:

   - Lighting the moving object with a lamp fed from two different out-of-phase AC supplies, or from two different phases of the same three-phase supply
   - Operating the lamps from high frequency supplies (electronic circuits operating at 32 kHz overcome the problem of flicker; Thorn Lighting, 1991)
   - Selecting a lamp with low flicker characteristics, e.g. high- and low-pressure mercury discharge lamps (low-pressure sodium lamps should be avoided, as they can give rise to flicker), or using an induction lamp
   - Using tungsten filament lamps fed from a direct current (DC) supply or a reduced AC supply.

Summary

It can be seen that there are numerous light sources to choose from. Table 8.4 gives a summary of the luminous efficacy, CCT, colour rendering characteristics and uses of the main types of light sources available. The manufacturers' literature should be consulted for further details and current data.

LUMINAIRES

Most light sources emit light in all directions, but this can be wasteful and cause visual discomfort. The functions of most luminaires are to (Thorn Lighting, 1991):

1. Redistribute the light from the lamp in preferred directions with the minimum of loss
2. Reduce glare from the source
3. Be acceptable in appearance, and in some cases make a definite contribution to the decor
4. Provide support, protection and electrical connection to the lamp.

Luminaires can take many different forms, but they all fulfil the above functions. Four methods of light control are commonly used (Figure 8.12):

1. *Obstruction.* The lamp is surrounded by an opaque enclosure with a limited size aperture. An example of this type is a downlighter in a refined metal tube with an open bottom.
2. *Diffusion.* The lamp is enclosed by a translucent

Table 8.4 Light sources for general lighting (courtesy of J. Baker, Electricity Association Services Ltd)

Name or type	Efficacy range	Approx. CCT (K)	Colour rendering characteristics	Typical applications
Incandescent filament lamps				
GLS	11–19	2700	Accuracy quite good but blues dull and reds bright	Homes, hotels, restaurants shop display, anywhere that sparkle is required
Tungsten halogen	17–25	3000–3200	As above, but blues brighter	Display and area lighting
Tubular fluorescent lamps (older T12 types)				
Artificial daylight	20–40	6500	Very good. BS 950 Part 1	Used for critical colour matching
Deluxe Natural	15–35	3600	Good. All colours bright but greens slightly yellow	Was widely used in food shops but low efficacy has led to its replacement
Northlight	20–40	6500	Good	Industrial colour matching
Deluxe Warm white	20–45	3000–3200	Good. Blues slightly dull	Blends well with filament lamps. Homes, hotels, etc.
Kolor-rite, Trucolour 37	20–45	4000 4200	Very good. Slight distortion to blues and greens	Were standard in hospital clinical areas. Museums, shops with special need
Natural	30–40	4000–4200	Good. Slight distortion but all colours bright	Offices and shops. Compromise between efficacy and rendering
Daylight	45–65	4300	Fair. Emphasizes yellows, reds dull	Used when colour not important
Warm white, White	45–65	3000–3500	Poor. Yellows bright most other colours dull	General purpose. Too often used in the home with poor results
Tubular fluorescent lamps (modern T8 types)				
Various, e.g. Pluslux	50–80	3000 3500 4000	Generally good	High efficacy versions of older T12 types
Various, e.g. Polulux, Colour 83/84	55–90	3000 3500	Very good. Some slight risk of metamerism	The modern high efficacy good colour rendering lamp
Compact, e.g. 2D, PL, SL, Lynx, etc.	40–55	2700–3500	Generally good. Most use TB phospors	Mainly used as replacements for filament lamps

continued

Table 8.4 *(continued)*

Name or type	Efficacy range*	Approx. CCT (K)†	Colour rendering characteristics	Typical applications
High pressure discharge lamps				
Mercury fluorescent (MBF)	35–50	circa 4000	Not good. Some distortion of of all colours	Mainly industrial. Cheap circuit
Metal halide (MBI/MBIF)	45–80	3000–4000	Good. Roughly equal to a Natural fluorescent lamp	Offices and shops with a crisp appearance, floodlighting
High pressure sodium (SON)	65–100	2000–2200	Poor. All colours distorted. Blues dull reds/yellows bright	Standard source for industry and city streetlighting, floodlighting
Deluxe high pressure sodium (SONDL)	50–80	2300	Fair. Roughly equal to a White fluorescent lamp	Offices, shops, leisure complexes (warm appearance)
Low pressure sodium (SOX)	70–135	Not applicable	None. Monochromatic output	Almost exclusively for street and security lighting

* A range is shown for efficacy to allow for differences between manufacturers and wattages (lm/W).
† A range is shown for CCT (correlated colour temperature) to allow for differences between manufacturers. Because of continuous improvement in products, manufacturers should be consulted for the latest data.

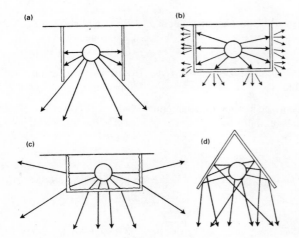

Fig. 8.12 *Four methods of light control: (a) obstruction; (b) diffusion; (c) refraction; and (d) reflection (courtesy of the Electricity Association Services Ltd 1990, previously The Electricity Council).*

material, which increases the apparent size of the light source. This will reduce the brightness of the source. Most diffusers also absorb light, as much as 60 per cent being lost. The diffusion is achieved by ribbing or stippling a specular reflector, providing a glass cover of diffusing material (such as acid-etched or sand-blasted glass), or using translucent glass or a plastic filter.

3. *Refraction*. This technique uses numerous prisms to deviate the rays of light and redirect them in the direction required. The luminaire is generally made of glass or plastic, and is highly suitable for general office lighting as it combines good glare control with reasonable efficiency.

4. *Reflection*. This technique makes use of reflecting surfaces, which may vary from a matt finish to a highly polished one. This type of luminaire is very efficient, as all the light can be directed where required. This is one of the oldest methods of controlling light and is seen in vehicle headlights, which have highly specular reflectors.

The methods described above are often combined in one luminaire. For example, a reflecting plate may be used above a lamp, whilst prismatic controllers are used at the sides and below.

The British Standard that covers most of the lumi-

Table 8.5 Classification of luminaires according to BS 4533/EN 60 598

Type of protection against electric shock	Level of insulation provided	Range from 0 to III (0 not permitted in UK)
Protection against dust and moisture, Ingress Protection (IP) system	1st digit – protection against dust system and objects 2nd digit – protection against moisture	Range from 0–6 (no protection to dust-tight) Range from 0–8 (no protection to continuous submersion)
Material of surface to which luminaire is fixed	Details of materials permitted for supporting surfaces	Five groups, including non-combustible, flammable

naires in the UK is BS 4533 (1990), and the equivalent European Standard is EN60 598-1 (1989). It is suitable for use with luminaires containing tungsten filaments and with tubular fluorescent and other discharge lamps running on supply voltages not exceeding 1 KV.

The luminaires are classified according to:

- Their type of protection against electric shock
- Their degree of protection against ingress of dust or moisture
- The material of the supporting surface for which the luminaire is designed.

For details, see Table 8.5.

Luminaire characteristics can be listed as follows:

1. Mounting position
2. Light distribution – polar curve shape, light output ratio, upward and downward light
3. Spacing to height ratio.

Mounting position

Luminaires can be recessed into the ceiling (R), fixed on the ceiling (surface-mounted, S), suspended from the ceiling (pendant-mounted, P), or free-standing or wall-mounted (F).

Light distribution

Polar curve shape

The distribution of light from a lamp or luminaire can be indicated graphically by a 'polar curve', which is the result of plotting the intensity of light in a series of directions within one vertical plane through the source. From the polar curve shown in Figure 8.13a, it can be seen that the maximum intensity of light is vertically down, although there is some upward light. For a symmetrical type of luminaire the polar curve will be virtually the same for all vertical planes. Filament lamps give a symmetrical distribution of light, and only one polar curve is required. Tubular fluorescent and other linear luminaires are known as non-symmetrical luminaires, as the distribution of light varies from one vertical plane to another. Manufacturers may therefore provide a split polar diagram with two polar curves for these non-symmetrical luminaires, one from the long axis and the other at 90° to it, i.e. axial and transverse (Figure 8.13b).

The polar curves can be used to calculate the total flux from a luminaire using the equation:

Light flux (1m) = intensity (cd) × solid angle (sr)

The intensity readings are taken at 10° intervals around the source. These intervals are described as 'zones', and the average intensity for each zone is then calculated. For example the average intensity for zone 4 shown in Figure 8.13a is:

$$\frac{290 + 260}{2} = 275 \text{ candelas}$$

The plane angles must be converted to their equivalent solid angles to obtain the 'zone factor'. Multiplication of the average intensity of each zone by the zone factor will give the total flux emitted from that zone. The zone factor will vary for each zone, being higher for zones nearer the horizontal than for those near the vertical (Table 8.6).

Hence, the total flux from zone $4 = 0.628 \times 275 = 172.5$ lm. The sum of all the zone factors gives the total flux (in lumens) from the lamp or luminaire (Table 8.6).

Light output ratio

The ratio of the flux from the luminaire to that from the lamp is called the light output ratio (LOR):

$$\text{LOR} = \frac{\text{Light from luminaire}}{\text{Light from lamp}}$$

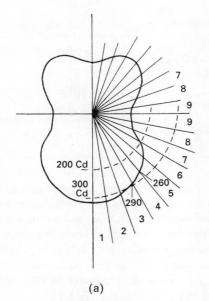

(a)

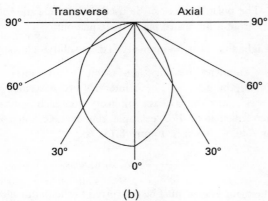

(b)

Fig. 8.13 *Polar curve: (a) symmetrical distribution of light; (b) non-symmetrical distribution.*

Upward/downward LOR

$$= \frac{\text{Upward/downward light from luminaire}}{\text{Light from lamp}}$$

Upward and downward light

The proportion of the total light output of the luminaire in the upper and lower hemispheres can be used to classify the luminaire. Luminaires providing most of their light downwards are called 'direct'; those whose light is mostly upwards are known as 'indirect' (e.g. an uplighter). A general diffusing luminaire gives

Table 8.6 Zone factors (courtesy EASL and LIF 1986)

Zone	Angle from vertical	Zone factor
1	0–10	0.095
2	10–20	0.284
3	20–30	0.463
4	30–40	0.628
5	40–50	0.774
6	50–60	0.897
7	60–70	0.993
8	70–80	1.058
9	80–90	1.091

approximately equal amounts of light in all directions. The flux fraction ratio is the percentage of the total light from the luminaire in an upwards direction divided by the percentage of the total light from the luminaire in the downwards direction:

Upper/lower flux fraction

$$= \frac{\text{Upward/downward light}}{\text{Total light from luminaire}}$$

$$\text{Flux fraction ratio} = \frac{\text{Upper flux fraction}}{\text{Lower flux fraction}}$$

Examples

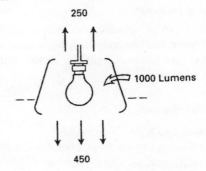

$$\text{LOR} = \frac{250 + 450}{1000} = 0.7 \text{ or } 70 \text{ per cent}$$

$$\text{Upward LOR} = \frac{250}{1000} = 0.25$$

$$\text{Downward LOR} = \frac{450}{1000} = 0.45$$

Upward LOR + Downward LOR = LOR

$$LOR = 0.25 + 0.45 = 0.7$$

$$\text{Upper flux fraction} = \frac{250}{250 + 450} = 35.71 \text{ per cent}$$

$$\text{Lower flux fraction} = \frac{450}{250 + 450} = 64.29 \text{ per cent}$$

Flux fraction ratio = 0.55

Table 8.7 CIE classification of luminaires

Luminaire	Flux above horizontal (%)	Flux below horizontal (%)
Direct	0–10	90–100
Semi-direct	10–40	60–90
General diffuse	40–60	40–60
Semi-indirect	60–90	10–40
Indirect	90–100	0–10

CIE classification of luminaries

The CIE classification of luminaires is based upon the luminous flux directed above and below the horizontal (Table 8.7).

Spacing to height ratio (SHR)

Manufacturers' data accompanying luminaires should include the maximum spacing to height ratio. This defines the spacing of the luminaires (centre to centre) in relation to their height above the work surface, which is generally taken as being 0.8 m above the floor. This information should then allow the luminaires to be positioned so that they provide an even illumination on the work surface. Luminaires that are placed too far apart will create some poorly lit areas.

LIGHTING DESIGN

So far, this chapter has discussed the different types of light sources and luminaires – i.e. how light is produced and its distribution. Now we need to discuss where and for what reason lighting is required. It can be used for several purposes:

1. To aid and facilitate the performance of a visual task

2. To create an appropriate visual environment, i.e. aesthetic appearance
3. To ensure the safety of people
4. To provide security for premises.

Lighting during the day can be provided by daylight, electric light, or a combination of both. People usually prefer to work in daylight, and dislike being in rooms with no windows. However, windows can create uncomfortably hot conditions when there is plenty of sunlight, and may also act as sources of glare. The most common approach to interior lighting is therefore to use daylight and artificial light sources together to produce the required task lighting; the artificial light acts as a supplement to daylight when and where it is insufficient.

Daylight

The extent to which daylight is available at a point inside a room is normally expressed as the 'daylight factor'. This is the illuminance received at a point on a plane in an interior expressed as a percentage of the illuminance outdoors.

Daylight factor

$$= \frac{\text{Daylight illuminance at point within room}}{\text{simultaneous illuminance on a horizontal plane outside from an unobstructed sky}} \times 100\%$$

When the average daylight factor is 5 per cent or more, the interior will appear to be well lit and lighting should be sufficient for most of the day. If the average daylight factor is between 2 and 5 per cent, then it may be worthwhile to consider using artificial light in addition to the available daylight so that when the daylight falls below the expected value the supplementary lighting can be used. For values of less than 2 per cent, the interior will be poorly lit and artificial light sources will be required nearly all the time.

Artificial lighting

There are several methods by which a task may be illuminated. The three most common in use are shown in Figure 8.14 (CIBSE, 1994) and are referred to as:

1. Generalized lighting
2. Localized lighting
3. Local lighting.

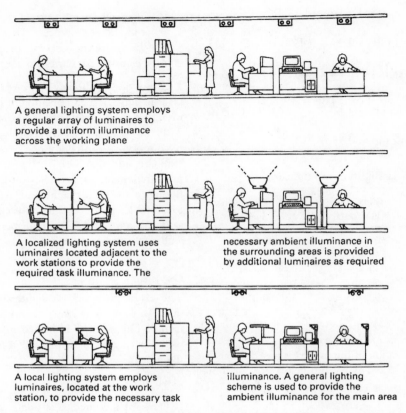

A general lighting system employs
a regular array of luminaires to
provide a uniform illuminance
across the working plane

A localized lighting system uses
luminaires located adjacent to the
work stations to provide the
required task illuminance. The

necessary ambient illuminance in
the surrounding areas is provided
by additional luminaires as required

A local lighting system employs
luminaires, located at the work
station, to provide the necessary task

illuminance. A general lighting
scheme is used to provide the
ambient illuminance for the main area

Fig. 8.14 *Lighting systems: (a) general; (b) localized; and (c) local (from CIBSE, 1994, reproduced courtesy of The Chartered Institution of Building Services Engineers).*

General lighting system

These are lighting systems designed to provide an approximate average illuminance over the entire working area. This has the advantage of allowing flexibility of workstations, as there is an even degree of illumination over the working area. However, energy is wasted because the whole area is illuminated to a level needed for the most critical task, and it is therefore more costly than it need be. The luminaires are generally arranged in a regular layout, which is easy to plan using the lumen method of lighting design. It is recommended that the uniformity of illuminance over the task area should be not less than 0.8 (ratio of minimum illuminance to average illuminance, CIBSE, 1994).

Localized lighting

This system is designed to provide the required illuminance on the working surface, together with a lower

level of illuminance for other general areas. The difference in illuminance between the task and general areas should be in the ratio of 3:1 or less (CIBSE, 1994). Great care must be taken at the design stage of this system to match the lighting to the workstations. If at a later date the workstations are relocated, there may be a problem with fixed luminaires. This can be overcome if uplighters (stand or desk-mounted) are used, as they can easily be moved to a new location.

Localized lighting will generally use less energy but may require more maintenance than generalized systems.

Local lighting

This has two separate lighting systems; one to provide the ambient background lighting and the other to provide supplementary lighting at the task. Local lighting is a very efficient method of providing high task illuminance and allows flexible, directional lighting for detailed tasks. It is also a method whereby additional lighting can be provided at the task, the luminaire usually being mounted at the workstation. Care must be taken when positioning the luminaire at the workstation so that it does not create veiling reflectances or shadows, or become a glare source for the surrounding workers. Local light should not be placed directly in front of the worker because it will reduce the visibility; the best position is to the left of the workstation or desk if the worker is right-handed and vice versa, so that the reflections will mainly go across the worker's line of sight. The task to background illuminance ratio should not be less than 3:1 (CIBSE, 1994).

This system has the advantage of providing the necessary level of lighting, but unfortunately the luminaires may be inefficient, rather expensive and have higher maintenance costs due to increased wear and tear.

Lumen method of lighting design

This is a method of lighting design that will provide uniform illumination of an area when the luminaires are arranged in a regular layout. If the lighting is to vary over the working area, then the point-by-point method should be used. The lumen method can be used to calculate the average illumination produced by a lighting installation, or the number of luminaires required to achieve the desired illuminance. The light received on a work surface will depend on the direct light and the reflected light. Therefore, when calculating the lighting to be installed to give a certain level of illuminance on the work surface, factors such as room size, reflectance of the surfaces and the type of lamp have to be taken into account. The number of luminaires (N) may be calculated from the equation (CIBSE, 1994):

$$N = \frac{E \times A}{F \times n \times MF \times UF}$$

where A = area of the work surface (m^2), E = average illuminance on the working surface (lux), F = lamp luminous flux (lumens), MF = maintenance, n = the number of lamps per luminaire, and UF = the utilization factor.

Illuminance (E)
The CIBSE Code for Interior Lighting (1994) recom-

mends levels of illumination for many tasks and occupations. It may be consulted to determine the value of **E** that should be provided for a specific task.

Utilization factor (UF)
The utilization factor may be published by the manufacturers for standard conditions of use of their luminaires, or it may be calculated as described in CIBSE Technical Memorandum No. 5 (1980). To use the UF tables correctly, it is necessary to know the room size (room index) and the room reflectances of the ceiling, walls and floor.

Maintenance factor
The new definition of the maintenance factor is 'the ratio of the maintained illuminance to initial illuminance'. This takes into account all losses, including decreased light output from an installation due to dirt and ageing and the reduction in light output from the lamp that occurs with time.

$$MF = LLMF \times LMF \times RSMF \times LSF$$

where LLMF = lamp luminance maintenance factor, LMF = luminaire maintenance factor, RSMF = room surface maintenance factor, and LSF = lamp survival factor.

LLMF is the proportion of initial light output that is produced after a specified time. The light output will decrease with time for most lamps, but the extent varies for the different types of lamp. The manufacturers' data should be consulted for the LLMF value for a specific number of hours for each lamp.

LMF takes into account the reduced light output that will occur due to dust and dirt being deposited on the luminaire. If the LMF is not available from the manufacturers, it can be estimated from tables in the CIBSE (1994).

RSMF takes into account the altered reflectance that will occur as surfaces collect dust and dirt, which will in turn alter the illuminance produced by the lighting installation. The reduction of reflected light will have less effect if the luminaires have a strong downwards distribution. Note that indirect lighting, which is dependent upon reflections, will have a far greater reduction of light reaching the work surface. This can also be calculated from graphs in the CIBSE (1994).

LSF is the percentage of lamp failures for a specific number of hours of operation, and is given in the manufacturers' data.

RECOMMENDED LEVELS OF ILLUMINANCE

In the UK, statutory instruments such as the Health and Safety at Work Act (1974) and the Factories Act (1961) require that lighting at places of work should be sufficient and suitable. This is normally taken to mean that the lighting on the tasks and in the areas where people circulate is adequate. The illuminance required for a particular task will depend on many factors, including the size of the detail, the contrast of the detail with its background, the accuracy and speed with which the task must be performed, the age of the worker, etc. Fortunately, recommendations that take these factors into account are given in the CIBSE Code for Interior Lighting (CIBSE, 1994), which provides levels of illuminance for a variety of tasks and occupations. The Code gives a scale of standard maintained illuminance, which increases as the visual task becomes more difficult (Table 8.8).

The standard maintained illuminance values assume that the task and/or interior is representative of its type in details, duration etc. However, it can be modified if the task concerned differs from the assumed typical circumstances. Modifying factors can include visual difficulty, duration of the work and the consequence of any mistakes. A flow chart permits these modifying factors to be taken into account so that the standard maintained illumination (from 200 lux to 750 lux) can be modified to give a value known as the design maintained illuminance (Figure 8.15). For standard maintained illuminance values of 150 lux or less, the modifying factors are not relevant.

A good lighting system must provide suitable lighting for all employees, whatever their task and whatever their age. Older employees require higher levels of illuminance to achieve the same levels of visual efficiency, and therefore the level of illumination may need to be increased; this is most easily achieved by the use of local lighting. Care must be taken to ensure that this additional lighting does not become a glare source to other employees working in the surrounding area. Older individuals are more sensitive to glare than the young, due to increased light scattering

within the eye, and also take longer to adapt from one lighting level to another.

Of particular interest to ophthalmologists and optometrists is the CIBSE LG2 (1989) guide, which recommends the following service illuminance levels:

Area	Illuminance (lux)
Ophthalmology	
Test room (working plane)	50–300
Consulting room (working plane)	300
Vision chart (vertical plane)	300
Bjerrum screen	100(maximum)
Chair (local)	1000
Operating theatre	
Operating cavity	10 000–50 000

When Ishihara charts are used, it is recommended that the colour temperature of the light source should be as near as possible to 6500 K.

The test rooms require blackout facilities and a means of dimming the general lighting.

GLARE

A good lighting system, as well as providing a suitable level of illumination, must avoid glare. There are two types of glare; disability glare and discomfort glare.

Disability glare

The term 'glare' is usually thought of as the presence of a very bright light source (such as car headlights or the sun) that prevents us from seeing the necessary detail. This type of glare is known as disability glare, which impairs the ability to see the detail without necessarily causing visual discomfort. It is nearly always associated with excessive light received by the eye, either directly from the light source or by reflection from bright shiny surfaces.

Discomfort glare

This is defined as glare that causes visual discomfort without necessarily impairing the ability to see detail. It is therefore a less obvious type of glare, and manifests itself in the form of discomfort. Lighting systems in most interiors are more likely to cause visual discomfort than disability. The discomfort may not be apparent, but its effects are cumulative and contribute to a sense of tiredness, especially towards

Table 8.8 Example of activities/interiors appropriate for each standard maintained illuminance (CIBSE (1994), reproduced courtesy of the Chartered Institution of Building Services Engineers)

Standard maintained illuminance (lux)	Characteristics of activity/interior	Representative activities/interiors
50	Interiors used rarely with visual tasks confined to movement and casual seeing without perception of detail	Cable tunnels, indoor storage tanks, walkways
100	Interiors used occasionally with visual tasks confined to movement and casual seeing calling for only limited perception of detail	Corridors, changing rooms, bulk stores, auditoria
150	Interiors used occasionally or with visual tasks not requiring perception of detail but involving some risk to people, plant or product	Loading bays, medical stores, plant rooms
200	Interiors occupied for long periods, or for visual tasks requiring some perception of detail	Foyers and entrances, monitoring automatic processes, casting concrete, turbine halls, dining rooms
300†	Interiors occupied for long periods, or when visual tasks are moderately easy, i.e. large details >10 min arc and/or high contrast	Libraries, sports and assembly halls, teaching spaces, lecture theatres, packing
500†	Visual tasks moderately difficult, i.e. details to be seen are of moderate size (5–10 min arc) and/or high contrast; also colour judgement may be required	General offices, engine assembly, painting and spraying, kitchens, laboratories, retail shops
750†	Visual tasks difficult, i.e. details to be seen are small (3–5 min arc) and of low contrast; also good colour judgements or the creation of a well lit, inviting interior may be required	Drawing offices, ceramic decoration, meat inspection, chain stores
1000†	Visual tasks very difficult, i.e. details to be seen are very small (2–3 min arc) and can be of very low contrast; also accurate colour judgements or the creation of a well lit, inviting interior may be required	General inspection, electronic assembly, gauge and tool rooms, retouching paintwork, cabinet making, supermarkets
1500†	Visual tasks extremely difficult, i.e. details to be seen extremely small (1–2 min arc) and of low contrast; optical aids and local lighting may be an advantage	Fine work and inspection, hand tailoring, precision assembly
2000†	Visual tasks exceptionally difficult, i.e. details to be seen exceptionally small (< 1 min arc) with very low contrasts; optical aids and local lighting will be of advantage	Assembly of minute mechanisms, finished fabric inspection

† 1 minute of arc (min arc) is 1/60 of a degree. This is the angle of which the tangent is given by the dimension of the task detail to be seen divided by the viewing distance.

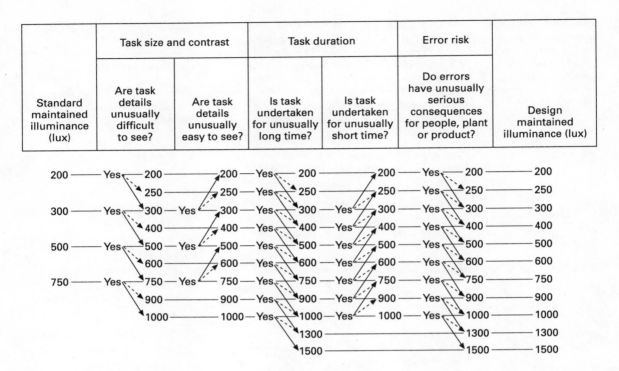

Standard maintained illuminance (lux)	Task size and contrast		Task duration		Error risk	Design maintained illuminance (lux)
	Are task details unusually difficult to see?	Are task details unusually easy to see?	Is task undertaken for unusually long time?	Is task undertaken for unusually short time?	Do errors have unusually serious consequences for people, plant or product?	

Fig. 8.15 *Flow chart for obtaining design maintained illuminance (from CIBSE (1994), reproduced courtesy of the Chartered Institution of Building Services Engineers). NB: Follow the horizontal path from the standard maintained illuminance until the answer to a question is 'yes'. If the yes is strong, follow the solid arrow; if moderate, follow the dashed line.*

the end of the day. People with poor health are particularly sensitive to visual discomfort caused by glare, as are elderly people. Discomfort glare (g) from a light source can be expressed (Electricity Council, 1990) as:

$$g = \frac{B_S^{1.6} \times W^{0.8} \times 0.478}{B_B \times P^{1.6}}$$

where B_S = luminance of source (cd/m^2), B_B = luminance of background (cd/m^2), W = angular size of source and P = position index, which indicates the effect of position of source on the eye.

The CIBSE Code (1994) also gives recommendations for the limiting glare index for the various tasks, etc. The limiting glare index specifies the degree of discomfort glare that is permissible from an overhead lighting installation (it is not applicable to local lighting installations). Calculation of the glare index is outlined in the CIBSE Technical Memorandum No. 10, and the value calculated should not exceed the limiting values suggested. The values of the limiting glare index usually lie in the range of 10 (low glare) to 30

(high glare). For example, the limiting glare index advised for general offices is 19, whereas for warehouse storage areas it is 25.

Control of glare
It is often possible to reduce or avoid glare by the following means:

1. The reflection factor of the object and the immediate background should be adjusted so that the contrast is adequate for seeing the task without being so high as to cause discomfort.
2. Where local lighting is provided the surrounding general illuminance should not fall too low, i.e. increase the background illuminance to reduce glare effects. The areas surrounding the task should be illuminated to not less than one-third of the task illuminance. Figure 8.16 shows the recommended illuminance and luminance ratios and surface reflectances (CIBSE, 1994).
3. Shiny or specular surfaces should be avoided

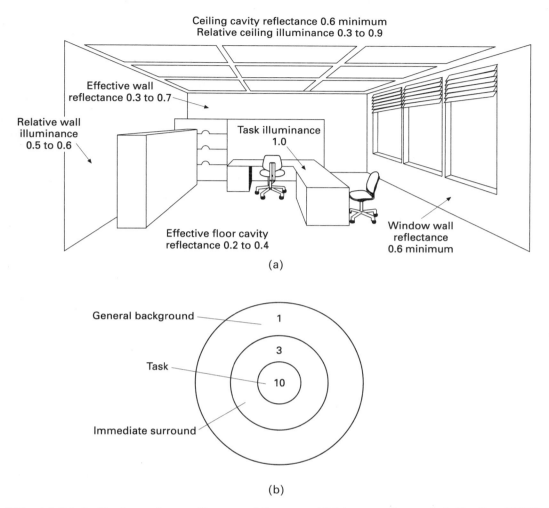

Fig. 8.16 *(a) Relative illuminances from a ceiling mounted direct general lighting system for a typical office (from CIBSE, 1994, reproduced by courtesy of The Chartered Institution of Building Services Engineers). (b) Recommended luminance ratios.*

where there is the possibility of bright images being reflected; use matt surfaces.

4. Luminaires should be installed at the correct mounting heights and spacing, otherwise uneven lighting will occur.
5. Source luminance should be kept at a minimum; use diffusers or screens.
6. The solid angle subtended by the source at the observer's eye must be kept at a minimum.
7. The glare source should be moved out of the line of sight (i.e. increase P). This is easy if the lamps are suspended.
8. Visual tasks should not be located so that a window is near the line of sight. If this cannot

be avoided, the window should be screened to reduce its brightness.

The most common cause of glare from lighting installations is due to the direct view of bare fluorescent tubes or incandescent lights from the normal viewing angle. Uplighters, which are luminaires that direct most of the light upwards onto the ceiling or upper walls to illuminate the working plane by reflection, are being used increasingly because they avoid glare by giving diffuse light. Several different types of light source are used in uplighters. Commonly used sources are the incandescent tungsten halogen, metal halide and high-pressure sodium deluxe discharge lamps. Most uplighters have a wide symmetrical light distribution, although this is reduced if they are wall mounted.

CHOICE OF LIGHTING EQUIPMENT
Light source
Once the lighting system has been designed, a list of suitable lamps should be made. The suitability of the lamp will depend on the nature of the task in the work place. Lamp selection should be based on the following factors (CIBSE, 1994):

1. Is good colour rendering required - either for accurate performance of the task or the aesthetic appearance of the area being illuminated?
2. Does the task require rapid provision of lighting? If the answer is yes, then most discharge lamps should be avoided, as they need a run up time.
3. Lamp life and luminous efficiency must be considered. If luminaires are difficult to access, then lamps requiring regular maintenance will be inappropriate.
4. Stroboscopic effects should be avoided if the work place has moving machinery.
5. The degree and accuracy of light control required for the task must be assessed. It is easier to control light from a small compact light source than a large one. The type of luminaires available must also be taken into account.

Luminaire
The following factors must be assessed regarding the work place and the specific task before a luminaire can be selected:

1. Environmental conditions. Does the luminaire have to withstand vibration, moisture, dust and extremes of temperature? Such factors must be taken into consideration - the luminaire must operate safely in the environmental conditions of the work place. The safety of the luminaire can be guaranteed by using equipment conforming to BS 4533(1990), which covers the electric, mechanical and thermal aspects of safety. The luminaires are classified according to the type of protection against electric shock, the degree of protection against dust and moisture (Ingress Protection (IP) System), and the material of the

supporting surface for which the luminaire is designed.
2. Light distribution of luminaires. This will influence the distribution of the light and the directional effects that will be achieved. The illuminance ratio charts of the CIBSE Technical Memorandum No. 15 can be used to assess the distribution of lighting and directional effects for a regular array of given luminaires. Illuminance ratio charts enable the effects of room size, reflectances of the surfaces, the luminaire direct ratio and flux fraction ratios to be assessed. The most useful way to use the charts is to identify the range of reflectances and luminaires necessary to provide the recommended conditions. Each chart is marked with the direct ratio along the horizontal axis and the flux fraction ratio along the vertical axis, while the recommended ranges are shown as unshaded 'safe areas'.
3. The utilization factor. The UF of the luminaire and the luminous efficacy of the lamp will allow the efficacy of the installation to be calculated. This is a measure of the amount of luminous flux that reaches the work plane for each watt of power supplied. The luminaires are all ranked according to the installed efficacy, so the most efficient may be chosen.
4. Other factors. Luminaire life, reliability, and the ease of maintenance should also be considered.

LIGHTING SYSTEM MANAGEMENT
The management must control the chosen lighting system so that it operates as efficiently as possible; it must also be maintained. Lights are often switched on in the morning and left on until the end of the work. This can be wasteful, as it may not be necessary for all the luminaires to be in use all the time. For example, luminaires near the windows can be switched off when daylight is adequate for the task, and local lighting can be switched off when the workstation is not being used. There are three methods by which lighting systems may be controlled (CIBSE, 1994; Electricity Council, 1990); manual, automatic, or processor control.

Manual control
The manual control of the lighting system, for example by a foreman, may appear to be a cheap method,

although this is not always the case. The lights will be switched on when the daylight is inadequate, but are less likely to be switched off when the daylight becomes sufficient. The control panel for work areas must be clearly marked so it is clear which switch controls which bank of lights or individual lights, and it must be easily accessible and located in a convenient place.

Automatic control

Automatic control may be provided by photocells, which can monitor the level of useful daylight. These can either be of the type that simply switch on or off at preset levels, or they may increase or decrease the electric light so that a certain level of illumination is maintained. The photo-electric type of control, which simply switches on or off, may control the whole working area or only the lighting near to the windows. To prevent the lights from switching on and off because of passing clouds, they are usually fitted with a time delay. If dimming control is required, it should be noted that this may be used only with filament or tubular fluorescent lamps (Electricity Council, 1990). This system is generally preferred by employees, as the light increases or decreases slowly - there is no sudden switching on or off. Time switches may also be used to switch lights on at the start of the day and, most importantly, off at the end of the day. All too often lights are left on overnight - a waste of money and energy. A manual over-ride should be available so that unexpected circumstances can be dealt with, such as maintenance or cleaning outside of normal hours. Other control devices can detect the presence of a person within an area and switch on the lights, and then turn them off after the area has been vacated for a set time. These devices include audio, ultrasonic and IR-sensitive systems.

Processor control

These systems, which are either computer- or microprocessor-based, are becoming more popular. They can not only control lighting but also building services such as air-conditioning, fire alarms and lifts. The great advantage of this system is its flexibility, in that the computer control programme can be adjusted to suit the work areas and modified as required. The system can monitor the building continuously so that it is operating at maximum efficiency and economy (CIBSE, 1994).

MEASUREMENT OF LIGHT LEVELS

The most common measurement required is the level of illuminance, i.e. the amount of light falling on a surface. The CIBSE Code (1994) and other lighting codes give recommended levels of illuminance (in lux) for various occupations and tasks; hence a method of measurement is required to check whether the level is appropriate. An illuminance meter usually consists of a light-sensitive cell, which is connected by an amplifier to a display; the display may be analogue or digital. The light-sensitive cell may consist of a selenium or silicon photovoltaic cell, although neither of these have a spectral response similar to that of the human visual system. One method of matching the spectral sensitivity of the cell to the spectral sensitivity of the eye is to superimpose a coloured filter. This is known as a 'colour-corrected' illuminance meter. The other method is to use correction factors, which are provided by the manufacturer for various light sources. It is also desirable to use a light meter which is 'cosine-corrected'. Ideally all the light falling on the photocell should be measured, but light falling on the cell at an oblique angle may be reflected and not measured. To reduce these reflections, a transparent hemisphere or diffusing cover is placed over the cell. Illuminance meters measuring illuminances from 0.1 to 100 000 lux (i.e. from moonlight to daylight) are available.

A luminance meter usually consists of an imaging system (some form of small telescope), a photoreceptor and a display. The imaging system is adjusted so that it forms an image of the object of regard on the photocell. Like the illuminance meter, the photocell must be colour-corrected. Luminance meters that can operate over the range of 10^{-4}–10^{8} cd/m^2, are available, and they can be used for areas varying in size from a few seconds of arc up to a few degrees.

Photographic light meters can be used to estimate light levels. Once again, the appropriate correction factors must be employed. For further details, see Long and Woo (1980) and Smith (1982).

SUMMARY

This chapter has attempted to outline the major types of light sources available, their characteristics, and the

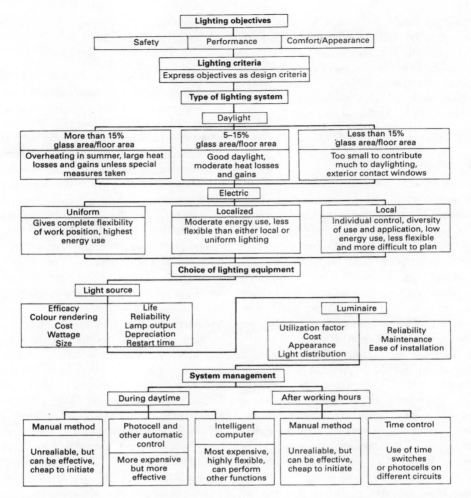

Fig. 8.17 *Lighting design flow chart (from the Thorn Lighting Technical Handbook, 1991, courtesy of Thorn Lighting Ltd).*

various methods of lighting design. As there are so many different types of artificial light sources, and a constant flow of new developments, the choice of light source and layout can be very difficult. Figure 8.17 shows a design flow chart that gives a sequence of steps to help simplify the planning of a lighting scheme (Thorn Lighting, 1991).

REFERENCES

BS 950 (1961) Artificial daylight in the assessment of colour, Part 1. BSI, London.

BS 950 (1967) Artificial daylight in the assessment of colour, Part 2. BSI, London.

BS 4533 (1990) Luminaires. BSI, London.

CIBSE (1994) Code for interior lighting. Chartered Institution of Building Services Engineers, London.

CIBSE LG02 (1989) Lighting guide number 2: hospitals and health care buildings. Chartered Institution of Building Services Engineers, London.

CIBSE Technical Memorandum No. 5 (1980) The calculation and use of utilization factors. Chartered Institution of Building Services Engineers, London.

CIBSE Technical Memorandum No. 10 (1985) Evaluation of discomfort glare – the IES Glare Index system for artificial lighting installations. Chartered Institution of Building Services Engineers, London.

CIBS Technical Memorandum No. 15 (1988) The multiple criterion design method: a design method for electric lighting installations. Chartered Institution of Building Services Engineers, London.

EASL and LIF (1986) *Interior Lighting Design*, 6th edn. Electricity Association Services Ltd and Lighting Industry Federation Ltd, London.

Electricity Council (1984) *Lighting for Visual Inspection*. Technical Information EC 4573/5, London.

Electricity Council (1990) *Better Office Lighting*. Technical Information EC 5212/ 1, London.

Factories Act (1961) HMSO, London.

Health and Safety at Work Act (1974) HMSO, London.

Long W.G. and Woo G.C.S. (1980) Measuring light levels with photographic meters. *Am J Optom Physiol Opt*, **57**, 51–5.

Pritchard D.C. (1999) *Lighting*, 6th edn. Longman Group Ltd, Harlow, Essex.

Smith G. (1982) Measurement of luminance and illuminance using photographic luminance light meters. *Aust J Optom*, **65**, 144–146.

Thorn Lighting (1991) *Thorn Lighting Technical Handbook*, 4th edn (ed. G. Williams). Borehamwood, Hertfordshire.

FURTHER READING

Smith N.A. (1999) *Lighting for Occupational Optometry*. HHSC Handbook No. 23. H and H Scientific Consultants Ltd, Leeds.

Other useful publications from the Chartered Institution of Building Services Engineers, 222 Balham High Rd, London SW12 9BS include:

Lighting guides for:
CIBSE LG01 The industrial environment
CIBSE LG02 Hospital and health care buildings
CIBSE LG03 The visal environment for display screen use
CIBSE LG04 Sports
CIBSE LG05 Lecture, teaching and conference rooms
CIBSE LG06 The outdoor environment
CIBSE LG07 Lighting for offices
CIBSE LG 08 Museums and art galleries

A series of pamphlets are available from the Electricity Association Services Ltd, 30 Millbank, London SW1P 4RD:

Lighting and You
Lighting and Low Vision.

9 Visual display units

Millions of people of all ages now use visual display units (VDUs) both at home and at work. Initially the introduction of VDUs caused concern about their use and possible health hazards. This chapter reviews the information regarding the health and welfare of VDU operators and the recommendations for the design of the workstation and environment.

The various health risks that have been suggested to be associated with the use of VDUs and that may affect the eyes are:

1. Asthenopia/eye strain
2. Facial rash/dermatitis
3. Epilepsy – photosensitive type
4. Radiation.

ASTHENOPIA

Asthenopia is a very common complaint amongst VDU operators, and some studies have estimated that up to 40 per cent of VDU operators suffer daily from asthenopic symptoms (Bergquist, 1984). These symptoms may be due to a variety of factors (Chakman and Guest, 1983), including:

- Ocular status
- Personal factors
- Workstation factors – glare, luminance, flicker, colour, contrast, alphanumeric design and postural factors
- Environmental factors – room temperature, relative humidity and air movement.

The symptoms of asthenopia may be ocular, visual, systemic or functional. The ocular symptoms are sore, tired, tender, itchy, dry, burning, throbbing or aching eyes. The usual visual symptoms are focusing problems, blurred or double vision, and fixation problems. The systemic symptoms are headaches and tiredness, while functional symptoms include behavioural changes.

Ocular status

Several studies have investigated the relationship between visual defects and asthenopia in VDU operators, and the results are somewhat conflicting. Gunnarson and Ostberg (1977) and Dain *et al.* (1988) found that workers with minor refractive errors, especially astigmatism, are likely to be predisposed to asthenopic symptoms. However, other studies investigating visual function and asthenopic symptoms have not shown a consistent relationship (Dainoff *et al.*, 1981; De Groot and Kamphuis, 1983).

Asthenopia can be caused by convergence and accommodation difficulties. Convergence insufficiency and low fusional reserves have been found to be a major cause of asthenopia amongst VDU operators (Gunnarson and Soderberg, 1980). Dain *et al.* (1988) found that the horizontal near heterophoria was significantly different between asymptomatic and symptomatic VDU operators. However, no basis for a standard could be established. Inadequate accommodation may lead to asthenopia, especially amongst presbyopic operators, who may not be able to focus the required distances without an appropriate spectacle correction.

The speed of accommodation decreases with age, and the layout of the VDU workstation should take this into account, as the viewing distances change rapidly from script to screen to keyboard. For data-entry tasks the viewing direction is estimated to alter once every 0.8–4 s, and ideally the keyboard, screen and script should be positioned at the same distance from the operator to avoid alteration of accommodation (Cakir *et al.*, 1980). The use of a document holder is particularly beneficial, especially for older operators.

The accommodative search system is thought to be affected during VDU operation, as blur is a stimulus to accommodation (Fincham, 1951; Phillips and Stark, 1977). Dot matrix characters, which have blurred edges, may cause the accommodative system to search in an attempt to produce a clear image. Hence, the focusing search with VDU displays may be higher than in non-VDU displays (e.g. script). This could lead to accommodative fatigue. However,

Rupp *et al.* (1984) found no significant difference in the accommodation stability between hard copy and VDU viewing.

Transient changes in accommodation have been encountered. Osterberg (1980) found an increase in the dark focus (i.e. resting point of accommodation) indicating an increase in ciliary tonus (spasm) after VDU work. Murch (1982) also found that the accommodative system does not focus as accurately on the display as on script. The accommodation system tends to move towards the dark focus, rather than focus accurately on the plane of the VDU screen. It has therefore been suggested that the VDU screen should be positioned at a distance approaching that of the dark focus, i.e. 100–66 cm, to allow for the under-accommodation of the visual system, thus maintaining a clearer focus.

After a work period of 4 hours on a VDU it can take up to 15 minutes for the induced myopia to relax and clear distance vision to return (Holler *et al.*, 1975). A study by Yeow and Taylor (1989) assessed both short- and long-term changes in visual functions of VDU operators. The study revealed a small but significant myopic shift in refractive error of 0.11 D following continuous VDU usage for periods up to 4 hours. This shift was seen in both presbyopic and non-presbyopic operators, and it rapidly returned to normal after the work was completed. VDU operators who were monitored for a period of 2 years did not appear to have any permanent myopic shift (Yeow, 1988).

Cole *et al.* (1989) engaged in a 6-year study of a group of VDU operators and a control group, to determine whether VDU work was a factor in the occurrence of visual symptoms, ocular abnormalities and ocular disease. During the initial examination of the two groups, the VDU operators were found to be significantly more myopic than the control group (difference in mean refractive error between the groups being 0.35 D). The most likely cause for this is felt to be self-selection – i.e. myopes have some characteristic(s) that have led them to select occupations involving VDU use. In 1996 Cole *et al.* reported their 6-year findings, and they did find differences between the groups, including the amount of myopia and the prevalence of symptoms. However, the differences were small and no clear trend or pattern was found to support the hypothesis that VDU work was a factor in the occurrence of visual symptoms, ocular abnormalities and ocular disease.

It appears from the above studies and others, including Gur and Ron (1992) and Mutti and Zadnik (1996), that there is no clear evidence that VDU users are more likely to develop myopia.

Type of work

Copy typists have a very visually demanding task, and reports indicate that they are more likely to complain of asthenopia than operators using only a VDU (Laubli *et al.*, 1980). It has been found that some copy typists prefer to view the copy from the right rather than the left side because their binocular co-ordination and binocular stability are better in this viewing direction. When reading, a person tends to take a head orientation that will bias the position of the text slightly to the right of the median plane. Therefore, if text to be copied is placed in any other position, the binocular stability may well be affected (Bedwell, 1978). It should also be noted that convergence is held more easily below the horizontal than above, and hence the screen and document holder should be situated below eye level.

Work breaks

The length of time spent by an operator at a VDU affects the incidence of asthenopia. For example, Gunnarsson and Soderberg (1980) found that increasing the time at the VDU from 3.5 to 6 hours produced an increase from 9 to 45 per cent in the number of operators reporting symptoms. This represents a five-fold increase in the number of people with problems, which were caused by less than twice the amount of exposure.

Frequent work breaks are strongly advised to reduce the incidence of asthenopia, especially for operators who have no variation in tasks during the work period. The US National Institute of Occupational Safety and Health (NOISH) recommends a 15-minute work break after 2 hours of continuous VDU work under moderate visual demands and/or moderate work loads, or after 1 hour of high visual demand, high work load, and/or repetitive work tasks (Miller, 1984).

Visual standards for VDU operators

The Association of Optometrists (AOP) has suggested a specific visual standard for VDU operators for the guidance of the profession (AOP, 2000a). This standard aims to increase the level of operator comfort and efficiency, and therefore should not be considered as inflexible or used to exclude people from working with VDUs. The recommendations are that operators should meet the following criteria:

1. The ability to read N6 throughout the range of 75–33 cm with adequate visual acuity for any task undertaken at a greater distance, if this is an integral part of the work.
2. Well-established monocular vision or good binocular vision. Phorias at working distances should be corrected unless well compensated or deep suppression is present.
3. No central (20°) field defect in the dominant eye.
4. Near point of convergence normal.
5. Clear ocular media checked by ophthalmoscopy.

Recommendations for minimum optometric tests have been set in other countries. In the USA, NIOSH has adapted two alternative methods, one given by the American Optometric Association and the other suggested by the National Society for the Prevention of Blindness. These recommendations, along with those of the New Zealand National Health and Medical Research Council and the Australian Optometric Association, are set out in a review by Chakman and Guest (1983). Table 9.1 summarizes some of the recommended screening procedures for VDU users (Taylor and Yeow, 1990).

Most of the recommendations do not include a measurement of the fusional reserves or fixation disparity. As asthenopia, or blurred vision, is often due to the inability to compensate for a heterophoria due to poor fusion, it would be of significant value to measure the fusional reserves and the fixation disparity. The latter can indicate the stress in the binocular system, and it has been reported to show an exo-shift after a day of close work (Yekta *et al.*, 1987). Whilst the various standards for VDU operators require the heterophoria to be within certain logical limits, they have not been based on clinical studies. Another point to note is that some of the recommendations do not include ophthalmoscopy, which is necessary for the early detection of ocular pathology.

Ideally, the vision screening should be carried out by a qualified person and should include ophthalmoscopy and retinoscopy either as part of a full

Table 9.1 Recommended screening procedures for VDU operators (reproduced by courtesy of Taylor and Yeow (1990) and *The Optician*)

	AOP	Australian Optometric Association	Australian National Health and Medical Research Council	UK VDU eye test Advisory Group	National Society for Prevention of Blindness	American Optometric Association
External examination of the eye	*	*				*
Ophthalmoscopy	*	*				*
Amplitude of accommodation	*	*		*		*
Suppression	*			*		
Muscle balance (distance)	*	*		*	*	*
Muscle balance (1 m)	*			*	*	*
Muscle balance (near)	*		*		*	*
Convergence	*	*		*		*
Refraction–distance	*		*	*	*	*
Refraction–intermediate	*			*		*
Refraction–near	*		*	*	*	*
Colour vision		*	*		*	*
Visual fields		*				*
Tonometry		*				*
Retinoscopy		*				*
Unaided acuity				*		
Stereopsis		*			*	*
Keratometry						*

examination or as a modified clinical technique. Although it is more expensive to employ a professional person, the number of false referrals will be reduced and the reliability of the results assured. Vision rechecks should be carried out at regular intervals; a 2-yearly period has been suggested by the Australian Optometric Association.

If an instrument screener is to be used for vision screening, then care should be taken to select one that includes an intermediate testing distance (for a summary of the available vision screeners, see Chapter 2). An alternative method of vision screening is to use a computer program. Software packages, such as the City University Vision Screener for VDU Users (see Appendix B), can be used by the operators at their own workstations (Thomson, 1994). The results of the vision screening are automatically evaluated, and a printout is provided. One advantage of this type of screening is that tests are carried out under the actual work conditions. Alternatively, there is the City VDU toolkit, which allows a variety of test targets to be displayed on a VDU and is designed to be used in the consulting room for assessing visual performance of VDU users and to help establish the optimal refractive correction under more realistic viewing conditions (Thomson, 1998).

Spectacle prescriptions

An emmetropic pre-presbyope should not have any problem in focusing the range of distances required for VDU work. The VDU screen is often situated at a distance of 50–70 cm, whilst the keyboard and the

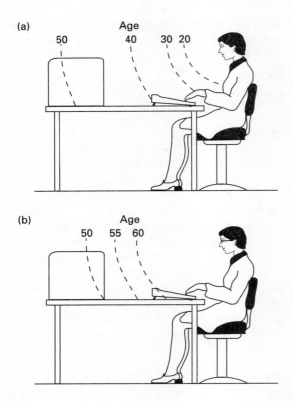

Fig. 9.1 *(a) The focusing ability varying with age. The dotted lines indicate the closest point at which near tasks can be viewed for prolonged periods of time without wearing spectacles prescribed for near. (b) The restricted range of clear vision of older operators wearing spectacles prescribed only for reading. The dotted lines indicate the point beyond which vision will be blurred (reproduced by kind permission of Grundy* et al. *(1991) and The Association of Optometrists).*

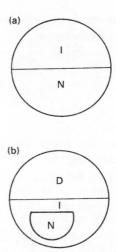

Fig. 9.2 *Examples of some of the lens forms available for presbyopic VDU operators: (a) executive bifocal; (b) trifocal. D, distance prescription; I, intermediate prescription; N, near prescription.*

script is usually at a closer distance of approximately 33–40 cm. Figure 9.1a shows the typical focusing abilities of various age groups. Whereas a 30-year-old can focus at all the necessary distances without any problem, operators in their mid-forties will be able to read the VDU screen easily but may have difficulty reading scripts/if they are positioned at a closer distance. A 50-year-old operator may have difficulty in focusing on both the VDU screen and the scripts without a spectacle prescription.

Problems occur for the presbyopic operator in that a conventional near correction for 40 cm is often too restrictive. Figure 9.1b shows the range of clear vision of older operators wearing spectacle prescription for reading only. For a 60-year-old, the keyboard and script will be in focus but the VDU screen will be blurred. To enable the older operator to read both the screen and the script, spectacles specially for use with a VDU may have to be prescribed.

Grundy and Rosenthal (1982) have found that the straight-line bifocals (i.e. so-called executive (E) or D segments) are superior to round or crescent-top bifocals (Figure 9.2). They provide a greater area of useful vision, and therefore minimize head and eye movements. Also, there is a reduction in 'jump' - displacement of objects which occurs when viewing is changed from one section of the lens to the other. However, operators up to the age of 50 years may find conventional bifocals suitable, although the bifocal segment height may need to be increased to correspond to the position of the VDU screen. It is suggested that the ideal situation for viewing the VDU screen is with the eyes depressed at an angle of 15–20° from the horizontal.

Older operators (over 50 years of age) may require an intermediate and a near prescription. This can be provided by bifocals, in which the upper part of the lens provides an intermediate prescription to focus the screen, and the lower segment contains a near prescription to focus the script if it is positioned nearer than the screen. However, if the screen and script are placed at the same distance then operators often cope well with an intermediate single-vision prescription.

Trifocal lenses can be used if clear distance vision is required. Particularly useful are trifocals with distance and intermediate executive lenses, with a D segment for the near prescription (e.g. SE 825, SE 1128).

The use of progressive lenses is controversial. Some authors consider them to be less suitable than bifocals, especially when a script to be copied is placed at the side of the VDU. They have a smaller reading area and can produce unwanted peripheral distortions. They also require considerable head movement for VDU work. When viewing the screen the operator usually looks through the intermediate zone of the lens, which is relatively narrow and set low, requiring the head to be tilted back. Whilst the width of the zone may be adequate for most visual needs of daily life, it is not entirely satisfactory for VDU work. Therefore, some reject progressive lenses because of the forced head posture, resultant neck cramp, and limitations of the intermediate and near portions' size upon vision. However, there are progressive lenses that have been designed specifically for VDU operators. These have larger intermediate areas, which are set higher than conventional progressive lenses. Lenses for VDU use include Technica (AO), Interview (Essilor), Zeiss Business 10 and 15, Zeiss Gradal RD, Sola Access and Cosmolit Office. Sanders (2000) gives a review of the characteristics of these lenses.

Hamard *et al.* (1987) studied emmetropic presbyopic VDU operators, who were given half-eye spectacles fitted with Varilux 2 lenses positioned so that the intermediate progression started at the upper edge of the frame. These were found to be particularly successful, allowing good horizontal and vertical scanning. Another study (Good and Daum, 1985) also investigated the use of half-eye spectacles fitted with progressive lenses. They recommended that emmetropes be fitted with progressive lenses incorporating a $+0.75\,\mathrm{D}$ addition to the distance power and with the near power appropriately reduced; this increases the intermediate and near focusing portions of the lens. After an initial adaptation period, most wearers reacted favourably to these lenses. A half-eye frame with a large vertical dimension is advised to allow full use of the near addition.

Contact lenses have an advantage over spectacles in that they give rise to fewer reflections and distortions. However, problems may occur due to the fact that concentration on the VDU (or any task for that matter) often results in a reduced blink rate, which

will cause symptoms resembling those of a 'dry eye'. The tear film can also be affected by high temperatures and low humidity, which may result in similar symptoms.

Several companies in the past have marketed VDU spectacles with tinted lenses. These lenses were designed to reduce asthenopia by reducing glare from overhead light sources, windows, or the VDU screen, and were reported to improve the contrast of the characters on the screen. Obstfeld and Thomson (1985) reviewed some of these tinted lenses introduced to reduce glare. They concluded that because VDUs do not emit much radiation in the UV or IR parts of the spectrum, tinted lenses that absorb these wavelengths will not be of much use. To reduce glare and hence enhance contrast, the spectral transmissions of the tinted lenses should be matched to the spectral emissions of the VDU screen phosphors. Figure 9.3 shows that the AO and Bolle Irex 90+ filters did not have transmission curves that match the commonly employed screen phosphors. The most likely effect of these filters was to diminish the contrast of the display.

Mousa (1986) studied the effects of tinted lenses (pink and UV-absorbing) on the spectral distribution from fluorescent lights. Results indicated that both lenses reduce the discomfort caused by stray light, but by different methods. The pink lenses reduce the overall illumination, which is suggested to be useful as most offices are over-illuminated for VDU operation, whilst the UV-absorbing lenses eliminate UV, which is scattered by the cornea and lens.

To conclude, it is generally agreed that it is best to try to control or eliminate the glare sources wherever possible before considering prescribing tinted VDU spectacles. The AOP state that tinted lenses would not normally be prescribed in spectacles specifically for VDU use, unless the tint is clinically necessary and also incorporated in the person's normal spectacles (AOP, 2000b). Some manufacturers do recommend anti-reflection coated lenses.

Personal factors

Factors such as general fatigue, ill health, the use of certain drugs and a tendency to migraine and photophobia are some of the physiological factors that may contribute to symptoms of eye strain. Psychological factors such as nervous or anxious personality, level of stress, motivation and interest in the work may

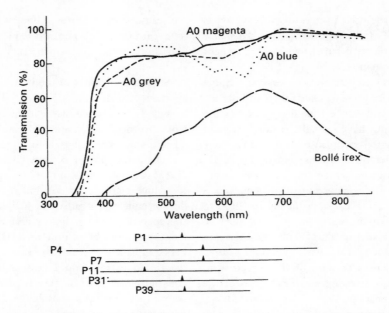

Fig. 9.3 *Spectral transmission curves of some VDU lenses. Phosphor colours: P1, P7, and P39, yellowish green; P4, white; P11, blue; and P31, green (reproduced by kind permission of Obstfeld and Thomson (1985) and* Optometry Today*).*

also be associated with eyestrain. Although these personal factors may increase the risk of asthenopic symptoms arising, the physical factors of the environment and task are generally the main cause.

Trainee VDU operators may well complain of asthenopia due to the high level of concentration and unfamiliar demands that are initially made upon the visual system. Once the operator has become acquainted with the VDU and its operation the symptoms will generally decrease, provided that the design, environment etc. of the VDU is correct.

It has been suggested that older VDU operators will complain more of asthenopia. The results of various studies are conflicting, some finding that the younger operators complain more of asthenopia (Starr *et al.*, 1982; Sauter, 1984), whilst others find the reverse or no difference (Rey and Meyer, 1980; Levy and Ramberg, 1987; Ong and Phoon, 1987). There are significantly more complaints regarding health and asthenopic symptoms from women operators (Knave *et al.*, 1985).

Several studies have investigated stress among VDU operators. Stress commonly arises when the person's perception of his or her own abilities are not matched by the job's demands. This is a frequent complaint reported by VDU operators, who perform repetitive, monotonous tasks. Data entry in particular seems to be responsible for many adverse health effects (Salvendy, 1982; Knave and Wideback, 1987; Levy and Ramberg, 1987). To minimize stress for the VDU operators, the task should therefore be designed to avoid or reduce repetitive elements by introducing variability in the workload, rather than long periods of concentrated work.

Workstation design

Factors to be considered in workstation design include lighting, glare, flicker, colour contrast, alpha–numeric design and ergonomics.

Lighting

The correct level of illumination is essential for a comfortable and efficient visual performance. Several investigators have suggested that illumination and its effects on the VDU are a possible cause of the high rate of asthenopic symptoms amongst the operators (Hultgren and Knave, 1974; Gunnarsson and Ostberg, 1977; Cakir *et al.*, 1980). A high level of illumination will improve the legibility of the script when there are dark characters on a light background, but the reverse occurs for a display with light

Table 9.2 Categories of downlighter luminaires for VDUs (from CIBSE 1989)

Category	VDU use	Luminance limitation angle (°)	Other uses
1	Intense	55	High density area of VDUs. Older types of VDUs. Highly specular surfaces
2	General	65	Positive contrast displays
3	Minimal	75	Low density area of VDUs. Positive contrast displays

The angles do not refer to cut-off angles but a sharp run back on the polar curve in all vertical planes. Above these angles the average luminance does not exceed 200 cd/m² (see Figure 9.4)

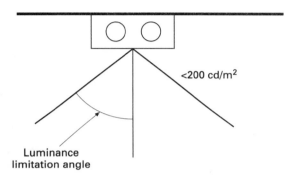

Fig. 9.4 *Downlight luminaires for VDUs. The angles do not refer to cut-off angles but a sharp run back on the polar curve in all vertical planes. Above these angles the average luminance does not exceed 200 cd/m².*

characters on a dark screen. Therefore, an optimum level of illumination is required to ensure that the legibility of the script and the screen characters are least impaired. The CIBSE Lighting Guide for visual display terminals (1989) recommends a background illuminance level of 300–500 lux. The lower end of the range should be used when the task is mainly screen-based, e.g. data retrieval, and the upper end of the range should be used when the task is mainly documentation-based, e.g. data entry.

Different illumination levels were assessed subjectively by VDU operators, and the majority found their task easiest at levels of around 300 lux (Varrall, 1983). Older VDU operators will require a higher level of illumination, which can be provided by local lighting, but it must be shielded from other operators, otherwise it will act as a glare source. In general, ambient lighting should provide about two-thirds of the required illuminance, and local lighting of the workstation should provide the rest.

The lighting needs to be designed to avoid direct and reflected glare, and this can be achieved by direct lighting from low-luminance downward-pointing luminaires, by indirect lighting from uplighters, or by a combination of the two systems.

The CIBSE (1989) guide defines three categories of luminaires for downlighters depending on the degree of VDU use; intense, general or minimal VDU. It is hoped that manufacturers will state the category into which their luminaires fall. Table 9.2 details the categories of downlighters, and Figure 9.4 illustrates the luminance limitation angle. The recommended room reflectances, with/without daylight, are: floor, 0.3/0.2; work surface, 0.4/0.3; walls, 0.5/0.5; and ceiling, 0.7/0.7.

When using uplighters, the ceiling is used as a large area of low luminance. This overcomes any problems of glare; any reflections from the VDU screen will be of low luminance. Uplighters can be free floor-standing, furniture-mounted, wall-mounted or suspended, and ideally they should be used where the ceiling height is at least 2.5 m. According to CIBSE (1989), the room reflectances, especially that of the ceiling, should be 0.8. The average luminance of the ceiling, or other major reflecting surfaces, should be less than 500 cd/m² and should not be greater than 15 000 cd/m² at any point. Various light sources are suitable for uplighters. The metal halide lamps and high-pressure sodium lamps can be used in all forms of uplighters; tubular and compact fluorescent lamps are large, and are therefore used in the furniture-mounted or suspended forms.

Glare

Glare, as already mentioned, is one of the main complaints made by VDU operators, and is caused by bright sources of light falling within the operator's field of vision. There are two types of glare; disability glare and discomfort glare. The former impairs the ability to see detail without necessarily causing visual discomfort, and the latter causes visual discomfort without impairing the ability to see detail. To avoid discomfort glare, a glare index of 19 is recommended for general office work (CIBSE, 1994). Values of this order or less can be achieved if the area is lit according to the recommendations in CIBSE (1989).

Glare may arise from direct light or indirectly from reflections. Direct glare is most frequently caused by the light from a window or an artificial light source that is too large or too bright. Other causes of glare are reflections from shiny, even surfaces such as gloss-painted walls, linoleum covered floor, polished wooden furniture, etc. Light may be reflected from the VDU itself, from the screen or the keyboard. Reflectances from the surface of the VDU screen can be very annoying. Screens are often slightly convex and act as a mirror, reflecting whatever is in front of the screen – e.g. the operator, or light sources.

Several methods of reducing or eliminating glare sources have been recommended (Birnbaum, 1978; CIBSE, 1989; Grundy *et al.*, 1991):

1. The position of the VDU screen should be adjusted so that the operator cannot see any reflections from the screen or other polished surfaces.
2. The position of troublesome light sources should be changed where possible.
3. Light sources should be fitted with the appropriate diffusers.
4. Fluorescent light fittings, if used, should be positioned with their length parallel to the side of the VDU.
5. The screen should be non-reflective and designed so that it can be tilted or rotated.
6. The keyboard should have a matt surround and the keys should have low reflectance surfaces.
7. Matt scripts should be used, preferably in pastel colours.
8. A light-coloured desk top should be used in preference to a dark one.
9. The VDU has contrast and brightness controls so that the legibility of the characters on the screen can be altered. The ratio of luminances between the workstation and the immediate surrounding should be within a range of 1–10 (CIBSE, 1989).
10. Windows should be fitted with blinds, e.g. vertical louvred blinds.

Several methods have been used to try and eliminate the screen reflections (Cakir *et al.*, 1980):

- Filter panels
- Polarization filters
- Micromesh filters
- Etching the glass screen
- Anti-reflection coats – vapour-deposited quarter-wavelength thin film
- Tube shields.

Each type of filter has advantages and disadvantages, which may vary depending upon the environment. Unfortunately, many of the techniques, whilst decreasing the amount of reflected light, also reduce the character brightness and resolution.

Cakir *et al.* (1980) have suggested that, in a normal office environment, filters can be ranked in decreasing order of effectiveness as: (i) anti-reflection coating; (ii) etching; (iii) polarization with additional anti-reflection layer; (iv) micromesh filters; and (v) polarization filter. The best method of providing an anti-reflection coating without losing the clarity of the characters is by the vacuum deposition of a thin film layer with a thickness of 0.25 of the wavelength of light. This technique is effective but expensive, as the coating is applied to a glass panel, which is then bonded to the screen surface. It is also very sensitive to dust and dirt, and shows up finger prints. Therefore, if the filter surface is not cleaned regularly the characters will appear to be smeared.

There is another glare filter, the Optique, which is very effective in reducing screen reflections. It consists of a curved sheet of tinted plastic mounted in a wide plastic housing. The housing reduces the viewing window, but it shields the screen from ambient light and acts as a light trap for specular reflections from the filter.

Flicker

A flickering image on a screen will diminish the legibility and can cause fatigue and asthenopia. The flicker on the VDU screen is dependent upon design characteristics of the display and personal factors. The design characteristics to be taken into account include the phosphor type, refresh rate, character size and colour, area of screen illuminated, and viewing angle.

The personal factors include the critical fusion frequency (CFF) and tolerance to a flickering display. The CFF is the lowest frequency at which a flickering stimulus is perceived as continuous. It varies between individuals, and is affected by such factors as pupil size, age and general health.

The characters on a VDU screen are generated by electrons. The screen is coated with phosphor, which, when bombarded with electrons, produces a spot of light. The intensity and position of the spot can be controlled so that characters can be formed. The rate at which the phosphorescent image decays (0.001–1 s) and the rate at which it is refreshed by the electronic pulse is very important. If the pulse refresh rate is slow (30–40 Hz) and the decay rate is fast due to a short duration phosphor, the normal saccadic and the minor oscillatory eye movements will interact with the intermittent image formation, causing different parts of the retina to be stimulated. This will result in the display appearing to 'jump' along the line in the case of saccadic eye movements and to 'dance' in the case of eye tremors (Birnbaum, 1978). Long persistence phosphors decrease the 'jump' and 'dance' of the display, but have a short life and produce 'smearing' of the characters. This smearing is caused by the persistent after-image when the character is changed. Research has suggested that refresh rates of up to 100 Hz may be needed to avoid flicker of some high luminance displays (Bauer *et al.*, 1983).

It has also been found that eye movements made in the direction of the field scan will cause a brief reduction in the refresh rate, which may result in bursts of flicker on an otherwise flicker-free screen (Thomson and Saunders, 1997). There are several methods available for calculating the refresh rate for a screen to appear flicker-free, which take into account such factors as the type of phosphor, luminance and size of the screen (ISO 9241). Using a simplified method, the International Standards Organization (ISO 9241) suggest that a 72-Hz display will appear flicker-free.

The use of dark characters on a light background (positive contrast or polarity) ensures good legibility, as reflections are less obvious and edges of the characters appear sharper. However, positive contrast tends to enhance the flicker effect and hence it is suggested that negative contrast displays should be used (Miller, 1984). These have another advantage in

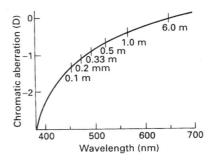

Fig. 9.5 *Axial chromatic aberrations of the eye (reproduced by kind permission of Sivak and Woo (1983): copyright, American Academy of Optometry).*

that the legibility is superior for people with low vision (CIBSE, 1989).

Colour contrast

Colour contrast is not essential in determining the legibility of a display; it is the overall contrast that is more important. The colour of the phosphors used for VDUs varies. Green phosphors are usually used for monochromatic displays, as they are most readily available. From surveys it appears that white, yellow or green on a neutral background are the preferred combinations, with green being favoured most of all. The preference for green phosphor is due to the relationship between accommodation and chromatic aberration. It has been shown that the wavelength in focus on the retina varies with the state of accommodation. When the eye is unaccommodated and fixating a distant target, a wavelength of about 650 nm is in focus (Millodot and Sivak, 1973). However, when the eye accommodates for targets at closer distances, the wavelength in focus gradually shifts towards the short wavelengths. At a distance of 0.5 m the wavelength in focus is about 520 nm, so green phosphors P1, P31 and P39 (max. 525–520 nm) would be most suitable (Figure 9.5). Blue phosphors, e.g. P11 (max. 460 nm) would induce a small amount of myopia if the operator accommodated by the amount normally appropriate for 0.5 m (Sivak and Woo, 1983).

Scrolling

It is possible to generate scrolling on a VDU screen so that the text moves rapidly up the screen. It has been suggested that increased rates of scrolling lead to poor performance and increased stress (Barfield, 1984).

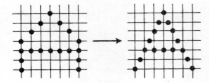

Fig. 9.6 *Character formation by dot matrices. The appearance can be enhanced by displacing some of the dots horizontally by a half dot separation.*

Alpha-numeric displays

The characters on the displays should be:

- Visible – characters should be readily detectable from the background
- Legible – it should be easy to identify each character
- Readable – spacing of characters, etc. should permit easy reading.

Careful consideration has to be given to the design of the various features of the characters and their arrangement. The following factors should be considered regarding the legibility of characters: character format and height, width to height ratio, stroke width to height ratio, and display luminance and contrast.

Character format

Each character is composed of a matrix of circular dots, and the greater the number of dots the better the quality of the character. Problems arise with a 5×7 (width to height) matrix, as it is difficult to distinguish between certain numerals and letters (e.g. U and V, S and 5) and therefore more operator errors are likely. For this reason the 7×9 matrix is most commonly used. The size of the dots is also important; if they are too small the character has a broken appearance, and if too large it is difficult to resolve. A technique for enhancing the characters and giving them a more rounded appearance is known as 'half-shift' (Figure 9.6), whereby some of the dots are moved in the horizontal plane by half a dot separation to the left or right (Reading, 1978).

BS EN 29241-3 (1993) provides the following recommendations regarding the character format. This standard has replaced BS 7179-3 (1990), which is now withdrawn, and is identical to ISO 9241-2 (1992).

1. A 7×9 matrix should be the minimum used for tasks requiring continuous reading for context, or in tasks such as proof reading, where legibility of each character is important.
2. A 5×7 matrix should be the minimum used for numeric and upper case only displays.
3. A 4×5 matrix should be the minimum used for superscripts and subscripts, and for numerators and denominators of fractions that are to be displayed in a single character position.

Character height

It is suggested that for most office tasks the viewing distance should be 40 cm or greater. The preferred character height for most tasks should be between 20 and 22 min of arc, with a minimum height of 16 min of arc.

Width to height ratio

The relationship between the width and height of a character is usually described as the width to height ratio. To provide maximum legibility and readability, a ratio of between 0.7 : 1 and 0.9 : 1 is advised. For other considerations, such as proportional spacing and line length, the ratio should be between 0.5 : 1 and 1 : 1.

Stroke width to height ratio

The stroke width is the width of the line forming the letter or symbol, and is usually expressed as the ratio of the thickness of the stroke to the height of the character. A stroke width of between 1/6 and 1/12 of the character height is advised. It is also suggested that wider strokes are preferred for dark characters on a white background (positive polarity). White characters on black (negative polarity) can have a thinner stroke width, as the white appears to spread to the adjacent black; the converse is not true.

The characters and lines should be well spaced for easy reading. The inter-character spacing must be such that an adequate number of characters can be viewed with a single fixation of the eye. It is suggests that:

- The between-character spacing should be a minimum of one stroke width or one pixel
- The between-word spacing should be a minimum of one character width
- The between-line spacing should be a minimum of one pixel.

Most VDUs have a line width of 80 characters, whereas a script has 60 characters per line. As the display should not cause unnecessary fatigue, over-crowding and cramming of letters within lines should be avoided. If the task involves continuous text, upper and lower case letters should be used (Reading, 1978).

Display luminance and contrast
The display should have a luminance of at least 35 cd/m^2, and the minimum luminance contrast of character details should be 3 : 1.

Ergonomics
To ensure that the design of the workstation is operational, the VDU operator should:

- Have easy access and egress
- Be able to reach and operate all controls with ease
- Be able to see and reach all the displays
- Be able to work comfortably.

The very common complaints of back- and neck-ache may be due to incorrect workstation design, perhaps due to chair position or the height/angle of the VDU being fixed without any method of adjustment/alteration.

The relationship between poor posture and asthenopia is controversial. Some argue that poor posture will cause fatigue of the neck and back, and hence lead to ocular fatigue/asthenopia. Others argue that visual difficulties lead to poor posture. Bergquist (1984) reviewed the literature on this subject, and concluded that musculoskeletal problems are not specific to VDU operators and are found in people doing other types of office work. However, the site of discomfort appears to be different. VDU operators appear to suffer more from discomfort in the neck, shoulders and upper arms, whilst non-VDU operators complain more of pain in the extremities. The occurrence of musculoskeletal pain is found more frequently in women, in people engaged in data entry, and after long periods of work.

Screen
BS EN 29241-3 (1993) suggests that screens should be viewed with the line of sight between the horizontal and 60° below. The screen should be at right angles to the line of sight, and it should be possible to rotate the screen laterally so that the operator is not disturbed by his or her own reflection. Ideally, the display should be legible from any direction of view up to at least 40° from the normal to the surface in any plane.

Keyboard
The keyboard height should be such that the operator's arms form angles of about 90° at the elbows and allow the wrists to be slightly flexed. The keyboard should be detachable, to allow the operator to find the best working position - for example, it should not be placed too far from the desk edge as this results in a cutting action by that edge on the wrists and forearms. Some operators may find a hand/wrist support useful. It should only be used intermittently while the hands are resting.

For tasks in which largely numeric data are being entered, an auxiliary numeric key set should be considered. The keyboard should have a slight slope and it should be as thin as possible. The keyboard should also have a matt surround and keys should have low reflectance surfaces (HSE, 1983; Miller, 1984).

Posture
The chair should have an adjustable seat height, adjustable backrest height and an adjustable tension on the backrest. According to ISO 9241-5 (1988), the seat height should be such that the operator's thighs are positioned in an approximately horizontal position with the lower legs vertical. The sole of the foot should make an angle of 90° with the lower leg. The angle between the upper and lower arms should also be at approximately 90°. Opearators should sit with a straight back and the line of sight in a relaxed seated position should be inclined by approximately 35° below the horizontal. Ideally, the optimum position for the most important part of the visual display should be 15° either side of the line of sight. There should also be an adequate knee clearance between the seat and the table. Figure 9.7 outlines some of the postural requirements for a VDU operator according to ISO 9241-5 (1998).

Work tables and desks
There should be sufficient space for documents, books and other ancillary equipment to be arranged as required. The work surfaces should also have a matt finish to prevent troublesome reflectances or glare. Document holders should be provided because they

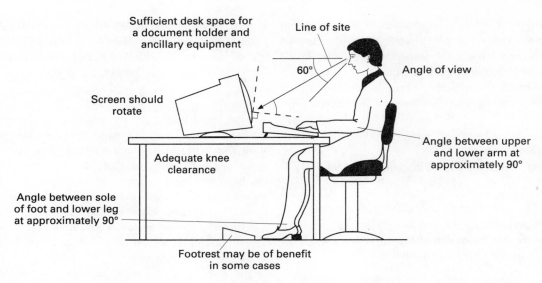

Fig. 9.7 *Some of the VDU workstation requirements according to ISO 9241 (1998).*

will prevent bending of the neck by the operator to read documents placed flat on the desk. The holders should be adjustable and can be placed next to the VDU screen at a similar angle, distance and height, to give visual comfort.

Environmental conditions

Office decor needs to be visually restful and glare-free. High reflectance walls, ceiling or floor surfaces may lead to glare, but low reflectance surfaces may create gloom. Therefore, large surface areas should be decorated in soft pastels or warm grey (i.e. have medium reflectance and low contrast). During extended periods of writing and reading, etc., unconscious involuntary relief for the eyes occurs by looking away from the task at distant objects. Paintings and foliage may be useful to provide visual relief.

Noisy equipment, such as printers, should be positioned away from the operator, or soundproofed.

VDUs and light sources inevitably produce heat, which, in warm weather or in confined spaces, can become a real problem if the ventilation system is inadequate. Many VDU operators complain of sore, dry eyes. This is generally due to a reduced blink rate, which occurs with intense concentration, and to the lack of humidity, which is quite prevalent in many offices, especially those with air conditioning. This is particularly problematical for contact lens wearers. Therefore, adequate ventilation and reasonable

humidity should be maintained to avoid such problems as drowsiness and dryness of the eyes. HSE (1983) and CIBSE (1989) also detail environmental conditions.

FACIAL RASH/DERMATITIS

There are several reports concerning facial rashes amongst VDU operators (Rycroft and Calnan, 1980; Tjonn, 1980). The complaints varied from itching of the skin to reddening with occasional minor desquamation and small papules. It usually occurs after a couple of hours at work and disappears a few hours after leaving work.

All VDUs generate a positively charged electrostatic field, which extends 2–3 m in front of the VDU. This field is generated by the interaction of the electron beam with the VDU screen, and attracts particles of smoke, pollen, dust etc. These particles are then drawn to the nearest negative charge, or ground, which may be the face or hands of the operator. Negatively charged particles will also be drawn to the screen, forming the commonly seen 'dusty' layer.

Various experiments have been carried out to prevent skin reactions amongst known cases. One method tried was to place a glass sheet between the operator and the screen. The results have been conflicting, with one case reporting the method to be successful whilst another found it of no use in preventing the facial rash. The most successful method appears to be the elimination of build-up of static electricity by replacing normal floor carpets with anti-static carpets and by the grounding of the display terminals (Cakir *et al.*, 1980; HSE, 1983). It is believed that the contact dermatitis is caused by irritating submicron dust particles precipitating on the skin of the VDU operator because they are accumulating static electricity. Manufacturers should try to design units so that the outside screen potential is as near to 0 V as possible. Periodic cleaning of the VDU screen with antistatic solution will control the dust accumulation, and maintaining a constant relative humidity of 50–70 per cent should also help (Canadian Occupational Environment Branch of the Ministry of Labour, 1983).

EPILEPSY

There has been concern in the past about people who suffer from epilepsy operating VDUs. In fact, VDU work does not cause epilepsy, and a person who suffers from this disorder should not be prevented from being a VDU operator (HSE, 1983). However, some people suffer from a relatively rare form of epilepsy, known as photosensitive epilepsy. In these people, a seizure may be triggered after stimulation by a flickering light source or after viewing striped patterns. The incidence of epilepsy in the population is estimated to be about 2 per cent, of whom approximately 4 per cent suffer from photosensitive epilepsy (Wilkins, 1978). Most people who are likely to suffer from an attack will have done so before the age of 20 years, and it will probably occur whilst watching television.

The possibility of a striped pattern triggering a seizure depends on various stimulus parameters, such as the area of the retina stimulated, the number of cycles of the pattern per degree (typically 1–4), luminance, and pattern stability (frequencies of 20 Hz should be avoided). Wilkins (1978) suggested that the epileptogenic factors of a television or VDU can be reduced by:

- Using a small screen to reduce the area of retina stimulated
- Using white alpha-numerics on a black background
- Limiting the amount of text on the screen
- Avoiding scrolling of the text

- Reducing the luminance of the display, either by the operator wearing tinted spectacles or by covering the screen with tinted perspex.

Despite this information, it is still difficult to give an accurate assessment of the risk of a photosensitive epileptic suffering a seizure when operating a VDU. Thus it would be wise for a known photosensitive epileptic to seek medical advice before using VDUs. In the UK, such advice can be given by the Employment Medical Advisory Service.

RADIATION

There has been a great deal of concern about dangerous radiation emissions from VDUs. According to Marriott and Stuchly (1986), radiation may be given off by:

- The screen (visible, UV and IR, depending on the phosphor)
- The cathode tube or electronic damper circuit (X-rays)
- The electronic components or circuit (microwave, UV, radiofrequency).

A number of surveys have been carried out to determine the levels of electromagnetic radiation emitted by the VDU (Weiss and Peterson, 1979; Cox, 1980; Terrana *et al.*, 1980; Elliot *et al.*, 1986). These surveys concluded that the measured values of electromagnetic radiation were at levels substantially below existing limits. The national and international limits for continuous exposure were not exceeded, and hence the radiation emitted from VDUs is not considered to be a health hazard. For reviews of these studies, see Cox (1983) and Rosner and Belkin (1989).

REGULATIONS REGARDING THE USE OF VISUAL DISPLAY UNITS

The EC has issued legislation regarding the minimum safety and health requirements for work with display screen equipment (EC Directive, 1990). Each member state can decide how the directive is implemented, and in the UK the Health and Safety (Display Screen Equipment) Regulations (1992) have been issued. A booklet, *Display Screen Equipment Work: Guidance on Regulations*, has been published by the Health and

Safety Executive, and this is exceedingly useful as it states the regulations and then gives further information and advice in relation to the specific requirements.

The legislation may be considered under six main headings:

1. Analysis of workstations
2. Workstation design
3. Daily work routines
4. Eyes and eyesight testing
5. Training
6. Health and safety information.

The Health and Safety (DSE) Regulations give definitions of 'display screen equipment', 'workstation' and 'user', which determine the application of the regulations. A 'user' is stated as being an employee who habitually uses display screen equipment (DSE) as a significant part of his or her normal work. The term 'operator' is used for self-employed workers. Display screen equipment covered by the regulations includes not only the conventional VDU, but also other displays such as the microfiche and liquid crystal; however, the regulations do not apply if the main use is for television or film display. There are exemptions to the regulations, such as DSE intended mainly for public use and those systems used in transport, cash registers and calculator displays.

The regulations apply to users whether they work at their own or other employer's workstations, or at a workstation at home. Employers have to decide which of their employees are 'users', and the guidelines and examples given will be of considerable help. Factors that should be taken into account are the dependence on the DSE, training required, time spent at DSE, intensity of use, and consequences of any errors. Examples of jobs are given, categorizing the workers as definite users and not users according to these factors.

Analysis of the workstations must be carried out by the employer to assess the risk to the health and safety of the user. The possible risks are listed in the Appendix of the regulations, and the main ones are considered to be musculoskeletal problems, visual fatigue and mental stress. Any potential risks that are identified have to be dealt with straight away. Records should be kept of workstation assessments and any alterations/modifications that are required.

In addition, the regulations detail employers' duties in the provision of health and safety training and

information to users of workstations. The employer must also organize the daily work routine so that users are not continually operating DSE but have periodic breaks.

The minimum requirements for the workstation are stated in the schedule of the regulations. It covers requirements for the DSE and the work environment, including details regarding the display screen, keyboard, the work surface, chair, lighting, glare, heating, humidity and noise. For example, the screen image must be stable and flicker-free, and reflections and glare should be avoided.

Of particular importance for optometrists is Regulation 5, which states that the employer must provide an appropriate eye and eyesight test to employees who are existing users or to those who are to become users. Further eye and eyesight tests should be provided at regular intervals, or if the user experiences visual problems which may be due to DSE work. The guidelines state that an 'eye and eyesight test' is a 'sight test' as defined by the Opticians Act. An employer may offer vision screening tests; however, if the employee requests a sight test this must be provided. There is no obligation for an employee to participate in any form of vision testing; it is entirely his or her choice.

The regulations also state that an employer must provide special corrective appliances for DSE work where a sight test has shown the need and where normal appliances cannot be used. For example, an intermediate prescription may be required for the screen to be seen clearly. It is estimated that only approximately 10 per cent of employees will require correction specifically for DSE use. The guidelines state that anti-glare screens and so-called VDU spectacles are not considered to be special corrective appliances.

The College of Optometrists (CO) (1993, 1994) and the Association of Optometrists (2000, see Appendix D) have each issued a statement of good practice for work with DSE. The guidelines to the DSE Regulations refer to the statement of the CO (1993). A report should be given to the employer, with a copy to the employee, stating whether or not a corrective appliance is required specifically for DSE work and when a retest is advised. The prescription for the corrective appliance can only be included in the report to the employer with the employee's permission. The College of Optometrists also states that clinical information should only be provided to an employer if it is relevant to the employee's DSE work, and then only with the employee's permission. The employer is responsible for the expenses incurred in the provision of eye and eyesight tests, and the provision of special corrective appliances if required. The guidelines state that the employer is liable for the costs of a basic appliance. If the employee wishes to have a more costly appliance, then the employer may contribute a portion of the total cost equivalent to the cost of the basic appliance.

SUMMARY

The use of VDUs can be of great benefit in the work situation, but the visual capabilities of the operator must be assessed and the workstation must be arranged in an appropriate manner to prevent the frequent complaints of asthenopia. Figure 9.8 gives a summary of some of the causes of asthenopia. If a VDU operator complains of asthenopia and requests an eye examination, then the following information will prove useful in ascertaining the cause (Grundy *et al.*, 1991):

- Date of last eye examination
- When VDU was work commenced
- How many hours per day the VDU is used
- Whether work breaks are provided, and their duration
- The character size and form (letters, numbers) on screen and documents
- The colour of characters and screen
- The distance of the screen, keyboard and documents

- The position of VDU screen (above or below eye level)
- The position of the document relative to the screen
- The type and colour of the background behind the screen
- Reflections or glare sources in view
- Whether the chair is adjustable.

Acknowledgement

Extracts from BS EN 29241-3 (1993) are reproduced with the permission of the BSI under licence number 2000SK/0408. British Standards can be obtained by post from BSI Customer Services, 389 Chiswick High Rd, London W4 4AL.

REFERENCES

Association of Optometrists (2000a) Guidance on visual standards for VDU/DSE users. *AOP Members Handbook C. AOP*, p. 4.

Association of Optometrists (2000b) Display screen equipment. *AOP Members Handbook C. AOP*, pp. 7–9.

Barfield W. (1984) Stress as a function of increased cognitive load at a VDT. In *Ergonomics and Health in Modern Offices, Proceedings of the International Conference, Turin, 7–November, 1983* (ed. Grandjean, E.). Taylor and Francis Ltd, London, pp. 181–186.

Bauer D., Bonacker M. and Cavonius C.R. (1983) Frame repetition rate for flicker-free viewing of bright VDU screens. *Displays*, **January**, 31–32.

Bedwell C.H. (1978) Assessment of eye strain and difficulty in viewing visual display units. Edited transcript of the one-day meeting on eyestrain and VDUs. The Ergonomics Society, Loughborough, p. 215.

Bergquist U.O.V. (1984) VDTS and health: a technical and medical appraisal of the state of art. *Scand J Work Environ Health*, **10**(Suppl. 2), 1–87.

Birnbaum R. (1978) *Health Hazards of Visual Display Units with Particular Reference to the Office Environment*. Review prepared for the Information and Advisory Service, TUC Centenary Institute of Occupational Health, London School of Hygiene and Tropical Medicine, London.

BS EN 29241-2 (1993) Ergonomic requirements for office work with visual display terminals (VDTs) – Part 2: Guidance on task requirements. BSI, London.

BS EN 29241-3 (1993) Ergonomic requirements for office work with visual display terminals (VDTs) – Part 3: Visual display requirements. BSI, London.

Cakir A., Hart D.J. and Stewart T.F.M. (1980) *Visual Display Terminals*. John Wiley and Sons, Chichester.

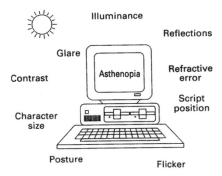

Fig. 9.8 *Summary of some of the causes of asthenopia.*

Canadian Occupational Environmental Branch of the Ministry of Labour (1983) Working with visual display terminals. *Can J Optom*, **45**, 134–140.

Chakman J. and Guest D.J. (1983) Vision and the visual display unit. A review. *Aust J Optom*, **66(4)**, 125–137.

CIBSE (1994) *Code for Interior Lighting*. Chartered Institution for Building Service Engineers, London.

CIBSE (1989) *Lighting Guide (LG3): Areas for Visual Display Terminals*. Chartered Institution for Building Service Engineers, London.

Cole B.L., Sharpe K., Slack A. and Maddocks J.D. (1989) The Sec-VDU Study. Comparison of refractive error and visual acuity of VDU users and non-VDU users. *Bulletin No. 3*, Victorian College of Optometry, University of Melbourne, Australia.

Cole B.L., Maddocks J.D. and Sharpe K. (1996) Effects of VDUs on the eyes – report of a six-year epidemiological study. *Optom Vis Sci*, **73**, 512–528.

College of Optometrists (1993) *Work with Display Screen Equipment. Statement of Good Practice*. College of Optometrists, London.

College of Optometrists (1994) *Work with Display Screen Equipment. Ethical Implications of Vision Screening by Optometrists*. College of Optometrists, London.

Cox E.A. (1980) Radiation emissions from visual display units. *Proceedings of the Conference on Health Hazards of VDUs*. Loughborough University, Loughborough, p. 27.

Cox E.A. (1983). Electromagnetic radiation emissions from visual display units: a review. *Display Tech Appl*, **4**, 7–10.

Dain S.J., McCarthy A.K. and Chan-Ling T. (1988) Symptoms in VDU operators. *Am J Optom Physiol Opt*, **65**, 162–167.

Dainoff M.J., Happ A. and Crane P. (1981) Visual fatigue and occupational stress in VDT operators. *Human Factors*, **23**, 421–438.

De Groot J.P. and Kamphuis A. (1983) Eye strain in VDU users: physical correlates and long-term effects. *Human Factors*, **25**, 409–413.

EC Directive (1990) Directive 90/270/EEC: the minimum safety and health requirements for work with display screen equipment. *Official J Eur. Comm.*, **L156**, 14–18.

Elliot G., Gies P., Joyner K.H. and Roy C.R. (1986) Electromagnetic radiation emissions from video display terminals (VDTs). *Clin Exper Optom*, **69(2)**, 53–61.

Fincham E.F. (1951) The accommodation reflex and its stimulus. *Br J Ophthalmol*, **35**, 381–393.

Good G.W. and Daum K.M. (1985) *The Use of Progressive Multifocals with Video Display Terminals*. Ohio State University College of Optometry, Ohio.

Grundy J.W. and Rosenthal S.G. (1982) VDUs on site. *Ophthal Optician*, **July 17**, 500.

Grundy J.W., Rosenthal S.G. and Seymour H. (1991) *Visual Aspects of VDU Usage*. Association of Optometrists, 233–4 Blackfriars Road, London SE1 8NW.

Gunnarsson E. and Ostberg O. (1977): *The Physical and Psychological Working Environment in a Terminal-based Computer Storage and Retrieval System*. National Board of Occupational Safety and Health, Stockholm, Sweden.

Gunnarsson E. and Soderberg I. (1980). *Eye Strain resulting from VDT Work at the Swedish Telecommunication Administration*. Stockholm National Board of Occupational Safety and Health, Stockholm, Sweden.

Gur S. and Ron S. (1992) Does work with visual-display units impair visual activities after work? *Doc Ophthamol*, **79**, 253–259.

Hamard H., Chevaleraud J.P., Trubert E. and Meillon J.P. (1987) Presbyopic correction by use of progressive half spectacles among users of video terminals. *J Fr Ophthal*, **10**, 505–513.

Holler H., Kundi M., Schmid H., Still H.G., Thaler A. and Winter N. (1975) Arbeitsbeansprachung und Augenbelastung an Bildschirmgetaten Wein: Verlag des OGB. Cited by Mah L.J. (1983) Aspects of visual stress in visual display terminal work. *Can J Optom*, **45**, 124–127.

HSE (1983) *Visual Display Units*. Health and Safety Executive, HMSO, London.

HSE (1992) Health and Safety (Display Screen Equipment) Regulations (1992). No. 2792. HMSO, London.

Hultgren G.V. and Knave B. (1974) Discomfort glare and disturbances from light reflections in an office landscape with CRT display terminals. *Appl Ergonom*, **5**, 2–8.

ISO 9241-5 (1998) Ergonomic requirements for office work with visual display terminals (VDTs) - Part 5 Workstation layout and postural requirements.

Knave B.G. and Wideback P.G. (1987) *Work with Display Units. 86. Selected Papers from the International Scientific Conference on Work with Display Units*. Stockholm, May 12–15, 1986. Elsevier Science Publishers, Amsterdam.

Knave B.G., Wibom R.I., Hedstrom L.D. and Bergquist U.O.V. (1985) Work with video display terminals among office employees. 1. Subjective symptoms and discomfort. *Scand J Work Environ Health*, **11**, 457–466.

Laubli T.H., Hunting W. and Grandjean E. (1980) Visual impairments in VDU operators related to environmental conditions. In *Ergonomic Aspects of Display Terminals* (eds Grandjean E. and Vigliani E.).Taylor and Francis Ltd, London, pp. 85–94.

Levy F. and Ramberg I.G. (1987) Eye fatigue among VDU users and non-VDU users. In *Work with Display Units. 86. Selected Papers from the International Scientific Conference on Work with Display Units*, Stockholm, May 12–15, 1986 (eds Knave B.G. and Wideback P.G.). Elsevier Science Publishers, Amsterdam, pp. 42–52.

Marriott I.A. and Stuchly M.A. (1986) Health aspects of work with visual display terminals. *J Occup Med*, **28**, 833–848.

Miller S.C. (1984) Meeting the eye care needs of video display terminal operators. *J Am Optom Assoc*, **55**, 611–618.

Millodot M. and Sivak J. (1973) Influence of accommodation on the chromatic aberration of the eye. *Br J Physiol Opt*, **28**, 169–174.

Mousa G.Y. (1986) Control of glare for VDT operators. 1. Transmission of fluorescent light through UV filters and pink lenses. *Can J Optom*, **48**, 47–49.

Murch G. (1982) How visible is your display? *Electro-Optical Sys Des*, **14**, 43–49.

Mutti D.O. and Zadnik K. (1996) Is computer use a risk factor for myopia? *J Am Optom Assoc*, **67**, 521–530.

Obstfeld H. and Thomson D. (1985) Visual display units, visual discomfort and VDU spectacles. *Optom Today*, **25**, 732–733.

Ong C.N. and Phoon W.O. (1987) Influence of age on performance and health of VDU workers. In *Work with Display Units. 86. Selected Papers from the International Scientific Conference on Work with Display Units*, Stockholm, May 12–15, 1986 (eds Knave B.G. and Wideback P.G.). Elsevier Science Publishers, Amsterdam, pp. 211–216.

Osterberg O. (1980) Accommodation and visual fatigue in display work. In *Ergonomic Aspects of Visual Display Terminals* (eds Grandjean E. and Vigliani E). Taylor and Francis Ltd, London, pp. 41–52.

Phillips S. and Stark L. (1977) Blur: a sufficient accommodative stimulus. *Documenta Ophthal*, **3**, 65–89.

Reading V. (1978) *Visual Aspects and Ergonomics of Visual Display Units*. Institute of Ophthalmology, London.

Rey P. and Meyer J.J. (1980) Visual impairments and their objective correlates. In *Ergonomic Aspects of Display Terminals* (eds Grandjean E. and Vigliani E.). Taylor and Francis Ltd, London, pp. 77–83.

Rosner M. and Belkin M. (1989) Video display units and visual function. *Surv Ophthal*, **33**, 515–522.

Rupp B.A., McVey B.W. and Taylor S.E. (1984) Image quality and the accommodative response. In *Ergonomics and Health in Modern Offices*, Proceedings of the International Scientific Conference, Turin, November 7–9, 1983. (ed. Grandjean E.). Taylor and Francis Ltd, London, pp. 254–259.

Rycroft R.J.G. and Calnan C.D. (1980) Facial rashes among VDU operators. *Proceedings of the Conference on the Health Hazards of VDUs 1*, Loughborough University, Loughborough, p. 15.

Salvendy G. (1982) Human computer communication with special reference to technology developments, occupational stress and educational needs. *Ergonomics*, **25**, 435–447.

Sanders P. (2000) Lenses for VDU use. *Optician*, **5741(219)**, 16–17.

Sauter S.L. (1984) Predictors of strain in VDT users and traditional office workers. In *Ergonomics and Health in Modern Offices*, Proceedings of the International Scientific Conference, Turin, November 7–9, 1983 (ed. Grandjean E.). Taylor and Francis Ltd, London, pp. 129–135.

Sivak J.G. and Woo G.C. (1983) Colour of visual display terminals and the eye. Green VDTs provide optimal stimulus to accommodation. *Am J Optom Physiol Opt*, **60(7)**, 640–641.

Starr S.J., Thompson C.R. and Shute S.J. (1982) Effects of video display terminals on telephone operators. *Human Factors*, **24**, 699–711.

Taylor S.P. and Yeow P.T. (1990) Visual display units – friend or foe? *Optician*, **5234**, 18–22; **5237**, 19–23; **5241**, 15–9.

Terrana T., Merluzzi F. and Giudici E. (1980) Electronic radiations emitted by visual display units. In *Ergonomic Aspects of Display Terminals* (eds Grandjean E. and Vigliani E.). Taylor and Francis Ltd, London, pp. 13–21.

Thomson D. (1998) The computerised office. Part 2 – the eye examination for VDU users. *Optician*, **5652(215)**, 28–31.

Thomson W.D. (1994) The City University Vision Screener for VDU users. *Br J Optom Disp*, **2(2)**, 61–74.

Thomson W.D. and Saunders J. (1997) The perception of flicker on faster-scanned displays. *Human Factors*, **39**, 48–66.

Tjonn H.H. (1980) Report on facial rashes among operators in Norway. *Proceedings of the Conference on Health Hazards of VDUs*. Loughborough University, Loughborough, p. 19–23.

Varrall G. (1983) The visual environment and new office technology. *Ophthal Optician*, **June 4**, 401–404.

Weiss M.M. and Peterson R.C. (1979) Electromagnetic radiation emitted from video computer terminals. *Am Ind Hygiene Assoc J*, **40**, 300–309.

Wilkins A. (1978) Epileptogenic attributes of TV and VDUs. Edited transcript of the one-day meeting on eyestrain and VDUs. The Ergonomics Society, Loughborough, pp. 27–35.

Yekta A.A., Jenkins T. and Pickwell D. (1987) The clinical assessment of binocular vision before and after a working day. *Ophthal Physiol Opt*, **7**, 349–352.

Yeow P.T. (1988) The effects of short-term and long-term VDU usage on visual functions and visual fatigue. PhD thesis, University of Wales.

Yeow P.T. and Taylor S.P. (1989) Effects of short-term VDT usage on visual functions. *Optom Vis Sci*, **66**, 459–466.

FURTHER READING

Cakir A., Hart D.J. and Stewart T.F.M. (1980) *Visual Display Terminals*. John Wiley and Sons, Chichester.

Grandjean E. (ed.) (1984) *Ergonomics and Health in Modern Offices*. Taylor and Francis Ltd, London, UK.

Grundy J.W., Rosenthal J.G. and Seymour H. (1991) *Visual Aspects of VDU Usage*. The Association of Optometrists, 61 Southwark Street, London SE1 0HL.

Pearce B.G. (ed.) (1984) *Health Hazards of VDTs?* John Wiley and Sons, Chichester.

Stewart T.F.M. (1980) Problems caused by continuous use of visual display units. *Ltg Res Tech*, **12**, 26–35.

10 Driving

Vision is the one human sense that is absolutely essential for safe driving. Although other senses relay important information to a driver, so that the appreciation of a situation is much improved, it is estimated that up to 90 per cent of the information received is visual. Clearly a blind person cannot be permitted to drive. However, as a person's vision can vary from blindness to 6/5, there must be a minimum standard below which it is inadvisable for anyone to drive.

There has been a marked increase in the volume of traffic on the roads in recent years but, despite the increasing demands made on the driver of today, the visual standards required in the UK have remained virtually unchanged since they first came into operation in 1935. It may well be that those standards are now inappropriate.

Surprisingly, there is very little evidence that relates the standard of vision to a driver's performance, and hence it is not easy to determine the minimum level of vision for safe driving. This situation also exists in other countries, as visual standards have never been internationally agreed. There are very obvious differences in the testing procedures and standards required by different countries. One of the simpler vision tests is used in the UK, involving only the reading of a number plate at a prescribed distance. In other countries more rigorous examinations are used to assess visual functions, such as measurements of visual field, dark adaptation, stereopsis and glare recovery.

Drivers need to cope with a wide range of confusing visual situations. For example, conditions when visibility is poor due to rain, mist or fog demand a good standard of vision for safe driving.

Some studies have failed to relate poor vision to accident rate. This may be due to the fact that accidents do not generally have one single cause but often result from a combination of events. There are believed to be over 1000 independent factors affecting driver behaviour, which relate to the road conditions, the vehicle and the driver. It is well understood that vision, fatigue, alcohol, vehicle visibility, road lighting, motor co-ordination, accident proneness and attention affect a driver's behaviour. Fortunately, there is a certain amount of self-selection, and some people give up driving when their vision deteriorates to a level they consider unsafe. This is particularly evident amongst the elderly, who 'do not like to drive at night' as they have reduced dark adaptation, and often restrict their driving to the daylight hours.

The Transport and Road Research Laboratory (1980) carried out a large study to identify the important factors that provoked accidents. They visited the site where the accident happened as soon as possible after the event and interviewed the driver at a later date (Staughton and Stone, 1977). This 'on the spot' study investigated a total of 2036 accidents. The results of the study showed that road user error was responsible for 95 per cent of the accidents, and 44 per cent of the drivers at fault were judged to have made perceptual errors. The vehicle and road/environment were responsible for only 9 and 28 per cent of accidents, respectively. The perceptual errors made were mainly due to distraction and misjudgement of speed and distance. The latter is often due to a lack of visual adaptation to speed. After driving at 70 mph, 30 mph seems very slow; however, travelling at 30 mph after being in a slow-moving traffic jam seems relatively fast. The visual adaptation is believed to occur due to the streaming of the visual field across the periphery of the retina. A method of reducing accidents at roundabouts, where many accidents are due to drivers entering too fast, is to paint transverse bars across the road with decreasing separation. The lines are intended to create the illusion of speeding up if the driver continues to drive over them at a constant speed, and hence the driver will slow down. They also act as a visual hazard warning. These transverse bars have reduced accidents due to cars entering a roundabout too fast by about 60 per cent at 50 trial sites (Hills, 1980).

RELATIONSHIP BETWEEN VISUAL FUNCTIONS AND DRIVING PERFORMANCE

Many studies have been carried out to try and relate visual abilities with driving performance (Burg, 1967, 1968; Keeney, 1968; Cashell, 1970; Liesmaa, 1973; Council and Allen, 1974; Hofstetter, 1976; Hills and Burg, 1977).

Static visual acuity

Good central visual acuity, and its associated clear retinal image, is necessary for the early recognition and reading of road signs. It also aids the early detection of small or hazardous objects, such as pedestrians, motorcycles, and other obstacles in the roadway. Good acuity allows the driver more time to make decisions about events, obstacles and signs, and in effect slows down the action. A driver with poor acuity requires the obstacle to be closer before its significance can be appreciated, leaving less time to react. He or she must be more alert, and will therefore fatigue faster and become more easily perceptually overloaded. For example, Allen (1969) states that someone with 6/6 vision driving at 60 mph has 3.9 s to read a road sign of 15-cm high (6-inch) letters; when the visual acuity is reduced to 6/12 there are only 1.95 s for this sign to be seen. This is reduced even further, to 0.78 s, when the acuity is 6/60.

Burg (1967, 1968) carried out one of the largest studies investigating the relationship between visual functions and driving ability. He assessed over 17 500 Californian drivers, and compared their visual ability with their 3-year accident record. This study showed a weak but statistically significant correlation between the vision scores and the driver accident rate. In 1977 this information was reanalysed with a view to establishing a new set of driver vision standards (Hills and Burg, 1977). The sample, of well over 14 000 drivers, was subdivided into four age groups: under 25 years; 25–39 years; 40–54 years; and over 54 years. It was found that static and dynamic visual acuity were the most important factors in the over 54-year-old age group, where there was a clear relationship between these factors and the accident rate.

However, the Road Research Laboratory (1963) analysed the results of four separate studies on drivers' vision and, surprisingly, concluded that the visual acuity has a relatively small, almost insignificant, correlation with accidents.

Liesmaa (1973) found a positive relationship between poor visual acuity and poor driving ability. He observed drivers' behaviour whilst overtaking or entering a major road, from an unmarked police car. Drivers considered to be dangerous were stopped and their monocular and binocular visual acuities were measured. The results obtained were then compared with a control group. In the group of people who were driving dangerously there were three times as many drivers who were monocular or who had visual acuities below the required level as there were in the control group.

Hofstetter (1976) analysed the number of accidents and the visual acuities of 13 786 drivers. He found that, amongst those drivers who had been involved in three or more accidents, twice as many had poor acuity. The proportion who had been in two accidents was about 50 per cent greater amongst the drivers with poor acuity. From this study it was not possible to determine a precise level of acuity at which a person could be considered safe to drive.

A report from Germany concluded that accidents did occur more frequently amongst drivers with considerably reduced photopic (daylight) vision ($< 6/9 +$ in one or both eyes) than in those with adequate or slightly reduced vision (Hebenstreit, 1984).

Several summaries of papers relating to visual ability and driving performance have been compiled, and they have all come to the same conclusion; in general, there is only a weak statistical association between static visual acuity and poor driving ability (Levitt, 1975; Davison, 1978; Hedin, 1980).

Dynamic visual acuity

The strongest and most consistent relationship between the visual functions and the driving performance was found to be dynamic visual acuity (Burg, 1967, 1968). This positive correlation indicates that good co-ordination and freedom from confusion and dizziness are very important when driving. Medical conditions that interfere with the vestibular mechanisms, such as Meniere's disease, or where there is a limitation of head movement, such as in arthritis, can affect the dynamic visual acuity. A reduction of dynamic visual acuity will also occur if the static visual acuity is defective. Burg's data (1967, 1968) were reanalysed by Hills and Burg (1977), who found that only the older age group (over 54 years) showed a consistent relationship between dynamic visual acuity and accident rate.

Colour vision

Various studies have been carried out to determine the relationship between the accident rate and colour vision defects. Norman (1960) studied a number of London bus drivers, but did not find a higher accident rate or traffic violation rate in 149 colour defective drivers than in the control group of 149 drivers with normal colour vision.

Colour vision defects may be hazardous if they cause confusion between the red, green and amber signal lights. According to Coles and Brown (1966), a protanope (red colour-blind) requires about four times the normal intensity to see a red light. People with red colour vision defects may also find it difficult when driving in fog or at night, as they are unable fully to appreciate a red tail/brake light. It would be advisable for them not to wear tinted spectacles when driving, as they reduce/modify the mount of light reaching the eyes.

Peripheral visual fields

With such a high volume of traffic on the roads today, good peripheral vision is essential. A restriction of the visual field can never be fully overcome, although increasing head and eye movements and adding extra mirrors to the car can be of help. The visual field is important for maintaining the driver's orientation and in establishing relationships between the many objects in the field of view. Central vision, important as it is, can only fixate the pavement once every 7 m (22 ft) at 95 km/h (60 mph). The remaining portions of the roadway between and to the left and right of the fixations must be taken in by peripheral vision (Allen, 1969).

There have been varied reports concerning the relationship between visual field defects and accident rate. North (1985) reviewed the studies, and the following reports are a few of those that showed a positive correlation:

- Johnson and Keltner (1983) screened 10 000 drivers and compared their driving record over the previous 3 years with their visual field. They found that drivers with binocular visual field loss had accident and conviction rates that were twice as high as those of a control group.

- Kite and King (1961) found that a gross reduction of the visual field on one side, or monocularity, is associated with seven-fold increases in crashes at road intersections and pedestrian injuries.
- Keeney (1968) noted that monocular drivers were four times more likely to be found in a group cited for multiple driving violations (80 out of 991) than in an ophthalmic practice patient population (424 of 21 000).

It would appear from the above research that visual field defects are related to accidents. Keeney (1968) suggests that a visual field of 140° is advisable for driving and defensible in court as a minimum standard. This standard can be met by a monocular person, but it is important to note that a driver who becomes monocular (perhaps due to an eye injury) should be allowed time to adapt to the loss of visual field, the reduced depth perception and the effect of the blind spot (which produces an absolute scotoma within the visual field). In Sweden, a driver is banned for 1 year after the loss of vision in one eye.

No evidence was found by Hills and Burg (1977), or by Council and Allen (1974), to support the 140° visual standard proposed by Keeney (1968). Council and Allen (1974) studied the driving performance and visual fields of 52 000 North Carolina drivers and concluded that, overall, the 2-year accident records of drivers with limited visual fields (< 140°) were no different from those of drivers with normal visual fields (> 160°). They did find that restricted visual fields may be slightly related to a higher proportion of side collisions, but overall these drivers had no higher accident rate.

A study by Wood and Troutbeck (1992) investigated the effect of simulated visual field defects on the driving performance of a group of young normal drivers. Constriction of the binocular field of vision to 40° or less significantly affected many aspects of driving performance; it increased the time taken to complete the driving course, and reduced the ability to detect and correctly identify road signs, avoid obstacles and manoeuvre through limited spaces. However, speed estimation and stopping distance were not affected. Interestingly the monocular condition did not significantly affect performance for any of the driving tasks assessed.

Visual fields can be artificially reduced by, for example, aphakic spectacle corrections, thick spectacle frames and sides, and car design. There are obvious pathological disorders that can also cause visual defects, such as glaucoma, retinitis pigmentosa and cataracts. Elkington and MacKean (1982) studied 214 patients suffering from open-angle glaucoma. They found that many of them experienced difficulty when driving and, in six cases, glaucoma was diagnosed as a result of the patient becoming aware of a visual field defect whilst driving. Of the patients who were still driving (61 out of the 214), only five were aware of their visual field defect and made allowances for it by head movements. This report was concluded by raising the question as to the duty of medical practitioners to advise their patients when they are considered to be unsafe to drive due to their visual field loss.

Stereopsis and oculomotor balance

Stereoscopic vision is the ability to appreciate depth by the superimposition of two slightly dissimilar objects. The position of objects can be located with one eye by monocular cues such as relative size, position relative to the horizontal, contrast, movement, brightness etc. Unfortunately, under conditions of poor visibility (e.g. at night) the majority of the monocular cues are missing, and stereopsis becomes the major cue in depth perception. Stereopsis is inoperative beyond 500 m and is therefore of little benefit in high speed driving, although it is valuable for nearer tasks such as parking a car or locating children around cars, buses etc. (Allen, 1969).

It seems that stereopsis is not related to safe driving, as no correlation has been found between defective stereoscopic vision and increased accident frequency (Burg, 1968). Keeney (1968) states that stereoscopic vision is not important for the distances found in traffic.

The absence of stereopsis can be due to a squint. The presence of a squint without double vision is no obstacle to driving because the peripheral visual field is normal. However, the presence of double vision does constitute an obstacle to driving.

A horizontal phoria, although known to be enhanced by fatigue, low illumination and alcohol, has not been shown to correlate with crash rate (Burg, 1967). However, a vertical phoria of greater than 1 prism dioptre was found to be associated with poor accident records, especially in the over-55 years age group (Davison, 1985).

Night vision

It is often found that the accident rate relative to distance travelled during the hours of darkness is greater than the rate during the hours of daylight. Accidents occurring at night are also more likely to result in fatalities or severe injuries, and the majority of accidents to pedestrians occur at night. The increase of potential accidents during the hours of darkness is partly due to poor street lighting and to the glare from oncoming headlights reducing visibility.

Studies by Allen (1969) have shown that night vision performance, measured by the ability to detect objects at night in a laboratory and a field situation, can be severely handicapped by a refractive error. A driver with 6/12 daytime acuity was found to require 5–100 times more illumination to detect a given target than he would have required if his daytime acuity was 6/6. This means that 6/12 acuity by day cuts the critical perception distance by half compared with 6/6, and at night it may cut it to one-tenth or less. Therefore, Allen suggests that drivers with a daytime visual acuity of 6/12 should not be permitted to drive at night at all.

According to Hedin (1980), static visual acuity or contrast sensitivity testing under night driving conditions is urgently needed. Hedin also suggests alterations to the regulations to allow the issue of a driver's licence valid only during daylight hours if deemed necessary.

Night myopia

A phenomenon known as night myopia may also influence night driving. People become relatively more short-sighted at night, and this myopic shift can be as much as 4 D (Leibowitz and Owens, 1978), although it varies from person to person and with the level of lighting. There may be quite marked short-term variations, and the dark focus can also be affected by non-visual factors such as psychological stress (Hope and Rubin, 1984). Hence there are problems in prescribing spectacles for night driving. Several refractions on different days may be required to determine the representative dark focus to take into account patient variability, and the prescription found will be appropriate only for a limited set of conditions.

The Association of Optometrists (AOP, 1990) has made a statement regarding night myopia and prescribing a correction. It suggests that the variable nature of the myopia induced at low levels of illumination creates a major problem in prescribing a correction. When driving at night there is never total darkness, as there is light from car headlights, street lamps etc. Under conditions of low illumination (mesopic level) the degree of myopia induced will be reduced and, as stated, it will vary according to the lighting level so that a single prescription will not be suitable. Also, if a correction is provided there may be problems for the driver when travelling into a well-lit area. The extra negative power of the correction may then become a hazard because it may induce confusion and misjudgement of distances, speeds, etc. The difficulties encountered by a driver at night are not just due to myopia; there are other factors, such as increased reaction time and increased glare recovery time. Therefore, the provision of a correction is not a simple answer to the difficulties experienced by many when driving at night.

Another possible reason for the high rate of road traffic accidents at night is that drivers appear to be less cautious. This was demonstrated when drivers were observed turning onto the main road at a T-junction. In the daylight most drivers waited for gaps of 6.5–7.5 s before pulling out, whereas at night they pulled out after gaps of only 3.5–5.5 s. Drivers therefore incurred a much higher risk of being involved in a collision. It is believed that there is a 40 per cent greater chance of collision on a busy T-junction at night because of the willingness of emerging vehicles to go for shorter gaps, and it is 12 times more likely that the collision will be serious (Transport and Road Research Laboratory, 1980).

Glare

Many drivers complain about glare during night driving. This is due mainly to dirt and scratches on the windscreen causing scattering of light. Smoke from cigarettes can cause an increase in glare from oncoming headlights at night, and will cause veiling glare during the day. Allen (1969) estimates that windscreens should be replaced every 50 000 miles due to wear and tear. Tinted windscreens and the use of tinted

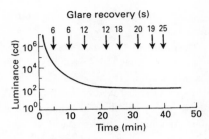

Fig. 10.1 *The influence of dark adaptation upon glare recovery. The curve represents the normal course of dark adaptation. It can be seen that the glare recovery time after dazzle, i.e. the time for readaptation, increases with duration of dark adaptation (after Papst, 1962, courtesy of the* New Scientist*).*

spectacles are detrimental to the following visual functions, which are important for night driving:

- Glare recovery, i.e. the speed of retinal recovery after being dazzled by glare
- Glare resistance, i.e. the ability to see against glare
- Visual acuity, i.e. the ability to see efficiently in low illumination.

Glare recovery

The recovery time of retinal sensitivity not only increases with age but also with the use of tinted spectacles or windscreens, and with the level of dark adaptation. Many elderly patients wear tinted spectacles to reduce the amount of light entering the eye, and thereby reduce the light scattering. Research shows that it takes longer to recover from glare when using tints. Although drivers feel more comfortable visually, tinted lenses do not improve performance. Phillips and Rutstein (1965) found that glare recovery increased by an average of 54 per cent, from 2.03 s to 3.02 s, with tinted spectacles. The colour of the tint is irrelevant, as the increase in retinal sensitivity depends upon the absorption of the lenses.

Tinted lenses increase the time required for dark adaptation (Davey and Sheridan, 1953; McFarland *et al.*, 1960; Wolf *et al.*, 1960). The time for readaptation also increases with increasing dark adaptation. For example, the recovery from glare took 6 and 25 seconds after 5 and 38 minutes of dark adaptation, respectively (Papst, 1962; Figure 10.1).

Glare resistance

This is the ability to see against glare. Visual recovery time during glare increases by about 25 per cent when wearing tinted spectacles (Davey, 1959; Phillips and Rutstein, 1967).

Visual acuity

Tinted spectacles reduce the visual acuity during day and night driving conditions (Richards, 1953; Wolf *et al.*, 1960). Visual acuity is found to decrease in proportion to the reduction in transmission of light, and is not affected by the colour of the tint (Sturgis and Osgood, 1982).

Yellow night-driving glasses are popular because they reduce glare. However, although the tint does diminish the amount of light entering the eye, and so reduces glare, other areas of the visual field can be covered with a dangerous level of darkness; their use is therefore not recommended. They give the subjective impression of brightening the overall scene whilst in fact they reduce the contrast of objects against an already dark background. Similarly, tinted windscreens are also detrimental to visual functions and are not recommended for night driving (Wolf *et al.*, 1960).

There are several theories as to the subjective preference for yellow tints (Phillips and Rutstein, 1965):

- Yellow is associated with the high luminous efficiency of sodium lamps, and hence implies good vision
- Glare is reduced by yellow headlights in foggy conditions; however, the reduction in glare is not due to the colour, but to the reduced intensity
- There is less glare from the yellow car headlamps used in France, but this is mainly due to the sharply cut-off beam pattern
- Yellow is associated with sunlight and a subjective impression of increased luminance.

No driver should wear tinted spectacles at night because of the reduction in visual function, which is further decreased by tinted or dirty windscreens and by age.

There is no real necessity to have a tinted windscreen. Although drivers will argue that their vision is more comfortable with the tint during the daytime, there is a potential night-time hazard caused by loss of light transmission. Even the angle at which the windscreen is mounted can reduce the amount of light transmitted. Most windscreens are at an angle of 60° which, apart from making them ideal dirt collectors, causes a 20 per cent loss of transmission due to reflection. A tinted windscreen is also supposed to absorb heat and reduce glare. However, it is very inefficient in performing both of these functions, absorbing only 25 per cent of solar heat. It would be better to paint the car in light colours and insulate the roof and floor, as this would reduce the heat by about 44 per cent (Allen, 1969). It should also be noted that there is not enough reduction in transmission of light to help reduce glare on a bright day. In bright conditions it would be better to wear tinted spectacles.

There are ways of reducing the number of road traffic accidents that occur at night. One survey (Sabey and Johnson, 1973) analysed the relationship between night-time accidents and street lighting, and found a considerable reduction in the number of accidents when street lighting was improved. Improving the standard of street lighting on trunk roads reduces the number of accidents and saves money, despite the cost of installation. An estimate of the saving in the cost of accidents on roads where a 70-mph speed limit applies was about three times the annual cost of the lighting. It appears that, in addition to reducing the number of road traffic accidents, the crime rate is reduced.

Road lighting is designed to provide a bright visual background against which drivers see a potential hazard as a dark silhouette. On a well-lit road the use of dipped headlights does not generally help drivers themselves for the following reasons:

- Dipped headlights act as a glare source to all road users
- Pedestrians and drivers can be dazzled by them
- The silhouette contrast is decreased, which in turn reduces the visibility of hazards, etc.

One advantage of a dipped beam is that road users are aware of the presence of a moving vehicle. The use of sidelights overcomes the problems of glare and reduced contrast, but they are so dim (one-hundredth the brightness of a dipped beam) that the vehicle is very difficult to detect.

Other factors

Alcohol

Alcohol impairs mental efficiency, acts as an anaesthetic, and slows the response to a hazardous situation. It also can cause diplopia and blurring of vision. Moreover, the effects of smoking are summative with the effects of alcohol.

The legislation making it an offence to drive with over 80 mg of alcohol per 100 ml of blood was introduced in 1967, and had a marked effect on the number of road casualties. In the UK in 1998 there were 16 000 casualties from road accidents involving illegal alcohol levels, 3 per cent of which were fatal (Matheson and Summerfield, 2000). The report highlights the fact that deaths have dropped markedly during the past decade, which is believed to reflect the success of long-standing drink-driving campaigns (Figure 10.2).

Age

As mentioned, visual functions change with age. There are changes in visual acuity, contrast sensitivity, visual fields, glare sensitivity and other visual capabilities (Rubin *et al.*, 1997, Haegerstrom Portnoy *et al.*, 1999). Many eye disorders that cause a reduction in visual acuity or visual fields are prevalent amongst the elderly – e.g. cataracts, open-angle glaucoma and macular degeneration. Therefore, one might expect to find a higher accident rate amongst the elderly. However, a higher accident rate may not be due primarily to poor vision, but to other factors. Burg (1975) found that accidents occur more frequently in drivers under 25 and over 54 years of age. There is little difference between the accident rates for males and females. Accidents occurring to younger drivers with good vision may have been due to inexperience, reckless driving or alcohol abuse. Older drivers may have poorer vision, but there are other factors, such as slower reaction times and poorer hearing, which confuse their assessment. As a result, Burg suggested that poor vision cannot be stated as being the major cause of accidents in the elderly, and improving their visual performance will therefore not necessarily improve the accident rate.

Rackhoff and Mourant (1979) investigated the eye movements of a group of young drivers (21–29 years) and a group of older drivers (46–60 years), and found that the older drivers made longer eye movements during a car-following task. One explanation for this

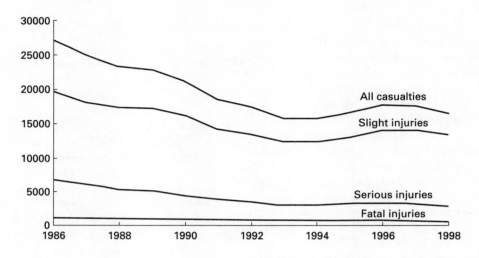

Fig. 10.2 *Casualties from road accidents involving illegal alcohol levels (After Matheson and Summerfield, 2000).*

is that older drivers have poorer parafoveal vision and so have to fixate foveally to acquire information, whereas younger drivers use their peripheral vision to gain the necessary information. Older drivers were found to have longer eye open times, which is presumably due to the fact that they need more time to acquire the relevant information. The ability to select relevant visual stimuli from an environment full of other distracting stimuli is impaired with age. This is an important factor in such tasks as driving, where the ability to select the relevant information quickly is necessary to avoid dangerous situations and accidents (Kahneman *et al.*, 1973; Mihal and Barrett, 1976).

Several surveys confirm the belief that older drivers travel at slower speeds and that they try to restrict their driving to low stress environments by, for example, avoiding driving at night or on icy roads (Case *et al.*, 1970; Rackhoff, 1974). However, despite this, accident rates for failing to give right of way, improper turning, or ignoring stop signs are higher for older drivers than for the middle-aged (McFarland *et al.*, 1964; Keltner and Johnson, 1987).

Keltner and Johnson (1987) conducted a survey of the Department of Motor Vehicles in 50 American states, studying the accident and conviction rates for different age groups. They found that although the elderly were responsible for a small percentage of traffic accidents, the type of accident in which they were involved could be related to peripheral and central visual field problems – for example, intersec-

tion collisions or failure to yield right of way. They concluded that, as age-related changes in visual functions occur at different rates for different people, licensing of the elderly should be based on functional abilities rather than age. Therefore, they suggested that evaluation of visual acuity and visual fields should be performed every 1–2 years in those drivers over 65 years of age.

Some recent studies have reported that the extent of the functional field for peripheral search and localization, known as the useful field of view (UFOV), had both a high sensitivity and specificity in predicting crash history of older drivers (Ball *et al.*, 1993; Owsley *et al.*, 1998). The UFOV is assessed by a computer-generated task that measures central and peripheral information processing. Subjects have to detect a centrally presented target and at the same time determine the location of targets in the periphery. These peripheral targets may be presented against a cluttered or an empty background. It appears that older drivers find it more difficult to derive relevant information in a cluttered view. One study found that older drivers with a 40 per cent or greater impairment in UFOV were 2.2 times more likely to have a crash in the 3-year follow-up period (Owsley *et al.*, 1998).

A study by Owsley *et al.* (1999) found that older drivers with cataracts experienced a restriction in their driving mobility and a decrease in their safety on the road when compared to those without cataracts. Drivers with cataracts were found to be 2.5 times more likely to have a history of at fault crash involvement in the previous 5 years (adjusted for distance and days driven per week).

Studies have investigated the effect of simulated visual impairment upon driving performance. Vision was impaired by goggles to simulate the effect of cataracts, binocular visual field restriction and monocularity (Wood *et al.*, 1995). Despite the induced visual impairment, the drivers still satisfied the legal requirement for driving. Driving performance was then assessed on a road circuit and was found to be significantly reduced. A significant relationship was also found between driving performance and contrast sensitivity and UFOV.

The proportion of older drivers is increasing year by year, and hence optometrists will have an increased responsibility to provide well-informed advice to their patients regarding their vision and driving performance. Advice that can be given to older drivers is summarized in an article by Grundy (1994). This includes the need to avoid tinted windscreens or spectacles, the use of anti-reflection coated lenses, the use of additional rear-view mirrors, avoiding fatigue, and the choice of travel time and route.

Summary

Many studies have failed to show that poor vision is an important cause of accidents. Burg (1967) pointed out the following difficulties in trying to relate driving performance to visual capabilities:

1. Vision is only one of many factors influencing driving performance
2. There may be disparity between the visual capabilities and the degree to which they are used when driving
3. Tests used may measure characteristics that are not closely related to the visual requirements of driving
4. Reliability of criteria used to measure driving performance may be low
5. Research methods may have shortcomings, such as an unrepresentative sample of the driving population.

A review by Owsley and McGwin (1999) of visual impairment and driving concluded that in order for older patients to be guided about their fitness to drive, valid and reliable methods of assessment must be developed and made widely available. From more recent studies it appears that there are several visual functions (including contrast sensitivity, dynamic visual acuity and UFOV) that may predict the driving ability/safety, and these need to be investigated further.

SPECTACLES FOR VEHICLE DRIVERS

This section makes a number of points regarding the dispensing of spectacles for motorists.

First, the frame should have thin rims and sides so that it does not restrict peripheral vision. The eye size chosen should be as large as possible, bearing in mind the prescription, again to allow the widest field of view. Lenses should be impact resistant, i.e. either plastic or toughened lenses should be used. If bifocals are required they should be dispensed with the smallest bifocal segment for driving spectacles. This is not to say that executive bifocals are unsafe – after all, many people wear them when driving without any problems – but they may not be ideal. Any bifocal or trifocal lens must be dispensed so that the reading portion does not encroach on the distance vision – i.e. fit the segment top low (Bateman, 1986). Varifocals do not appear to be a problem for drivers if they are correctly dispensed. In fact, many drivers find them very useful when parking, as they can see the car bonnet clearly through the intermediate portion of the lens.

Ideally, tinted spectacles should not be worn for night driving unless they are proven to be clinically necessary; nor should they be worn in conditions of poor visibility.

Tinted lenses for daytime driving may be considered under the following headings:

1. *Photochromics*. These do not work very well in vehicles, as the UV light that activates them is absorbed by the windscreen and windows of the car. Heat also lightens the lenses, and hence the lenses will not darken to their full potential inside a warm vehicle. They are most frequently made of glass, although plastics are available. Photochromics perform better than uncoated white crown glass by day, but are worse at night (Allen, 1979).
2. *Polarizing lenses*. These are particularly effective in reducing the glare from the road surface when driving towards the sun. They give the greatest benefit in the evening and winter months, when

the sun is low and the roads may be wet. However, problems may arise if the driver has a toughened glass windscreen or Triplex laminated glass, as the strain pattern will be clearly visible. Some drivers do not object to this pattern, but others do not like it. Polarizing lenses are often thought to absorb the UV/blue end of the spectrum, but this is not necessarily true.

3. *UV/blue-absorbing lenses.* These lenses, which absorb wavelengths up to 500 nm, are useful for drivers. UV light is important because it causes fluorescence of the crystalline lens proteins, and the visible light produced is then scattered over the retinal surface and reduces visibility. Examples of UV-absorbing lenses include UV 400 and UVPLS 530, 540, 550 from Norville, Essilor's UVX coating, or Zeiss Clarlets with Super ET coating.

A driver who wears sun spectacles with a deep tint is relatively more dark-adapted than the driver without sun spectacles. This means that if the sun spectacles are removed on entering a tunnel, the driver will be able to see more clearly than the more light-adapted driver (Davey, 1974).

There is a British Standard (BS 4110, 1999) that recommends various types of impact resistant eye-protectors for vehicle users, including visors, goggles and spectacles. It also states the transmission of the lenses and the minimum field of vision that should be present when wearing eye-protectors.

VISUAL STANDARDS FOR DRIVING LICENCES

National Standards for private motorists

Since 1935 it has been necessary for drivers of private vehicles in the UK to satisfy a minimum visual standard. Drivers are required to read a number plate, in good daylight (with glasses or contact lenses if worn), containing letters and figures 79.4 mm high, at a distance of 20.5 m (Statutory Instrument No. 1378, 1987). These symbols subtend a visual angle of 31.4 mm of arc at the eye. The number plate test is not considered to be a good test. One major point of criticism is that test conditions are poorly controlled with regard to lighting, distance, and the type and cleanliness of the number plate. The standard of visual acuity required to read the

number plate is greater than the nominal Snellen equivalent of 6/15. On examination of those who failed the number-plate test, the visual acuity was found to be equivalent to a clinical Snellen value of about 6/9–2 (Drasdo and Haggerty, 1981). The number-plate test is often considered to be irrelevant to the driving situation, as it is a static test in good daylight. Other tests of visual competence should be checked, such as visual field, dynamic visual acuity and contrast sensitivity.

It has been suggested recently that drivers applying for a provisional licence should be tested, and that drivers over 50 years of age should be examined at regular intervals. At present the driving licence is valid until the age of 70 years, with renewal every 3 years thereafter. Most people are not good at assessing whether their vision is up to standard, which was one reason why a number plate was used – to enable self-checking. However, various studies show an alarmingly high percentage of drivers who are ignorant of the visual standard required. A survey by McCaghrey (1986) showed that 59 per cent of drivers, when asked the distance of the number-plate test, either did not know or gave the wrong answer. Another survey by Guest and Jennings (1983) showed that 12 per cent of drivers fail to meet the driving standard test, and this shows no sign of improvement as a more recent survey in 1996 found that 16 per cent of the 8000 drivers screened could not read the number plate. The pass rate varied with age, with 7.3 per cent of the 17–20 years age group failing and 57.7 per cent of 71–75 years age group (Anon, 1996).

The decline of visual acuity with age (Davison and Irving, 1980; Rubin *et al.*, 1997) also supports the need for regular re-checks amongst the older driving population.

The booklet *What You Need to Know about Driving Licences* (D100 DVLA 12/1998) provides details about the health and eyesight requirements. It states that the DVLA must be informed if an applicant or licence holder has any of a number of health problems, such as epilepsy, angina, Parkinson's disease, any other chronic neurological condition, a major or minor stroke, diabetes controlled by insulin or tablets, or any visual disability that affects both eyes (not short/long sight or colour blindness).

There are two publications available that provide guidance on the medical standards for drivers;

Table 10.1 Guidance regarding fitness to drive – visual disorders (DVLA, 1999 Crown copyright is reproduced with the permission of the Controller of HMSO)

The law states that: A licence holder or applicant is suffering a prescribed disability if unable to meet the eyesight requirements, i.e. to read in good light (with the aid of glasses or contact lenses if worn) a registration mark fixed to a motor vehicle and containing letters and figures 79.4 millimetres high at a distance of 20.5 metres. If unable to meet this standard, the driver must not drive and the licence must be refused or revoked.

VISUAL DISORDERS	GROUP 1 ENTITLEMENT	GROUP 2 ENTITLEMENT
VISUAL ACUITY Severe bilateral cataract, failed bilateral cataract extraction.	Must be able to meet the above requirement. (In practice this corresponds to between 6/9 and 6/12 on the Snellen chart.)	New applicants are barred in law if the visual acuity using corrective lenses if necessary is worse than 6/9 in the better eye or 6/12 in the other eye or the uncorrected acuity in either eye is worse than 3/60. */*** Grandfather Rights below
MONOCULAR VISION	Need not notify DVLA if able to meet the visual acuity standard *and* has adapted to the disability.	Applicants are barred in law from holding a Group 2 licence. **/*** Grandfather Rights below
VISUAL FIELD DEFECTS e.g. homonymous hemianopia and homonymous quadrantanopia, severe bilateral glaucoma, severe bilateral retinopathy, diabetes, retinitis pigmentosa, complete bitemporal hemianopia and other serious bilateral eye disorders.	Driving must cease unless confirmed able to meet recommended national guideline for visual field.	Normal binocular field of vision is required.
DIPLOPIA	Cease driving on diagnosis. Resume driving on confirmation to the Licensing Authority that it is controlled by glasses or a patch which the licence holder undertakes to wear while driving.	Recommended permanent refusal or revocation if insuperable diplopia.
NIGHT BLINDNESS	Cease driving if unable to satisfy visual acuity and visual field requirements at all times.	Driving not permitted unless able to fully meet the Group 2 eyesight requirements.
COLOUR BLINDNESS	Need not notify DVLA. Driving may continue with no restriction on licence.	Need not notify DVLA; as for Group 1.
BLEPHAROSPASM	Subject to satisfactory medical reports able to retain licence but should inform DVLA of any change or deterioration in condition.	Refuse or revoke licence.

* Must have held the Group 2 licence on either 01.04.1991 or 01.03.1992 and be able to complete a satisfactory certificate of experience to be eligible. If obtained first Group 2 licence between 02.03.1992 and 31.12.1996 uncorrected visual acuity may be worse than 3/60 in one eye.

** Group 2 licence must have been issued prior to 01.01.1991 in knowledge of monocularity.

*** C1 applicants who passed the ordinary driving test prior to 01.01.1997 only need to satisfy the number-plate test. Monocularity is acceptable for these drivers also.

Table 10.2 Guidance regarding fitness to drive – diabetes mellitus (DVLA, 1999 Crown copyright is reproduced with the permission of the Controller of HMSO)

DIABETES MELLITUS	GROUP 1 ENTITLEMENT	GROUP 2 ENTITLEMENT
INSULIN TREATED Diabetic drivers are sent a detailed letter of explanation about their licence and driving by DVLA.	Must recognize warning symptoms of hypoglycaemia and meet required visual standards. 1,2 or 3 year licence.	New applicant on insulin or existing drivers are barred in law from driving HGV or PCV vehicles from 1/4/91. Drivers licensed from 1/4/91 on insulin are dealt with individually and licensed subject to satisfactory annual Consultant certification. From 11/9/98 some professional licence holders will be able to retain their entitlement to drive class C1 vehicles (3500–7500 kg lorries) subject to annual medical examination.
Commencement of insulin treatment following myocardinal infarction.	Notify DVLA. May retain licence but should stop driving if experiencing disabling hypoglycaemia. Notify DVLA again if treatment continues for more than 3 months.	
MANAGED BY DIET AND TABLETS Diabetic drivers are sent a detailed letter of explanation about their licence and their driving by DVLA.	Will be able to retain Till 70 licence unless develop relevant disabilities e.g. diabetic eye problems affecting visual acuity or visual field or if insulin required.	Drivers will be licensed unless they develop relevant disabilities e.g. diabetic eye problem affecting visual acuity or visual fields, in which case either recommended refusal or revocation or short period licence. If becomes insulin treated will be recommended refusal or revocation.
MANAGED BY DIET ALONE Diabetic drivers are sent a detailed letter of explanation about their licence and driving by DVLA.	Need not notify DVLA unless develop relevant disabilities e.g. diabetic eye problems affecting visual acuity or visual field or if insulin required.	Drivers will be licensed unless they develop relevant disabilities e.g. diabetic eye problem affecting visual acuity or visual fields, in which case the application will be refused or the licence revoked.
DIABETIC COMPLICATIONS	GROUP 1 ENTITLEMENT	GROUP 2 ENTITLEMENT
Frequent hypoglycaemic episodes	Cease driving until satisfactory control re-established, with GP/consultant report.	See above for *insulin treated*. Recommended permanent refusal or revocation.
Loss of awareness of hypoglycaemia	If confirmed driving must stop. Driving may resume provided reports show awareness of hypoglycaemia has been regained, confirmed by GP/consultant report.	See above for *insulin treated*. Recommended permanent refusal or revocation.
Eyesight complications (affecting visual acuity or fields)	See section: VISUAL DISORDERS.	See above for *insulin treated* and section: VISUAL DISORDERS.
Renal disorders	See section: RENAL DISORDERS	See section: RENAL DISORDERS
Limb disability	See DISABLED DRIVERS	As group I
Gestational diabetes	NOTIFY DVLA. May retain licence but should stop driving if experiencing hypoglycaemia. Notify DVLA again 6 weeks after delivery, if remains on insulin - see above.	Notify DVLA. Legal bar to holding a licence while insulin treated. Re-apply following delivery provided not on insulin.

Table 10.3 Field of vision requirements for Group 1 licence (DVLA, 1999 Crown copyright is reproduced with the permission of the Controller of HMSO)

The minimum field of vision for safe driving is defined as a field of at least 120° on the horizontal measured by the Goldmann perimeter using the III4e settings (or equivalent perimetry). In addition there should be no significant defect in the binocular field which encroaches within 20° of fixation above or below the horizontal meridian. This means that homonymous or bitemporal defects which come close to fixation whether hemianopic or quandrantinopic are not accepted as safe for driving.

The standard is not equipment specific and permits other equivalent perimeters including auto-perimeters. The list below (not exclusive) will satisfy the standard isolated scotomata represented in the binocular field near to the central fixation point. It may also be inconsistent with safe driving. The test must monitor the central area as well as its outer perimeter.

The majority of the charts received at DVLA are Esterman binocular charts. Central fields and monocular charts may also be requested. The advice to DVLA from the Secretary of State's Visual Panel is for an Esterman binocular chart to be considered reliable for licensing, the false positive score must be 20% or less. Other factors will be taken into account when considering acceptability of charts such as fixation loss. When a single missed point has been demonstrated within 20° of fixation on an Esterman binocular chart, the Panel advise that this may represent a significant central defect and, in these circumstances, central charts should be undertaken. *

a. The Gultron Biotronics Autofield 1 and the Fieldmaster perimeters using their basic programmes.
b. The Humphrey perimeter (3 zone, 61 point programme).
c. The Dicon perimeter AP2000 (target 2500 Asb. Bowl 31.5 Asb).
d. The Octopus perimeter 500EZ (programme No 7).
e. The Tubinger TAP 2000ct (programme No 6).
f. The Henson perimeter 4000, 5000 and 3500.
g. Medmont automatic perimeter.
h. Dicon LD400 equipment.
i. The Esterman test.

* Signifies amendments/additions to previous edition.

For Medical Practitioners – At a Glance Guide to the Current Medical Standards of Fitness to Drive (DVLA, 1999) and *Medical Aspects of Fitness to Drive* (Medical Commission on Accident Prevention, 1995). See Tables 10.1 and 10.2 for guidance about fitness to drive for drivers or applicants who have visual disorders or diabetes mellitus (DVLA, 1999).

The minimum visual field for safe driving is defined as a field of vision of at least 120° along the horizontal and at least 20° above and below the horizontal, measured by Goldmann perimetry using the III4e settings (or equivalent perimeter). A list of perimeters considered appropriate for use is given in DVLA (1999); see Table 10.3. This means that homonymous or bitemporal defects which come close to fixation, whether hemionapic or quadrantinopic, are not accepted for safe driving. For further details on driving standards, see Appendix D.

Large goods and passenger-carrying vehicle licences

Large goods and passenger-carrying vehicles are licensed by the DVLA from the Driver and Vehicle Licensing Centre at Swansea. The eyesight standard for those who applied on or after 1 January, 1997 is acuity (with the aid of corrective lenses if necessary) of at least 6/9 in the better eye and at least 6/12 in the worse eye and, if corrective lenses are needed to meet that standard, uncorrected acuity of at least 3/60 in both eyes.

Due to stricter vision standards being introduced, drivers who held a licence before 1 January 1997 may not be able to comply with this new eyesight standard and will need to check their licensing position with the DVLA (see Table 10.1 and Appendix D for further details). Licences are normally renewed at the age of 45 years, and after that renewals are required every 5 years until the age of 65 years, when they are required annually.

There are also stricter rules about the health of drivers of larger vehicles. When applying or renewing an existing licence, a medical report has to be provided. For example, the DVLA needs to be notified about any heart condition or heart operation, insulin-treated diabetes, and any visual problem affecting either eye. Currently insulin-treated diabetics may not drive large vehicles unless they held a licence to drive lorries or buses on 1 April 1991, and the Traffic Commissioner who issued the licence (or in whose area they lived) was aware of the insulin treatment before January, 1991 (DVLA D100, 1998). For further details see DVLA (1999) and Medical Commission on Accident Prevention (1995).

SUMMARY

This chapter has attempted to show how difficult it is to set standards of vision associated with safe driving, and suggests that other factors, such as driver education, should also be assessed and that street and vehicle lighting should be improved. Charman (1986) suggests that changing drivers' attitudes through education is the simplest way to reduce accidents. For example, the average driver's behaviour and road speed apparently change very little, regardless of the time of day and the level of visibility. Although it will be expensive to provide education for drivers, including the increasing number of elderly, and to improve road and vehicle lighting, the cost in human suffering and the estimated cost of road traffic accidents must be taken into account.

REFERENCES

Allen M. J. (1969) Vision and driving. *Traffic Saf Res Rev*, 8, 8–11.

Allen, M.J. (1979) Highway tests of photochromic lenses. *J Am Optom Assoc*, 59, 1023–1027.

Anon (1996) Survey shows 16 per cent of all UK drivers fail number plate test. *Optom Today*, **October 21**, 10.

Association of Optometrists (1990) AOP statement on night myopia. *Optom Today*, **November 19**, 13, 19.

Ball K., Owsley C., Sloane M.E., Roenker D.L. and Bruni J.R. (1993) Visual attention problems as a predictor of vehicle crashes in older drivers. *Invest Ophthalmol Vis Sci*, **34(11)**, 3110–3123.

Bateman N.F. (1986) Dispensing to car drivers. *Disp Opt*, **March,** 28.

BS 4110 (1999) Eye-protectors for vehicle users. BSI, London.

Burg A. (1967) The relationship between vision test scores and driving record: general findings. *Report 62–74.* University of California, Los Angeles.

Burg A. (1968) Vision test scores and driving record: additional findings. *Report 68-21.* University of California, Los Angeles.

Burg A. (1975) The relationship between visual ability and road accidents. In *Prevention Routiere Internationale, First International Congress on Vision and Road Safety*, Paris, 3–12.

Case H.W., Hulbert S. and Beers J. (1970) Driving ability as affected by age. *Final Report No.70-18.* Institute of Transportation and Traffic Engineering, University of California, Los Angeles.

Cashell G.T.W. (1970) Visual functions in relation to road accidents. *Injury*, 2, 9–10.

Charman W.N. (1986) Vision and driving. *Optician*, **192**, 27–32.

Coles B.L. and Brown B. (1966) Optimum intensity of red road-traffic signal lights for normal and protanopic observers. *J Optom Soc Am*, **56**, 516–522.

Council F.M. and Allen J.A. (1974) *A Study of the Visual Fields of North Carolina Drivers and their Relationship to Accidents*. Highway Research Safety Centre, University of North Carolina.

Davey J.B. (1959) Seeing times with yellow glasses – preliminary report. *Optician*, **136**, 651.

Davey J.B. (1974) Sunspectacles for drivers. *Ophthal Optician*, **March 2**, 154–167.

Davey J.B. and Sheridan M. (1953) Night driving spectacles and night vision. *Optician,* **July 31**, 33–38.

Davison P.A. (1985) Inter-relationships between British driver's ability, visual abilities, age and road accident histories. *Ophthal Physiol Opt*, 5, 195–204.

Davison P.A. and Irving A. (1980) Survey of visual acuity of drivers. *Transport and Road Research Laboratory Report No. 945.* Transport and Road Research Laboratory, Crowthorne, Berkshire.

Drasdo N. and Haggerty C.M. (1981) A comparison of British number plate and Snellen vision tests for car drivers. *Ophthal Physiol Opt*, 1, 39–54.

DVLA D100 (1998) *What You Need to Know about Driving Licences.* DVLA, Swansea.

DVLA (1999) *For Medical Practitioners – At a Glance Guide to the Current Medical Standards of Fitness to Drive.* Drivers Medical Unit, DVLA, Swansea.

Elkington A.R. and MacKean J.M. (1982) Glaucoma and driving. *Br Med J*, **285**, 777–778.

Grundy J.W. (1994) Vision and the older driver. *Optom Today*, **December 19**, 20–25.

Guest D.J. and Jennings J.B. (1983) A survey of drivers vision in Victoria. *Aust J Optom*, **66**, 13–19.

Haegerstrom Portnoy G., Scheck M.E. and Brabyn J.A. (1999) Seeing into old age: visual function beyond acuity. *Optom Vis Sci*, **76**, 141–158.

Hebenstreit B.V. (1984) Visual acuity and road accidents (Sehvermogen und Verkehrsunfalle). *Klin Montsbl Augenheilk*, **185**, 86–90.

Hedin A. (1980) Retesting of vehicle drivers' visual capacity. *J Traffic Med*, **8**, 18–21.

Hills B.L. (1980) Vision, visibility and perception in driving. *Perception*, **9**, 183–216.

Hills B.L. and Burg A. (1977) A reanalysis of California driver vision data: general findings. *Transport and Road Research Laboratory, Report No. LR768*. Transport and Road Research Laboratory, Crowthorne, Berkshire.

Hofstetter H.W. (1976) Visual acuity and highway accidents. *J Am Optom Assoc*, **47**, 887–893.

Hope G.M. and Rubin M.L. (1984) Perspectives in refraction: night myopia. *Surv Ophthal*, **29**, 129–136.

Johnson C.A. and Keltner J.L. (1983) Incidence of visual field loss in 20 000 eyes and its relationship to driving performance. *Arch Ophthalmol*, **101**, 371–375.

Kahneman D., Ben-Ishai R. and Lotan M. (1973) Relation of a test of attention to road accidents. *J Appl Psychol*, **58**, 113–115.

Keltner J.L. and Johnson C.A. (1987) Visual function, driving safety and the elderly. *Ophthalmology*, **94**, 1180–1188.

Keeney A.H. (1968) Relationship of ocular pathology and driving impairment. *Trans Am Acad Ophthal Otol*, **72**, 737–740.

Kite C.R. and King J.N. (1961) A survey of the factors limiting the visual fields of motor vehicle drivers in relation to minimum visual field and visibility standards. *Br J Physiol*, **18**, 85–107.

Leibowitz H.W. and Owens D.A. (1978) New evidence for the intermediate position of relaxed accommodation. *Documenta Ophth*, **46**, 133–147.

Levitt J.G. (1975) Vision and driving. *Ophthal Optician*, **December 13**, 1109–1016.

Liesmaa M. (1973) The influence of drivers' vision in relation to his driving. *Optician*, **166**, 10–13.

Matheson J. and Summerfield C. (eds) (2000) *Social Trends 30*. Office for National Statistics, The Stationery Office, London.

McCaghrey G.E. (1986) Vision and driving. Motorfair Survey, 1985. *Optom Today*, **March 1**, 132–136.

McFarland R., Domey R.G., Warren A.B. and Ward D.C. (1960) Dark adaptation as a function of age: I. A statistical analysis. *J Gerontol*, **15**, 149–154.

McFarland R.A., Tune G.S. and Welford A.T. (1964) On the driving of automobiles by older people. *J Gerontol*, **19**, 190–197.

Medical Commission on Accident Prevention (1995) *Medical Aspects of Fitness to Drive a Guide for Medical Practitioners*, 5th edn. The Medical Commission on Accident Prevention, 35–43 Lincoln's Inn Fields, London.

Mihal W.L. and Barret G.V. (1976) Individual differences in perceptual information processing and their relation to automobile accident involvement. *J Appl Psychol*, **61**, 229–233.

Norman L.G. (1960) Medical aspects of road safety. *Lancet*, **1**, 989–994, 1039–1045.

North R.V. (1985) The relationship between the extent of the visual field and driving performance. *Ophthal Physiol Opt*, **5**, 205–210.

Owsley C. and McGwin G. (1999) Vision impairment and driving. *Surv Ophthalmol*, **43**, 535–550.

Owsley C., Ball K, McGwin G., Sloane M.E., Roenker D.L., White M.F. and Overley E.T. (1998) Visual processing impairment and risk of motor vehicle crash among older adults. *J Am Med Assoc*, **279**, 1083–1088.

Owsley C., Stalvey B., Wells J. and Sloane M.E. (1999) Older drivers and cataract: driving habits and crash risk. *J Gerontol A Biol Sci Med Sci*, **54(4)**, M203–211.

Papst W. (1962) Dazzle and night driving. *New Scientist*, **314**, 436–438.

Phillips A.J. and Rutstein A. (1965) Glare – a study into glare recovery time with night driving spectacles. *Br J Physiol Opt*, **22**, 153–164.

Phillips A.J. and Rutstein A. (1967) Amber night driving spectacles. A further study. *Br J Physiol Optics*, **24**, 161–205.

Rackoff N.J. and Mourant R.R. (1979) Driving performance in the elderly. *Accid Annal Prev*, **11**, 247–253.

Richards O.W. (1953) Yellow glasses fail to improve seeing at night driving luminances. *Highway Res Abstr*, **23**, 32–36.

Road Research Laboratory (1963) Research on Road Safety. HMSO, London.

Road Vehicle Lighting Regulations (1989) Statutory Instrument SI 1989/1796. HMSO, London.

Rubin G.S., West S.K., Munoz B., Bandeen Roche K., Zeger S. and Schein O. (1997) A comprehensive assessment of visual impairment in a population of older Americans – the SEE Study. *Invest Ophthalmol Vis Sci*, **38**, 557–568.

Sabey B.E. and Johnson H.D. (1973) Road lighting and accidents: before and after studies on trunk road sites. *Report No. LR586*. Transport and Road Research Laboratory, Crowthorne, Berkshire.

Statutory Instrument No. 1378 (1987). Road traffic. Motor vehicles (driving licenses) regulations. HMSO, London.

Staughton, G.C. and Stone, V.J. (1977). Methodology of an in-depth accident investigation survey. *Report No. LR762.* Transport and Road Research Laboratory, Crowthorne, Berkshire.

Sturgis S.P. and Osgood D.J. (1982) Effects of glare and background luminance on visual acuity and contrast sensitivity: implications for driver night vision testing. *Human Factors*, 24, 347–350.

Transport and Road Research Laboratory (1980). Gap acceptance and traffic conflict simulation as a measure of risk. *Report No. SR 776*. Transport and Road Research Laboratory, Crowthorne, Berkshire.

Wolf E., McFarland R.A. and Zigler M. (1960) Influence of tinted windshield glass on five visual functions. *Highway Res Board Bull*, 255, 30–46.

Wood J.M. (1997) Vision and driving. Current standards and recent research. *Optom Today*, **January 24,** 29–32.

Wood J.M. and Troutbeck R. (1992) Effect of restriction of the binocular visual field on driving performance. *Ophthal Physiol Opt*, 2, 291–298.

Wood J.M. and Troutbeck R. (1995) Elderly drivers and simulated visual impairment. *Optom Vis Sci*, 72, 115–124.

Appendix A: Guidelines for the suitability of colour vision defects for certain occupations

(Courtesy of J. Voke and Keeler Ltd, 1980)

Jobs, careers and industries where defective colour vision is a handicap and in which important consequences might result from errors of colour judgement:

Air traffic controller

Buyers – textile, yarns, tobacco, food (e.g. fruit, cocoa), timber

Car body resprayer, retoucher

Cartographer

Ceramics – painter/decorater of pottery

Ceramics – inspector (quality control)

Chemists and chemicals (laboratory analysis, food chemist, teacher of chemistry, manufacturer of chemicals and polishes and oils)

Colour printer, etcher, retoucher

Colour photographer

Colour TV technician

Coloured pencils/chalks/paints manufacturing

Colourist/colour matcher in paints, paper, pigments, inks, dyes, wallpaper

Cotton grader

Coroner

Forensic scientist

Market gardener, e.g. fruit

Meat inspector

Oil refining

Paint maker and distributor

Paper making

Pharmacist

Plastics

Restorer of painting/works of art

Safety officer
Tanner
Tobacco grader

Jobs and careers where good vision is desirable but in which defective colour vision would not necessarily cause a handicap:

Accountant
Anaesthetist
Architect
Artist – graphic, commercial, advertising
Auctioneer
Barmaid/barman
Bacteriologist
Baker
Beautician
Botanist
Brewer
Builder/bricklayer
Carpenter
Carpet/lino fitter/planner
Chiropodist
Clothes designer
Cook or chef
Confectioner
Cosmetics director (stage, film, TV)
Dental surgeon and technician
Draughtsman
Dressmaker
Driving instructor
Driver in public services, e.g. bus
Engineer (various)
Farmer
Fishmonger
Florist
Forester
Furrier
Gardener and landscape gardener
Geologist
Gemmologist, e.g. setting stones, diamond grader
Grocer
Hairdresser
Horticulturist
Illuminating engineer
Interior decorator/designer/planner
Jeweller
Librarian

Lighting director (state/film TV)
Manicurist
Metallurgist
Milliner
Miner
Nurse
Optometrist/ophthalmologist
Osteopath
Painter
Pharmacy assistant (counter service)
Physician
Physiotherapist
Post Office counter assistant
Potter
Salesman/woman (fabrics, drapery, yarns, wool, carpets, garments/footwear, china and glass, linen, cosmetics/toiletries, jewellery, confectionery, stationery, storekeeper)
Shoe repairer
Surgeon
Tanner
Tailor
Telephone switchboard operator
Theatre/stage props manager
Veterinary surgeon
Waiter
Zoologist

Jobs and careers requiring perfect colour vision:

Armed forces – certain grades
Civil aviation
Colour matcher in dyeing, textiles, paints, inks, coloured paper, ceramics, cosmetics
Carpet darner/inspector, spinner, weaver, bobbin winder
Electrical work (electrician, electronics technician, colour TV mechanic, motor mechanic, telephone installer)
Navigation (pilot, fisherman, railways)
Police – certain grades
Radio – telegraphy

Appendix B: List of some of the suppliers of vision screeners

Model	Supplier
Essilor: Ergovision, Visiotest	Central Safety Equipment Ltd, 1 Myring Drive, Sutton Coldfield, West Midlands B75 7RZ, UK
Titmus II Vision Tester	Norville Optical Co. Ltd, Magdala Road, Gloucestershire, GL1 4DG, UK
	Parmelee Ltd, Middlemore Lane West, Aldridge, Walsall, West Midlands W59 8D7, UK
	Bolle (UK) Ltd, Brunel Close, Ebblake Industrial Estate, Verwood, Dorset BH31 6BA, UK
R10 (drivers), R11 (children), R12 (industrial)	Rodenstock (UK) Ltd, Springhead Road, Northfleet, Kent DA11 6HJ, UK
Topcon Screenoscope SS-3	Tinsley Medical Instruments, Kennet Side, Bone Lane, Newbury, Berkshire RG14 5PX, UK

Keystone VS-2, DVS-11 Driver Vision Screen	Warwick-Evans Optical Co. Ltd, 22 Palace Road, Bounds Green, London N11 2P5, UK	City University Vision Screener for VDU users	CITY Visual Systems Ltd, 35 Brackley Square, Woodford Green, Essex IG8 7LJ, UK
Optec 2000	Grafton Optical Co. Ltd, Unit D, Penfold Trading Estate, Imperial Way, Watford, Hertfordshire WD2 4YY, UK	City VDU Toolkit	Thomson Software Solutions, 49 Wroxham Gardens, Potters Bar, Hertfordshire EN6 3DJ, UK
Binoptometer	Oculus Optikgerate GmbH, Munchholzhauser Stralle 29, Dutenhofen, D-6330 Wetzlar 17, Germany		

Appendix C: Photometric units and the conversion factors necessary to change them to SI units

Quantity	Unit	Dimensions	Conversion factor
Illuminance	Lux	$lumen/m^2$	1.0
	Metre candle	$lumen/m^2$	1.0
SI unit = Lux	Phot	$lumen/cm^2$	10 000
	Footcandle	$lumen/ft^2$	10.76
Luminance	Nit	$candela/m^2$	1.0
	Stilb	$candela/cm^2$	10 000
SI unit = $candela/m^2$	Apostilb	$lumen/m^2$	0.32
	Lambert	$lumen/cm^2$	3183
	Footlambert	$lumen/ft^2$	3.43

Appendix D: Vision standards for various occupations

The following standards have been reproduced by kind permission of the Association of Optometrists and the Civil Aviation Authority. For information on other standards, please refer to the *AOP Handbook*.

1. Motorists
2. Royal Navy
3. Royal Air Force
4. Police
5. Army
6. Visual display unit operators
7. Civil Aviation Authority.

MOTORISTS
Changes to licence requirements
On 1 January 1999 new arrangements were introduced for the licensing of drivers of vehicles carrying passengers (PCV) or goods (LGV). These new rules require that, in general, drivers of these vehicles must hold a professional driver's licence, whereas before that date many of these vehicles could be driven on a car licence. The visual standards requirements are now more complex. There are however many exemptions to the requirements.

Holders of a full car licence (B) may drive some heavy vehicles, and a shortened version of the list follows. Drivers should consult DVLA for the definitive list and definitions.

a. Vehicles propelled by steam
b. Road construction vehicles
c. Engineering plant
d. Works trucks (e.g. dump trucks and forklift trucks)

e. Haulage tractors mainly used off road and under 7370 kg

f. Agricultural vehicles which are not tractors (e.g. crop sprayers and combine harvesters)

g. Digging machines travelling to and from sites

h. Vehicles used occasionally on public roads (precise requirements apply)

i. Any vehicle, other than an agricultural vehicle, which is used for agriculture and is used on a public road occasionally (precise requirements apply)

j. Haulage of lifeboats

k. Vehicles manufactured before 1960, without a trailer

l. Articulated goods vehicles under 3.5 tonnes

m. Some military vehicles

n. Special vehicles for the transport of disabled vehicles

o. Mobile project vehicles (e.g. for transport of educational exhibitions) (precise requirements apply).

Some passenger-carrying vehicles are exempt from the licensing requirements. Holders of category B (car) licences may drive any of the following vehicles:

a. A PCV manufactured over 30 years before the date driven, not used for hire or reward and with less than eight passengers

b. A minibus with up to 16 passengers provided that:

   i. The vehicle is used for social purposes by a non-commercial body but not for hire or reward

   ii. The driver is aged 21 or over

   iii. The driver has held a category B licence for at least 2 years

   iv. The driver is providing the service on a voluntary basis

   v. The minibus weight is under 3.5 tonnes (or 4.25 tonnes including specialist equipment for the carriage of disabled passengers)

   vi. If the driver is aged 70 years or over, the driver meets the health requirements of a category D1 licence.

Drivers of exempted LGVs must be at least 18 years of age, and of exempted PCVs or any vehicle over 7.5 tonnes at least 21 years.

Categories C1 and D1 were issued as a matter of course with Group 1 (ordinary) entitlement to all drivers who passed the ordinary driving test prior to January 1st 1997. Any driver who passed their ordinary test after that date did not have these entitlements issued. These C1 and D1 entitlements continue until the licence expires or is medically revoked after 1st January 1998. A driver who had C1 entitlement issued with a Group 1 licence before 1st January 1997 is known as an 'exempted licence holder'.

Ordinary driving licence provisions

It is a criminal offence for a driving licence holder or applicant to fail to notify Drivers Medical Branch, Driver and Vehicle Licensing Centre, Swansea, immediately they become aware of any eyesight condition which is likely to cause them to be a source of danger to the public when driving. Failure to notify can also have serious motor insurance implications. Awareness is normally regarded in law as starting as soon as the person has knowledge that a danger exists, and this includes when they have received professional advice that their condition represents an immediate or potential danger when driving.

Static visual acuity

The standard for ordinary drivers is the ability to read in good light (with the aid of glasses or contact lenses, if worn) a registration mark fixed to a motor vehicle and containing letters and figures 79.4 millimetres (31/8 inches) high at a distance of 20.5 metres (67 feet), or 12.3 metres (40 feet) in the case of an applicant for a licence for authority to drive vehicles confined to Group K (milk floats and pedestrian-controlled mowing machines). There is no precise Snellen equivalent to the number-plate standard. Drasdo and Haggerty found that applying a standard of 6/9-2 (6/10) resulted in a **mathematical** equivalent to this (i.e. this standard failed the same proportion of people, but not necessarily the same individuals). The normal number-plate test found on many test charts is NOT equivalent and should not be relied upon. It must be emphasized that the statutory standard of visual acuity for drivers is the practical test, which has to be taken in good light. The number-plate test is prescribed in the Motor Vehicles (Driving Licences) Regulations and the Road Traffic Act 1988, which makes it an offence for anyone to drive a motor vehicle on a road while his eyesight is such (whether through a defect which cannot be or one which is not for the time being sufficiently corrected) that he cannot comply with the standard quoted above.

Visual fields

There is no **statutory** requirement for fields of vision for Group 1 drivers, but the following standard is usually applied when there is evidence that a defect exists. Ordinary drivers are required to have a field of vision of at least 120° within the horizontal measured by the Goldmann perimeter using the III4e settings (or equivalent perimetry). In addition, there should be no significant defect in the binocular field that encroaches within 20° of fixation above or below the horizontal meridian. By these means homonymous or bitemporal defects that come close to fixation, whether hemaniopic or quadrantopic, are not accepted as safe for driving. Isolated scotoma represented in the binocular field near to the central fixation point may also be inconsistent with safe driving. The DETR has issued a list of perimeters which equate to this standard, and the Esterman test is recommended.

Diplopia

Insuperable diplopia causes unfitness to drive. Late onset sudden diplopia due to a minor stroke precludes driving for 1 month, then if persisting and superable with a prismatic lens or masking, driving is permitted providing the driver gives an undertaking 'always to wear the lens or patch when driving'.

Colour vision

Impaired colour vision is not a bar to driving.

Vision under adverse lighting conditions

Patients who have cataracts and those having undergone refractive surgery may be unable to meet the required standards under conditions of poor light or glare. A history of inability to see effectively when driving at night with headlights due to a night vision defect such as retinitis pigmentosa or advanced choroidoretinitis precludes issue of a driving licence. Patients with inability to see in the glare of sunlight or oncoming headlights at night may fail to read a number plate at the prescribed distance in good light.

Monocular drivers

Recent loss of an eye may require a period off driving for adaptation, but then driving may be resumed subject to meeting the above standards.

Diabetic retinopathy

Treatment of proliferative diabetic retinopathy by pan-retinal photocoagulation (laser ablation of the retina) can cause reduced visual field and jeopardize the right to drive.

Duration of ordinary driving licences

The Licensing Authority would require progressive conditions affecting both eyes such as glaucoma, high myopia, cataract, diabetic retinopathy, macular degeneration etc. to be notified.

Advice to patients

Optometrists are frequently asked by patients whether they are visually fit to drive. Statutory law and the tort of negligence makes it unwise to give advice purely on the basis of the Snellen acuity. If acuity only is in question, it is safer to advise patients to satisfy themselves that they can read a number plate at 20.5 m (67 feet) in good light with correction if worn, emphasis being given to the proper measurement of the distance. If there is any doubt, they should be advised to report their condition immediately to the Licensing Centre and they will be sent to their local Driving Test Centre for the test to be conducted by a driving examiner, measuring the distance correctly. Also, the other aspects of vision outlined above should be taken into account when considering advice to the patient. It is an optometrist's duty, if a patient of driving age does not meet the requirements above, to ask if they drive and, if so, to advise accordingly. An appropriate entry should be made on the patient's record card. Patients should be warned that failure to report the condition to DVLA could jeopardize their motor insurance. If it becomes clear that a patient who is manifestly and clearly visually dangerous is continuing to drive in spite of professional advice to the contrary, it is suggested that the optometrist should discuss the matter with the legal department at the Association.

Frames and lenses

Care should be taken in frame selection not to obscure lateral vision. Advice should be given on the limitations of high power lenses and the dangers of wearing tinted lenses at dusk or at night and of photochromic lenses when entering road tunnels and roads shaded by trees from good daylight conditions. Patients with borderline acuity should be advised not to drive vehicles with tinted windscreens, or be prescribed tints. Muscle imbalance must be corrected unless well compensated.

Follow-up

The AOP recommends that drivers and riders should have a retest at the most every 3 years up to the age of 70 years and annually thereafter, and be advised to report immediately any visual symptoms. Any pathological eye disease should, of course, be referred for investigation.

Professional and vocational driving licence provisions

Vocational licences include those for a large goods vehicle (LGV, previously HGV), and passenger-carrying vehicle (PCV, previously PSV). Professional driving implies that a person has employment driving, and the majority of employed time is spent riding or at the wheel. Hackney carriage and private hire licences come within this group. These standards may also be applied by other employers of professional drivers, such as ambulance drivers etc.

Licence requirements for some vehicles were changed in January 1999. Vehicles that could previously be driven with a Group 1 licence may now need a Group 2 licence.

Visual field

The second EC Directive states that a Group 2 driver should have a normal binocular field of vision (see above for definition of normal field). Therefore a pathological field defect in one eye may not preclude driving.

Visual acuity

A. New eyesight standards for drivers of large goods vehicles (LGVs) and buses and coaches (passenger-carrying vehicles or PCVs) apply to all applicants who obtain their first Group 2 licences on or after 1 January 1997.

B. Revised rules apply for those drivers who already hold a Group 2 licence on that date and whose eyesight would not, when their licences fall for renewal, meet the new standard. There are two such categories of drivers:

   i. Drivers who can comply with the outgoing standard, but who would not be able to comply with the application of the uncorrected visual acuity standard of 3/60 to both eyes in the new standard.
   ii. Drivers who cannot comply with the outgoing standard, and who first obtained their entitlements some time ago (mostly before 1983) when eyesight requirements were less stringent, and who have been allowed to continue to drive by virtue of provisions in existing national legislation, the so-called 'grandfather rights'.

Drivers in category (i) above will be entitled to renew their Group 2 licences, as long as they can continue to comply with the outgoing (i.e. pre-second European Directive) eyesight standards. In particular, they will be required to meet the uncorrected visual acuity standard in only one eye, rather than both.

Drivers in category (ii) will retain their existing 'grandfather rights' to continue driving and have their licences renewed, as long as they can certify at the time of renewal:

A. That they have driven LGVs or PCVs on at least 10 occasions within the preceding 5 years, three occasions of which were in the previous 18 months
B. That they have not been involved in an accident in the preceding 10 years, in which their eyesight might have been a factor.

The eyesight requirements for Group 2 drivers are produced here in summary.

London bus drivers

London Transport buses were privatized in September 1994. There is therefore no visual standard for London bus drivers, other than that included in the PCV requirements.

Vehicle type	Licence requirement	Visual standards applied
Passenger-carrying vehicles		
A driver of a passenger-carrying vehicle which has 9–16 seats	PCV licence category D1	Full vocational standards (no grandfather rights)
A driver of a passenger-carrying vehicle which has more than 16 seats	PCV licence category D	Full vocational standards
Goods vehicles		
For other vehicles it is the maximum authorized mass (i.e. vehicle + authorized load) that determines the driving licence requirement		
For a maximum authorized mass that is over 3.5 tonnes but less than 7.5 tonnes	LGV licence category C1 issued before 1 January 1997	Car acuity standard but visual field requirement is mandatory
	LGV licence category C1 issued after 1 January 1997	Full vocational standards
For a maximum authorized mass that is over 7.5 tonnes	LGV licence category C	Full vocational standards

Invalid carriages

There are three classes of invalid carriages defined in **The Use of Invalid Carriages on Highways Regulations 1988**:

Class 1 — Manual wheelchair, i.e. self-propelled or attendant-propelled, not electrically powered

Class 2 — Powered wheelchairs and scooters for footway use, with a maximum speed limit of 4 mph

Class 3 — Powered wheelchairs and other outdoor powered vehicles, including scooters, for use on roads/highways, with a maximum speed of 8 mph and the facility to travel at 4 mph on footways

Class 3 — Vehicles are not legally defined as motor vehicles and therefore do not need licensing or MoT testing, and the user does not need a driving licence or insurance. However, they can (in general) be driven only by disabled people over 14 years of age.

There is no legal eyesight standard, but it is recommended that riders should be able to read a car number plate at 12.3 metres (40 feet).

Licensing authority

The Licensing Authority in the case of Ordinary driver licences is the Secretary of State for the Department of Environment, Transport and the Regions (DETR). The Driver and Vehicle Licensing Agency at Swansea acts as his or her agent.

Large goods and passenger-carrying service vehicles are licensed by the Driver and Vehicle Licensing Agency (DVLA) from the Driver and Vehicle Licensing Centre (DVLC) at Swansea.

Taxi drivers are normally licensed by local authorities or, in the Metropolitan Police area, by the Public Carriage Office.

Right of appeal

If a driving licence is refused or revoked, a driver has a right to appeal to a magistrate's court in England or Wales or to a sheriff's court in Scotland. The Department's medical advisers will always be prepared to

Table 1

Person holding Group 2 licence or obsolete vocational licence on:	Standard of visual acuity applicable:
1 January 1983 and 1 April 1991	Acuity (with the aid of corrective lenses if necessary) of at least 6/12 in the better eye **or** at least 6/36 in the worse eye **or** uncorrected acuity of at least 3/60 in at least one eye
1 March 1992, but not on 1st January 1983	Acuity (with the aid of corrective lenses if necessary) of at least 6/9 in the better eye **or** at least 6/12 in the worse eye, **or** uncorrected acuity of at least 3/60 in at least one eye

Table 2

Person holding Group 2 licence on:	Standard of visual acuity applicable
31 December 1996, but not on 1 March 1992	Acuity (with the aid of corrective lenses if necessary) of at least 6/9 in the better eye **and** at least 6/12 in the worse eye **and**, if corrective lenses are needed to meet that standard, uncorrected acuity of at least 3/60 in at least one eye
On or after 1 January 1997 but not on 31 December 1996*	Acuity (with the aid of corrective lenses if necessary) of at least 6/9 in the better eye **and** at least 6/12 in the worse eye and, if corrective lenses are needed to meet that standard, uncorrected acuity of at least 3/60 in both eyes

consider any fresh medical evidence without recourse to the Courts.

Driving instructors
In order to pass the qualifying (ADI) examination to register as a driving instructor under the Road Traffic Act 1988, Part 5, amended by the Motor Cars Driving Instruction regulations 1989, 5(2), the candidate is required to read a motor car number plate at a distance of 27.5 metres (90 feet) where the letters and figures are 3 1/8 inches high, in good light, with the aid of glasses if worn. The general regulations regarding motorists' vision (see above) also apply.

Drivers of metropolitan motor cabs
Drivers of Metropolitan cabs are required to meet the Professional Drivers Group 2 licence standards applying to PCV drivers as above, including the 'grandfather rights' clauses. Medicals are undertaken on entry, and then at ages 50, 56, 62, 65 years, and then annually. The eyesight check will be performed as part of this medical by a general practitioner, but if there is any doubt the driver will be referred to an ophthalmologist or optometrist for completion of the relevant form.

Other professional drivers
Taxi drivers (with the exception of the London taxis above) are usually licensed by a local authority, who will determine the standards to be imposed. These will

normally be the Group 2 standards, but the recertification intervals may vary. Other drivers (such as ambulance drivers) have standards applied by the employer, and are usually the Group 2 standard. Some individual employers may set vision standards to be applied in respect of their employees driving company vehicles (such as delivery vans, cars) which do not have specific requirements in law.

Visual field testing on behalf of the DVLA

Optometrists who wish to undertake visual field testing on behalf of the DVLA and have the appropriate equipment can apply for an application form and information sheet by telephoning 01792 788410.

Useful references

British Standard 4274 (1968) test charts for determining distance visual acuity. British Standards Institution, London.

Drasdo N. and Haggerty C.M. (1977) *A Comparison of the British Number-plate and Snellen Vision Tests for Car Drivers*. Leaflet LF 676. Transport and Road Research Laboratory, Crowthorne, Berkshire.

Drasdo N. and Haggerty C.M. (1980) A comparison of the British number-plate and Snellen vision tests for car drivers. *Ophthal Physiol Opt*, 1, 39–54.

First Council Directive on the introduction of a Community driving licence (1980) *Official J Eur. Comm*, 31 **December**, No. L375-11–15.

For Medical Practitioners – At a Glance Guide to the Current Medical Standards of Fitness To Drive (1999) incorporating Jan 2000 amendments. Drivers Medical Unit, DVLA, Swansea.

Highway Code. London, HMSO.

Taylor J.F. (ed.) (1995) *Medical Aspects of Fitness to Drive – A Guide for Medical Practitioners*. The Medical Commission on Accident Prevention, 35-43 Lincoln's Inn Fields, London WC2A 3PN.

Motor Vehicles (Driving Licenses) Regulations (1986).

Road Traffic Act (1988) London, HMSO.

Taylor J.F. (1987) Vision and driving. *Ophthal Physiol Opt*, 7(2), 187–189.

ROYAL NAVY

Method of recording: PULHEEMS equivalents (PE)

For medical standards the Navy uses a form of shorthand, the PULHEEMS equivalents, and in vision these are as follows:

Snellen figures:

6/6	6/9	6/12	6/18	6/24	6/36	6/60	< 6/60

PER:

1	2	3	4	5	6	7	8

Right eye	Left eye
PE: unaided	
PE: with spectacles	

Thus unaided vision of 6/24 and corrected visual acuity of 6/6 would be recorded as PE: 5/1.

Eyesight and colour perception standards
Visual acuity (VA)

The following standards are applicable to all personnel on the Active and Reserve Lists of the Royal Navy, Royal Marines and QARNNS who joined the service before 1 January 1995.

There are three standards of visual acuity, graded as follows:

Requirements	Better eye	PE	PE	Worse eye
Standard 1 Visual acuity to be achieved without correcting lenses	6/9 N5	2	3	6/12 N5
Refraction limit				
Total hypermetropia	+ 2.50 sphere			+3.50 sphere
Astigmatism	+ 0.75 cyl			+1.00 cyl
Myopia	− 0.25 sphere or cyl			− 0.75 sphere or cyl

Requirements	Better eye	PE	PE	Worse eye
Standard 1A Visual acuity to be achieved without correcting lenses	6/12 N5	3	3	6/12 N5
Visual acuity to be achieved with correcting lenses	6/6 N5 1	1	1	6/6 N5
Refraction limit (in any meridian)				
Total hypermetropia	+ 3.50 sphere			+ 3.50 sphere
Astigmatism	+ 1.00 cyl			+ 1.00 cyl
Myopia	− 0.75 sphere or cyl			− 0.75 sphere or cyl
Standard 2 Visual acuity to be achieved with or without correcting lenses	Either 6/6 N5 or 6/9 N5 or 6/12 N5	8/1 8/2 8/3	8/5 8/4 8/3	6/24 N10 6/18 N10 6/12 N10
Refraction limit spectacle correction (in any medication)	±7.00 sphere or cyl			±7.00 sphere or cyl

The following standards are applicable to all personnel on the Active and Reserve Lists of the Royal Navy, Royal Marines and QARNNS, who join the service on or after 1 January 1995.

There are four standards of visual acuity, graded as follows:

Requirements	Right eye	PE	PE	Left eye
Standard I Visual acuity to be achieved without correcting lenses	6/12 N5	3	3	6/12 N5
Visual acuity to be achieved with correcting lenses	6/6 N5	1	1	6/6 N5
Refraction limit (in any meridian)				
Total hypermetropia	+3.00 sphere			+3.00 sphere
Astigmatism	+1.25 cyl			+1.25 cyl
Myopia	−0.75 sphere or cyl			−0.75 sphere or cyl
Standard II – Entry Standard Visual acuity to be achieved without correcting lenses	6/24	5	6	6/36
Visual acuity to be achieved with correcting lenses	6/6 N5	5/1	6/2	6/9 N5
Refraction limit (in any meridian)	+3.00 sphere −2.50 sphere or cyl			+3.00 sphere − 2.50 sphere or cyl

(*continued*)

Requirements	Better eye	PE	PE	Worse eye
Standard II – Serving Personnel (on the trained strength)				
Visual acuity to be achieved without correcting lenses	6/60	7	8	<6/60
Visual acuity to be achieved with correcting lenses	6/6 N5	5/1	6/2	6/9 N5
Refraction limit (in any meridian)	± 6.00 sphere or cyl			± 6.00 sphere or cyl
Standard III				
Visual acuity to be achieved without correcting lenses	6/60	7	8	<6/60
Visual acuity to be achieved with correcting lenses	Either 6/6 N5 or 6/9 N5 or 6/12 N5	7/1 7/2 7/3	8/5 8/4 8/3	6/24 N10 6/18 N10 6/12 N10
Refraction limit spectacle correction (in any meridian)	± 6.00 sphere or cyl			± 6.00 sphere or cyl

Standards required:

Specialization/Branch	Visual acuity standard Before 1 Jan 1995	After 1 Jan 1995	Colour perception
Officers			
Aircrew GL, SL, SD	1A	I	1
Other seamen	1A	II	1
S&E officers in SSBNs and SSNs (max correction ± 3.00 D)	1A	II	1
SD(AV), ATC and FDO	2	III	3
RM officers			
GL/SS	2	III	3
Pilots	1A	I	1
Bridge watchkeepers	1A	II	1
All other officers	2	III	4
Ratings			
Operations branch			
Seamen Group	2	NA	3
Missile aimers	1	NA	3
Communications	2	NA	3
Tactical sub branch	2	NA	3
Warfare branch	NA	II	3
except AW/AWW	NA	I	3
WSM	NA	II	4
FAA			
Aircrewmen	1A	I	1
Air Engineer Mechanics	2	III	2
Air Engineer Artificers	2	III	2
FAA other	2	III	3
Survey recorders	1A	II	3

Specialization/Branch	Visual acuity standard Before 1 Jan 1995	After 1 Jan 1995	Colour perception
Sub specializations			
Regulating	2	III	4
Diver			
Photo interpreter	2	III	3
Other RN ratings		III	4
RM other ranks			
Aircrew	1A	I	1
Snipers	1A*	I*	3
Landing Craft	1A*	I*	3
Swimmer canoeists	1A*	I*	3
All other	2	III	4
QARRNS	2	III	4

* Corrective lenses not permitted.

Method of testing

1. Distance visual acuity is tested using Snellen charts viewed directly at a distance of 6 metres (20 feet) or in a properly adjusted mirror at 3 metres. Specifications, including general recommendations on lighting, are contained in British Standard 4274 (1968).
2. Before being given an appointment for an initial medical examination, the recruit is to be questioned as to whether he or she wears glasses or contact lenses and the following procedure adopted.
   a. Recruits who wear spectacles are to be instructed:
   (1) to bring their spectacles with them when attending the medical examination; and
   (2) to bring a written spectacle prescription, which can be obtained from any optician.
   b. Recruits who wear contact lenses (hard or soft) and already have spectacles are:
      (1) to be given an appointment at a date no earlier than that which will allow them not to wear contact lenses for 2 weeks before the medical examination;
   2. to bring their spectacles with them when attending the medical examination;
   3. to bring a written spectacle prescription, which can be obtained from any optician.
   c. Recruits who wear contact lenses but do not own spectacles are:
      (1) to be given an appointment at a date no earlier than that which will allow them not to wear contact lenses for 2 weeks prior to the examination, but to bring them to the examination, if their civilian appointment allows;
   (2) to have their VA checked and recorded unaided first, then to fit their contact lenses and have their aided VA checked and recorded;
   (3) to be warned that should other selection procedures prove successful they will be required to be in possession of spectacles and an appropriate prescription at their initial medical examination;
   (4) Serial 83 of F Med. 1 is to be annotated 'VA checked with CL only'.

Ocular pathology

1. The following previous ocular pathology or surgery are a bar to acceptance for entry to the Royal Navy:
   a. Intra-ocular transplants in young persons
   b. Post-penetrating injuries to either eye
   c. Post-keratotomy (RK) surgery for myopia
   d. Post-photorefractive keratectomy
   e. Post-retinal detachment surgery
   f. Keratoconus.
2. If the examining doctor is in any doubt as to the candidate's acceptability, he is to seek the opinion of the Adviser in Ophthalmology.

NB: Refractive surgery:

- Personnel are to be informed that surgical and laser keratotomy is not available from service sources, and if carried out privately could well have an adverse effect on their future career by rendering them unfit for duty, due to potential side effects.
- Service personnel who have had corneal surgery carried out at their own expense are to be referred to a service consultant ophthalmologist for assessment, when the highest medical category awarded will normally be P3. If serving personnel undergo LASIK then they will be categorized as P3 (Remedial) until seen by a Consultant Adviser in Ophthalmology and assessed, then reviewed by the medical panel, but are unlikely to be rated higher than P3 (Permanent). In selected cases, however, the Consultant Adviser in Ophthalmology may consider higher grading to be more appropriate.
- As new refractive surgery techniques are introduced these will be evaluated. Currently no one is accepted into the Navy having undergone refractive surgery of any type.

Near-vision testing

Near visual acuity is tested using Times Roman print on reading charts approved by the British Faculty of Ophthalmologists (1951–1952).

Colour perception (CP)

1. There are four standards of colour perception graded as follows:

Standard Test specification

(1) The correct recognition of coloured lights shown through the paired apertures on the Holmes-Wright lantern at LOW BRIGHT-NESS at 6 metres (20 feet) distance in complete darkness

(2) The correct recognition of 13 out of the first 15 plates of the Ishihara Test (24-plate abridged edition 1969) shown in random sequence at a distance of 75 cm under standard fluorescent lighting supplied by an artificial daylight fluorescent lamp (British Standard 950, 1967)

(3) The correct recognition of coloured lights shown through the paired apertures on the Holmes-Wright lantern at HIGH BRIGHT-NESS at 6 metres (20 feet) distance in complete darkness

(4) The correct recognition of colours used in relevant trade situations, and assessed by simple tests with coloured wires, resistors, stationery tabs etc.

2. Personnel who fail to reach the minimum standard of colour perception are to be graded CP5 – failed trade test and colour expanses.

Methods of testing colour perception – Ishihara test

1. Ishihara plates are used as a screening for all entries.
2. Candidates who pass the Ishihara test are graded CP2 and require no further testing except for those whose critical visual task requires a categorization of CP1.
3. Candidates who fail the Ishihara test are further tested for CP3 or CP4 according to requirement.

Methods of testing colour perception – Holmes-Wright lantern

1. The Holmes-Wright Lantern is constructed to simulate, in controlled conditions, the critical visual task of seamen.
2. The test must be carried out at a distance of 6 metres (20 feet) in a completely darkened room. The candidate may wear spectacles if he wishes and may be 'dark adapted' if necessary. The colour pairs may be changed by rotating the colour setting flange at the rear of the lantern, the colour pairs presented being indicated by the code number visible in windows on each side and at the rear of the lantern.
3. Full Naval instructions on the operation of the lantern are available from the AOP office.

Retesting of colour perception

1. Colour perception does not normally change

Function	Efficiency	Applicable
Maddox Rod @ 6 m	Esophoria 6Δ Exophoria 6Δ Hyperphoria 1Δ	a) SD(X) b) Observers FL(X), SL, SD c) Engineering/S&S Officers and ratings d) RM pilots and aircrew
Maddox Rod @ 33 cm	Esophoria 6Δ Exophoria 16Δ Hyperphoria 1Δ	a) Observers FL(X), SL, SD b) RM pilots and aircrew
Other functions	Recovery on cover test must be rapid, convergence must be maintained at less than 10 cm, stereopsis must be present	a) Observers FL(X), SL, SD b) RM pilots and aircrew

significantly throughout life. It will require re-testing, therefore, only in certain circumstances:

a. Before employment in a specialization requiring a different colour perception standard as shown in the regulations, and
b. If there is any doubt concerning the existing grading.

2. Retesting is to be carried out by a Naval eye specialist at the request of a Medical Officer.

Binocular efficiency

Bifoveal fixation and perfect binocular functions are not essential requirements unless specified, but a squint must be cosmetically acceptable. Limits to heterophoria where applicable are shown in the table above.

Spectacles and contact lenses

1. There is in general no restriction on the wearing of spectacles or contact lenses (including on board submarines) provided that the required corrected standards of visual acuity are met. Contact lenses may not, however, be worn under AGRs or by Aircrew. Those who may wear contact lenses and chose to do so must always have a pair of Defence spectacles to wear as an alternative. Defence spectacles are provided from public funds if required for the efficient performance of duties; contact lenses are not.

Use of contact lenses

1. Contact lenses may well provide advantages over spectacles, enhancing peripheral vision and reducing reflection and aberration. They are also more compatible than spectacles with specialist equipment such as night vision goggles. Gas-permeable hard contact lenses cannot be recommended for military use as they cannot be worn on an extended wear basis should the need arise. Tinted lenses are also not permissible. The decision whether or not to wear contact lenses must remain with the individual. The individual must also be responsible for ensuring proper care of contact lenses. The vast majority of complications and ocular pathology arising from contact lens wear are associated with inadequate care of the contact lenses. Lenses must be of a soft type and are to be used on a daily wear basis but to have the facility for extended wear if required; that is to say that in normal working they should be inserted at the start of the working day and removed before any periods of sleep but could be left in for an extended period should the operational need arise. The extended period should not be more than 7 days.

2. At all times a pair of spectacles of up-to-date prescription must be available to the individual. If either eye becomes red or painful the individual must remove both contact lenses and return to wearing his or her spectacles and report to a MO within 24 hours.

3. Contact lenses are not permitted in operational service diving.

Deterioration of eyesight in service

Any serving personnel whose unaided vision in the better eye falls below 6/60, or who requires correction of greater than ± 6.00 dioptres, is to be referred for ophthalmic opinion and then to MBOS for determination of permanent medical category.

1. *Application of Revised Standard (1 Jan 1995).* Revised eyesight standards, which came into operation with effect 1 Jan 1995, apply to all personnel joining after that date and serving personnel on application for change of branch or Upper Yardsman/Special Duties List commission.

2. *Bridge watchkeepers.* Officers with bridge watchkeeping responsibilities are required to remain within VA Standard II (corrected) and should be tested annually to ensure that this standard is maintained. Those with the following restrictions must be referred to the Consultant Adviser in Ophthalmology and thence to Medical Board of Survey (MBOS) to determine permanent medical category.
   a. Those whose VA cannot be corrected to VA II
   b. Those who require greater than 6 dioptres correction to achieve VA II
   c. Those whose uncorrected vision is worse than 6/60 in either eye.

3. *Aircrew.* Aircrew who are found for the first time to require corrective lenses are to be refracted and then referred to Central Air and Admiralty Medical Board (CAAMB) for assessment of their flying medical category.

4. *Submarine seaman specialists.* Submarine seaman specialists whose correction is greater than ±3.00 dioptres (i.e. outside the range of periscope optical correction) are to be referred for an ophthalmic opinion and thence to the Senior Medical Officer Submarines, Institute of Naval Medicine.

5. *Seaman ratings.* Applicants for entry must meet Visual Standard II. However, OM ratings for AW/AWW specialization must achieve Visual Standard I in service.

Refraction

These eyesight standards set limits to the amount of refractive error allowed, and it is essential that this is determined at the entry medical examination:

a. Hypermetropia. In a young person, considerable hypermetropia may be present without any apparent effect on either near or distance vision. To detect its presence and the amount, plus spherical lenses of successively increasing strengths should be placed in a trial frame in front of both eyes together and the effect on the candidate's distance vision is an approximate measure of the manifest hypermetropia present. Borderline cases should be referred to an ophthalmic specialist.

b. Myopia. Short sight affects distance visual acuity and its presence is obvious. The candidates should be asked to provide a spectacle prescription, which will show the degree of myopia present.

Other abnormalities of the eyes or visual system

Any abnormalities of the eye or visual system (congenital, traumatic or pathological) may be cause for rejection even though visual function is within the standard limits; a decision regarding visual fitness for duty must then be made by a consultant ophthalmologist.

Royal Marines GL/SS officer entrants

Royal Marines GL/SS Officer entrants who are CP4 may be accepted at the discretion of CGRM after advice from the Consultant Adviser in Ophthalmology.

ROYAL AIR FORCE
Visual standards applicable for acceptance for flying and non-flying personnel

The following are the minimum visual standards for acceptance for service in the Royal Air Force. These standards are subject to alteration without notice and no responsibility for consequences arising as a result of these changes can be accepted by the Ministry of Defence (Air). The decision as to the individual's fitness is the prerogative of the Medical Board which examines him/her.

Definitions of colour perception

CP2   No errors are made using Ishihara plates in daylight or artificial light of equivalent quality. Tests carried out under normal tungsten or fluorescent lighting are not acceptable except where the ADLAKE lamp is used

CP3 Although errors are made using Ishihara plates the candidate is readily able to recognize the colours used in aviation. At present the Holmes-Wright lantern is the only recognized test.

CP4 Unable to pass Standard 3.

Artificial aids as a means of passing a colour vision test (e.g. colour correction contact lenses such a XChrom and Chromagen) have not been assessed and currently would not be permitted.

Definitions of acuity

The RAF uses code numbers for acuity measurement (e.g. 5/2), where the upper number is the unaided vision and the lower is the corrected visual acuity.

The codes are:

1	6/6	2	6/9	3	6/12	4	6/18
5	6/24	6	6/36	7	6/60	8	< 6/60

Thus 5/2 is unaided vision of 6/24, corrected acuity of 6/9.

Trade group numbers (TG)

TG	Trade
1	Aircraft engineering
2	Electronic engineering (Air)
3	Electronic engineering (Ground)
4	Obsolete
5	General engineering
6	Mechanical transport
7	Marine Craft
8	Gunner/fireman/police
9	Air traffic control
10	General Services (admin, GD and PTIs)
11	Telecommunications/radio operators
12	Aerospace systems operators
13	Safety and surface (survival equipment, and painter/finisher)
14	Photography
15	Medical
16	Dental
17	Accounting and secretarial
18	Supply and movements
19	Catering
20	Obsolete
21	Music

Refractive surgery: A history of refractive surgery of any type is a bar to entry into the RAF.

Pathology: As part of the examination the fundus will be viewed by the medical examiner, who will refer the applicant to an ophthalmologist for an opinion in the event of any defects being found.

Visual standards at selection: ground trades

Visual acuity

All RAF ground trades require 8/2 8/2 at entry except:

a. Sentry mission crew, TG9 and TG12 and SNCO fighter controllers, who require 8/1 8/1

b. Aerial erectors, RAF police (aerial erectors refraction range −0.25 to +2.00 D)

c. RAF PTIs – 5/1 5/1

d. Steward – 5/2 5/2

e. MT drivers – 7/2 7/2 with no allowance for amblyopia

f. Photographic interpreters and air cartographers – 7/1 7/1. In addition the following apply:

   (1) No history of migraine, blepharitis or ocular allergy
   (2) Refraction range − 2.00 to +2.00 dioptres, astigmatic component W 1.50 dioptres
   (3) Convergence 10 cm or better
   (4) Eso 5 Δ to exo 10 Δ , ±1 Δ vertical
   (5) Normal stereoscopic vision.

g. Fire-fighter – 1/− 1/− (Correction not allowed on entry).

Colour perception

Colour perception requirements for the ground trades are as follows:

a. CP2: Trade Groups 1, 2, 3, 5, 6, 9, 12, 13, 14, 18 (Q-sup-F, Q-sup-X and Movs Con AER appointments)

b. CP3: Trade Groups 8, 10, 11 (TCO), 18 Movs Cont and Movs Op in non-AER appointments, 19 Steward

c. CP4: All other ground trades.

Visual standards at selection: regular air crew

	Visual Acuity (minimum)			Refraction Range[1]		Muscle Balance Maddox Ros	Converg	Accomodation (with correction)	CP	Stereopsis TNO Test
	Uncorr[2]	Corr[2]	Near[3]	Spherical Component	Cylinder					
Pilot	6/12[4]		N5	Plano to +1.75 DS (Army & RN −0.75 to +1.75)	+0.75 DC (RN +1.25 DC)	Dist eso 6Δ to exo 8Δ ≤ 1Δ Vertical	≤ 10 cm			120 secs of arc
Navigator	6/24	6/6		−1.25 to +3.00 DS		Near eso 6Δ to exo 16Δ ≤ 1Δ Vertical		Age 17–20: ≤ 11 cm	3	120 secs of arc
ALMI (inc SAR duties)[5]	6/9			−0.25 to +3.00 DS	+1.25 DC					
ALM2 (Exc SAR duties)	6/24			−1.50 to +3.00 DS		No standard[6]		Age 21–25: 11–13 cm	2	
Sentry Mission Crew	/60[7]			−4.00 to +4.00 DS	+2.00 DC					
Air Signaller	6/60[7]					Laid down			4	
Air Engineer				−2.00 to +3.00 DS	+1.25 DC					
Air Electronics Operator										
Air Electronics Officer									3	

1. All aircrew: Manifest hypermetropia < + 2.50 DS (Initial Medical Board only).
2. If the examiner considers the candidate requires corrective flying spectacles (CFS) he is to be assessed A2 and awarded the appropriate restriction (see leaflets 2-03 and 5-14E). Pending delivery he may continue to fly unless it is considered unsafe to do so.
3. Each eye separately at the appropriate distance for age, with spectacles if applicable, as determined from the appropriate Duane scale or RAF binocular gauge test. The spectacles prescribed should enable the examinee to achieve an adequate standard of near vision for the aircraft he operates.
4. Tri-service minimum entry V/A standard. Single service refraction limits may demand a better uncorrected V/A.
5. An in-service deterioration of 3/1, 3/1 is permissible. CFS may be worn in the aircraft but must be removed before descending on the winch wire. Contact lenses are permissible in the cabin and on the wire when worn in accordance with the policy detailed in leaflet 5-14E.
6. Alternating strabismus which is cosmetically satisfactory and where each eye sees 6/6, with correction if necessary, may be accepted. However, if the examiner considers any candidate has an abnormality that may affect the full performance of his duty, he should be referred for assessment by the CA in ophthalmology.
7. Visual acuity worse than 6/36 requires referral to the CA in ophthalmology.

Visual standards at selection: non-regular aircrew (civilians, UAS, ATC and ground branch)

	Visual acuity (min)			Refraction range[1]		Muscle balance (Maddox Rod)	Converg	Accommodation (with correction)	CP	Stereopsis TNO Test
	Uncorr	Corr[2]	Near[3]	Spherical component	Cylinder					
Non Regular Aircrew* Civil Servants Contractors' pilots DHFS P/T Reserve Aircrew AEF Staff pilots	6/36	6/6	N5	−0.75 to 3.00 DS DHFS/Reserve aircrew (non pilot) – see note 4	+1.25 DC	Dist; eso 6Δ To exo 8Δ/ ≤ Δ Vertical Near: eso 6Δ to Exo 16Δ/1Δ Vertical	≤ 10 cm	Age 17–20: ≤11 cm Age 21–25: 11–13 cm	3 3/4[5]	120 secs of arc
Gliding Instructors	6/12			−0.75 to +3.00 DS		No standard for DHFS/Reserve aircrew			3	
Flight Medical Officer	6/60[6]	6/12[6]		5.00 D in any axis[7]						
UAS Flying Branches	As Regular Aircrew[8]									
UAS Ground Branches (RAFVR, bursars & cadets limited flying training)	6/60[9]	6/12	N5	5.00 D in any axis[7]					3	
Air/CCF Cadets		6/9	–	–	–				4	–
Air Stewards	6/24					–			3	
Passengers (inc research subjects)	No visual standards laid down									

1. *Aircrew: manifest hypermetropia < + 2.50 DS (Initial Medical Board only)
2. If the examiner considers the candidate requires CFS he is to be assessed A2 and awarded the appropriate restriction (see leaflets 2–03 and 5-14E). Pending delivery he may continue to fly unless it is considered unsafe to do so.
3. Each eye separately at the appropriate distance for the age, with spectacles if applicable, as determined from the appropriate Duane scale or RAF binocular guage test. The spectacles prescribed should enable the examinee to achieve an adequate standard of near vision for the aircraft he operates.
4. The refractive range for DHFS/Reserve aircrew (non-pilot) at selection is the same as that required for the equivalent regular crew position (leaflet 4–02 Annex A). Waivers for acceptance outside these limits may be granted by the CA in ophthalmology.
5. CP3 required for staff of the Central Gliding School and by any pilot who carries out ferry duties. CP4 is acceptable for all other pilots.
6. The limitation 'fit flight medical officer flying only' (Code 071) is to be awarded if the V/A in either eye tested separately is worse than 6/12 (uncorrected) or 6/6 (corrected). If the flight medical officer is unable to meet the minimum visual standard for the award of 'fit flight medical officer flying only', but is otherwise fit, he is to be referred to a service ophthalmologist for assessment of his fitness to fly.
7. Candidates outside this limit are to be referred for ophthalmic assessment.
8. Pilots with a V/A of 6/9 in one or both eyes, and navigators with a V/A of 6/24 in one or both eyes are to be referred for ophthalmic assessment.
9. Candidates who are otherwise fit for flying who have a V/A in one or both eyes are to be referred for ophthalmic assessment.

Visual standards at selection: officers of ground branches

Branch	Right eye[1]	Left eye[1]	Colour vision (CP)
Engineer[2]			
Photography	4/1	4/1	2
All other branches	8/2	8/2	2
Supply and movements[3]	8/2	8/2	2
Administration			
Secretarial	8/2	8/2	4
Physical education	5/1	5/1	3
Catering	8/2	8/2	4
Training	8/2	8/2	4
Security – Provost	7/2	7/2	4
Operations support			
RAF Regiment	8/2	8/2	4
Air traffic control	8/1	8/1	2
Fighter control[4]			
Aviation officer grade			
Flight operations	8/1	8/1	2
Intelligence[5]	7/1	7/1	2
Medical, dental, nursing[6, 7]	8/2	8/2	4
Legal	8/2	8/2	4
Chaplains	8/2	8/2	4
Director of music	8/2	8/2	4

Notes:

1. Candidates for branches in which the minimum uncorrected vision is 8/ 8/ (i.e. less than 6/60 in each eye) may not be accepted unless the following conditions are met:

   a. The fundi are normal
   b. There is no other pathological condition of the eyes
   c. Considering each eye separately, the spherical correction lies within the range −7.00 to +8.00 dioptres, and the astigmatic correction is ≤ 5.00 dioptres.

2. The colour perception standard required of officers appointed to all types of commission in the engineering branches is CP2. However, officers with a colour perception of CP4 may be appointed under certain conditions.
3. Officers in the Supply & Movements Branch employed on explosives or fuel duties must have colour perception standard CP2.
4. Candidates will not be accepted with a history of migraine, and serving individuals who develop migraine are referred for consultant opinion.
5. The minimum visual standards for Operations Support (Intelligence) are as follows:

   a. No history of migraine, blepharitis or ocular allergy
   b. Refractive limits − 2.00 to + 2.00 in any meridian
   c. Astigmatic error ≤ 1.50 dioptres
   d. Convergence 10 cm or better
   e. Muscle balance (Maddox Wing) Eso 5Δ to Exo 10 Δ, 1Δ vertical
   f. Normal stereoscopic vision (orthoptic stereo slide, Wirt, JSPI stereo card).

6. Many drugs and medical materials are colour coded, and some laboratory tests involve the use of colour comparators. Restrictions are applied on those in the medical branches with defective colour vision.
7. Medical Officers selected for Flight Medical Officer training must meet the same standards as regular pilots and have a corrected VA of no worse than 6/12 in each eye. If the uncorrected VA is worse than 6/60 or the required correction is greater than 5.00 dioptres, he or she is to be referred to a service ophthalmologist for assessment.

POLICE

The following are guidelines issued by the Home Office. However certain police forces, including Cambridgeshire, Hampshire, Humberside, Kent, Lincolnshire, Metropolitan*, Surrey, Sussex, Warwickshire, West Midlands, Scotland** continue to set their own standards. In addition many forces set different standards for the Mounted Branch. Practitioners are advised to seek clarification from the force concerned. The decision to recruit an individual lies with the Chief Constable.

System	Reject	Consider carefully	Comments
Vision	Squint; History of detached retina; History of glaucoma; Radial keratotomy; Photorefractive; Keratoplasty	Latent squint; Lens implant; Corneal graft with good uncorrected visual acuity	
Visual acuity unaided	Worse than 6/24 in either eye (binocular worse than 6/6 requires correction)	Between 6/18 and 6/24. Following the change in age restrictions, consider the effects of age on acuity	Some current Force standards are more strict than this where there may be special circumstances e.g. firearms in RUC. An independent specialist eye opinion may be helpful on occasions
Aided	Worse than 6/12 in either eye, with binocular worse than 6/6		
Colour vision	Failure on City University Test	Failure on Ishihara test	Current City University Test rationale states 7 out of 10 correct responses is within NORMAL limits

NB: The use of colour vision correcting lenses (e.g. x-chrom, chromagen) is not acceptable.

In addition, some police forces require visual fields to be checked. The standard is that applying to holders of a driving licence, but a confrontation test is considered adequate.

- 120° horizontal
- 20° above and below the horizontal throughout the 120°
- No isolated binocular scotoma close to fixation.

*Metropolitan Police:

Unaided vision	RE 6/24	LE 6/24	BE /24
Correction required if worse than	Better eye 6/6	Worse eye 6/12	BE 6/6
Corrected:	Better eye 6/6	Worse eye 6/12	BE 6/6

**Scotland:

As above table except:

System	Reject	Consider carefully
Vision	History of detached retina;	Latent squint; Lens implant;

Scotland continued:

	History of glaucoma; Radial keratotomy	Corneal graft with good uncorrected visual acuity; Congenital eye defects; Photorefractive keratoplasty – consider 1 year after successful surgery

ARMY
Minimum visual standards
Candidates for the Royal Military Academy, Sandhurst, who are to join the Infantry, Foot Guards or Parachute Regiment may be accepted with a visual acuity of 6/9 or above in the right eye; otherwise candidates for the Royal Military Academy, Sandhurst, Army Scholarships and University Cadetships require a minimum visual acuity with spectacles of 6/6 in one eye and not less than 6/36 in the other. Normally the right eye must be correctable to 6/6 except in the R. Sigs, RAChD, Army Medical Service, REME, AGC and Int Corps, where the right

eye may be the worse. Officer cadets for RLC must have the vision in the left eye correctable to 6/12.

Soldiers are accepted with a minimum corrected visual acuity between 6/6 and 6/12, depending on the regiment or corps, in the right eye, and 6/36 in the left eye. Driving grades require vision in the left eye to be correctable to 6/12, and certain safety critical trades require vision to 6/6 bilaterally with spectacles.

Myopia exceeding 7 dioptres in any meridian in either eye or hypermetropia exceeding 8 dioptres precludes acceptance even if vision is correctable to the required standard.

Diseases of the eye
Any pathological condition is liable to be a cause of rejection of military service.

Any form of refractive surgery, including radial keratotomy, PRK and excimer laser surgery is a bar to military service.

Colour perception (CP) standards
Three classifications are applied:

CP2	No errors made on Ishihara plates in daylight or using artificial light source of equivalent quality
CP3	Inability to achieve CP2 standard, but able to recognize signal colours on the approved lantern test. This is normally Holmes-Wright lantern
CP4	Inability to achieve Grade 3

Failure to achieve CP2 will restrict employment to certain grades.

Contact lens users
Candidates who normally wear contact lenses (hard or soft) and who are due to attend for medical examination for entry into the Army are required to refrain from wearing their lenses for 2 weeks prior to the examination. They should bring their spectacles to the examination, if in possession, and a written copy of their prescription obtained within the last year. They are not required to obtain spectacles in advance of the examination if they do not already have them, but will require to obtain them if they are successful in any selection procedures.

These notes are for guidance only. Each case must be judged on its merits, and the final decision as to a candidate's fitness will be made by the appropriate Army Medical Board.

GUIDANCE ON VISUAL STANDARDS FOR VDU USERS
The Association of Optometrists recommends the following guidance to practitioners on visual standards for VDU users:

- The ability to read N6 throughout the range 75–33 cm with adequate visual acuity for any task undertaken at a greater distance, if this is an integral part of the work.
- Well-established monocular vision or good binocular vision. Phorias at working distances should be corrected unless well-compensated or deep suppression is present.
- No central (20°) field defects in the dominant eye.
- Near point of convergence normal.
- Clear ocular media checked by ophthalmoscopy.

The above guidance is intended to increase the level of operator comfort and efficiency. It is not a set of inflexible criteria, and should not be used to exclude persons from working with VDUS.

Display screen equipment (DSE)/visual display unit (VDU) eye examinations
The following advice sheet can be issued to employers, together with the VDU/DSE report form.

The Regulations
The Health and Safety (Display Screen Equipment) Regulations came into force on 1 January 1993. Many employers find that the Regulations are beneficial in improving employee morale and reducing stress, but the take up of the eye examination provision is considerably lower than originally anticipated. There are still misunderstandings concerning the regulations by employers, employees and optometrists.

Employer's responsibility: what is expected of you
The employer is responsible for the health and safety of all who work in his or her premises. The Display Screen Regulations 1992 impose on management

specific responsibilities for the care of direct employees, who in the Regulations are termed 'users'. These duties are additional to the general duties of care required to satisfy other legislation.

All employed habitual users of Display Screen Equipment are entitled to eye examinations paid for by their employer. It is normally agreed that 'habitual' means regularly using a terminal for spells of over 1 hour – less if mistakes can have a critical effect, e.g. in situations where errors can have serious consequences. The acceptance by the user of a visual screening check, whatever the result, does not remove the entitlement to a full eye examination. Vision screening, if carried out annually, may have a useful role to play in identifying users who need a re-examination.

The employer is also required to pay for any spectacles *specifically* required for VDU use. The employer does not have to pay for spectacles which were not prescribed under the employer's arrangements, nor for the provision or updating of normal spectacles, even if these are used for display screen work. The employer can, when making arrangements for employees, choose a suitable range of basic frames to satisfy the requirements of the Regulations and to provide some choice to the employee.

Optometrist's responsibility: what you should expect

The purpose of the examination is to increase comfort and accuracy when using a display screen, and covers all aspects of workstation use. The optometrist requires some detail of the workstation design, lighting, ventilation, work routine and training. All these can affect symptoms, and in undertaking an eye examination the optometrist will keep in mind the other requirements of the DSE Regulations. The user should provide workstation measurements such as the distance at which the screen is viewed, the distance of the keyboard and that of any written or printed papers used at the workstation. These should be measured in each case. Documents supplied which specify pre-printed rather than individual measurements for that workstation are not adequate.

The examination will include the provisions of the Sight test as defined by the Opticians Act 1989, but will be extended to take into account the needs of the individual user in relation to the DSE Regulations. To ensure that all the requirements of the DSE Regulations are satisfied, the optometrist should know, at the outset, that he/she is conducting an examination under the DSE Regulations. The employer should not try to make arrangements retrospectively. Adequate time should be allowed by the optometrist for the discussion of problems and methods of alleviating them. The extra time needed will probably be reflected in the fee charged for this work. An examination carried out without reference to DSE will probably not record sufficient detail for subsequent advice relating to DSE work. Additional charges should be expected for detailed reports. (A suitable form follows this section.) Such reports cannot be given without the consent of the employee. The findings of the eye examination remain confidential even when paid for by the employer, unless the employee specifically gives permission for this information to be divulged.

It is preferable for the employee to choose the examining optometrist rather than have a practitioner preselected by an employer. This has the advantage of permitting continuity of eye care and maintaining the confidence of the user. Such arrangements fit well into the requirements of the Display Screen Regulations. Employers should be wary of selecting an optometrist purely on the basis of the lowest fee being charged, as an examination carried out without reference to DSE will probably not record sufficient detail for subsequent advice relating to DSE work.

It needs to be emphasized that failure to meet the recommended visual standards does not constitute an automatic debarment to continue with DSE or VDU work.

VDU spectacles

In a minority of cases, 'specific' spectacles are required. The employer pays for such basic appliances, but should not be expected to pay for any fashion element. It is very rare for a first correction or replacement near vision spectacle to be required solely for display screen use. In some countries 'specific need' is more broadly interpreted as a 'a major use of the spectacles'. The Health and Safety Executive, in consultation with the major optometry bodies, has taken the view that 'specific' is based upon correcting the screen range with possible additional help for closer or further objects as appropriate.

In order to be appropriate for the work undertaken, it may be necessary to prescribe spectacles in multifocal form for some older users. These will normally incorporate an intermediate (screen distance) upper lens together with a reading section. Often these spectacles will be inappropriate for use other than with display screens. If the work includes visual tasks at distances away from the workstation, trifocals or varifocals may be necessary to achieve these tasks. A tinted lens would not normally be prescribed in spectacles specifically for VDU use, unless this tint is clinically necessary and also incorporated in the person's normal spectacles. However many employers' schemes offer to pay sufficient to cover the cost of single vision lenses only, e.g. to pay for a proportion of the total cost involved. Such schemes are likely to be in breach of the Regulations and the employer cannot be absolved from the obligation to provide for more costly lenses, should the optometrist consider them a necessity. Even if the paper work is in copyholders at screen distance, the lighting requirements for screen and paper work differ widely and may not be resolved satisfactorily with single vision lenses.

Most VDU users do **not** need specific spectacle correction for workstation use. The eye examination offers the opportunity to advise how the user can increase comfort. The person's own spectacles will normally cope satisfactorily with the work until the user is well into middle age. Where a younger person requires a specific correction it is not unreasonable for the employer to expect the prescribing optometrist to state the reasons.

CIVIL AVIATION AUTHORITY

The following are excerpts from the standards issued by the Joint Aviation Authorities. They should not be taken as a definitive statement of the full regulations. For further information contact the CAA medical department at Aviation House, Gatwick Airport South, West Sussex, RH6 0YR; tel. 01293 573683; fax 01293 573995.

These standards apply to all new applicants in applicable categories from April 1999 and the renewal of medical certificates from 1 July 1999.

Under the new system, the Joint Aviation Requirements (JAR), there are two classes of medical assessment as follows:

Class 1   Commercial pilot (aeroplane and helicopter) Airline transport pilot (aeroplane and helicopter)
Class 2   Private pilot (aeroplane and helicopter)

The visual standards for air traffic control officers, flight engineers, flight navigators, balloon operators (passenger carrying) and microlight pilots are still covered by UK guidelines, which are unchanged from the previous UK standards.

JAR Class 1

a. There shall be no abnormality of the function of the eyes or their adnexae, or any active pathological condition, congenital or acquired, acute or chronic, or any sequelae of eye surgery or trauma, which is likely to interfere with the safe exercise of the privileges of the applicable licence.

b. A comprehensive ophthalmological examination is required at the initial examination.

c. A routine eye examination shall form part of all revalidation and renewal examinations.

d. A comprehensive ophthalmological examination is required in conjunction with revalidation and renewal examinations at the following intervals:
   (1) Every 5 years to the 40th birthday
   (2) Once every 2 years thereafter. CAA appointed doctors (Authorised Medical Examiners) can undertake ophthalmological assessments on pilots up to the age of 50 years, after which slit lamp examination and tonometry will be required.

e. Distant visual acuity, with or without correction, shall be 6/9 or better monocularly, and 6/6 or better binocularly.

f. If the visual requirement is met only with the use of correction, the spectacles or contact lenses must provide optimal visual function and should be suitable for aviation purposes.

g. At initial examination the refractive error shall not exceed ± 3.00 dioptres along the most ametropic meridian with no more than ± 2.00 dioptres astigmatic component and no more than 2.00 dioptres of anisometropia.

h. If the refractive error is within the range −3/−5 dioptres, the Aeromedical Section may consider Class I certification if:

VDU eye examination report
Name and Address of Employer
EMPLOYER:

The employee named below is a VDU user as defined under the DSE regulations. Please complete the following form and return to me after undertaking the eye examination:

Name of employee:	Distance from eye (in cm) to: Keyboard: Screen:
Type of Work Involved:	
	Documents:
Other relevant factors:	Position of top of screen relative to eye level: _____ cm above/below.

OPTOMETRIST:

I confirm that I am acquainted with the Association of Optometrists guidelines on the visual requirements of VDU users as defined in the current edition of the AOP handbook and the following is the result of my examination.

Result of examination	Tick one only	See note
Satisfies the standard without visual correction	☐	
Satisfies the standard with the current visual correction	☐	
Satisfies the standard with a new visual correction specifically for VDU use	☐	a
Satisfies the standard with a new visual correction but not specifically for VDU use	☐	
Does not satisfy the standard	☐	b
Further VDU examination required in _____ years	☐	

Notes:

a Spectacles specifically for VDU use should only be supplied when these are necessary and when spectacles for any other use (such as driving, TV or reading) cannot be used. This will apply, for example, when the layout of the screen and/or documents is such that an intermediate focus is required and the user cannot see at this distance with any other spectacles. If you have ticked box 3, please indicate below the lens type advised and your reasons for prescribing spectacles *specifically* for VDU use.

Type of spectacle required:

Single vision	Bifocal	Progressive	Other identify
Reason for supply:			

b The aim of the standard in the guidelines is to ensure comfortable vision and is not proscriptive. Established VDU users who are symptomless, or whose symptoms can be alleviated with appropriate measures, who can undertake the work required, and yet who do not meet the standard should not be prevented from continuing to work with a VDU even if they do not meet the standard suggested.

Name of optometrist:	Name and address of practice:
Signature of optometrist:	
Date:	

(1) No significant pathology can be demonstrated
(2) The refraction has remained stable for at least 4 years after the age of 17 years
(3) Visual correction by contact lenses has been considered
(4) Experience satisfactory to the Authority has been demonstrated.

i. An applicant shall be able to read N5 at 30–50 cm and N14 at 100 cm with correction if prescribed.

j. An applicant with diplopia or significant defects of binocular vision shall be assessed as unfit. There is no requirement for stereopsis.

k. Monocularity entails unfitness for Class I certificate. Central vision in one eye below the limits may be considered for Class I *re-certification* if binocular visual fields are normal and the underlying pathology is acceptable according to ophthalmic specialist assessment. A satisfactory flight test is required and operations limited to multi-pilot only.

l. An applicant with convergence which is not normal shall be assessed as unfit.

m. An applicant with heterophorias exceeding limits (see Table) shall be assessed as unfit unless the fusional reserves are sufficient to prevent asthenopia and diplopia.

n. An applicant with visual fields which are not normal shall be assessed as unfit.

o. An applicant shall have normal perception of colours (defined as no mistakes on Ishihara plates (24-plate version) tested in daylight or in artificial light of the same colour temperature such as that provided by illuminant C or D) or be colour safe. Applicants who fail Ishihara shall be assessed as colour safe if they pass extensive testing with methods acceptable to the Aeromedical Section (Holmes-Wright lantern or anomaloscope).

p. An applicant who fails the acceptable colour perception tests is to be considered colour unsafe and shall be assessed as unfit.

JAR Class 2

a. There shall be no abnormality of the function of the eyes or their adnexae, or any active pathological condition, congenital or acquired, acute or chronic, or any sequelae of eye surgery or trauma, which is likely to interfere with the safe exercise of the privileges of the applicable licence.

b. At examination, an applicant requiring visual correction to meet the standards shall submit a copy of the current spectacle prescription.

c. At each aeromedical renewal examination, an assessment of the visual fitness of the licence holder shall be performed and the eyes shall be examined with regard to possible pathology. All abnormal and doubtful cases shall be referred to a specialist in aviation ophthalmology acceptable to the Aeromedical Section.

d. Distant visual acuity, with or without correction, shall be 6/12 or better monocularly, and 6/6 or better binocularly. No limits apply to uncorrected visual acuity.

e. If the visual requirement is met only with the use of correction, the spectacles or contact lenses must provide optimal visual function and should be suitable for aviation purposes.

f. At initial examination the refractive error shall not exceed ± 5.00 dioptres along the most ametropic meridian with no more than ± 3.00 dioptres astigmatic component and no more than 3.00 dioptres of anisometropia.

g. If the refractive error is within the range −5/−8 dioptres, the Aeromedical Section may consider Class II certification if:

(1) No significant pathology can be demonstrated
(2) The refraction has remained stable for at least 4 years after the age of 17 years
(3) Visual correction by contact lenses has been considered.

h. An applicant shall be able to read N5 at 30–50 cm and N14 at 100 cm with correction if prescribed.

i. An applicant with diplopia or significant defects of binocular vision shall be assessed as unfit. There is no requirement for stereopsis.

j. In an applicant with amblyopia, the visual acuity of the amblyopic eye shall be 6/18 or better and may be accepted as fit provided the visual acuity in the other eye is 6/6 or better. In the case of reduction of vision in one eye to below the limits, **re-certification** may be considered if underlying pathology and the visual ability of the remaining eye are acceptable following ophthalmic evaluation acceptable to the Aeromedical Section and subject to a satisfactory medical flight test, if indicated.

k. An applicant with visual fields which are not normal shall be assessed as unfit.
l. An applicant shall have normal perception of colours (defined as no mistakes on Ishihara plates (24-plate version) tested in daylight or in artificial light of the same colour temperature such as that provided by illuminant C or D) or be colour safe. Applicants who fail Ishihara shall be assessed as colour safe if they pass extensive testing with methods acceptable to the Aeromedical Section (Holmes–Wright lantern or anomaloscope).
m. An applicant who fails the acceptable colour perception tests is to be considered colour unsafe and shall be assessed as unfit.
n. A colour unsafe applicant may be assessed by the Aeromedical Section as fit to fly within the flight information region of Joint Aviation Authority member states, visual flight rules by day only.

All JAR licence holders

Any spectacles necessary must be available for immediate use, and so there is no time to take them on or off. An applicant who needs a correction to meet the near visual acuity will require look-over or multifocal lenses in order to read the instruments and a manual held in the hand, and also to make use of distance vision through the windscreen without removing the lenses. The CAA does not proscribe any type of visual correction except a single vision full lens near correction. All types of contact lenses except bifocal are permissible.

An applicant is expected to advise the optometrist of relevant reading distances for the flight deck. The occupational needs may then be fulfilled by bifocal, trifocal or varifocal lenses. On occasions an intermediate correction in the upper field may be required, which may be accomplished by a segment of the relevant power in addition to the bifocal or varifocal design. Flip-up spectacles are also acceptable.

Sunglasses may often be required, and their use is encouraged. Tints should be neutral grey, but polarized lenses are not permitted and photochromic lenses are discouraged. An additional pair of untinted spectacles must be carried.

Contact lenses are permissible, but if soft lenses are used they should not be high water content due to the low relative humidity of the cockpit (often < 15 per cent). Bifocal contact lenses are not approved.

Colour vision enhancement lenses

Congenital (colour) defects are unaltered with age and cannot, contrary to what is sometimes claimed, be treated in any way. Tinted filters, e.g. the so-called X-Chrom lens, make possible a better discrimination of some confusion colours, but do not improve colour perception. Applicants passing a colour test by use of such a device are not colour safe.

Note: Refractive surgery entails unfitness. Re-certification for class I and certification for class II may be considered by the Aeromedical Section 12 months after the date of refractive surgery provided that:

a. Pre-operative refraction was less than 5 dioptres (myopia)
b. Satisfactory stability of refraction has been achieved (less than 0.75 dioptres variation diurnally)
c. Glare sensitivity is not increased.

To achieve uniformity in the measurement of visual acuity, the following shall be adopted:

a. In a lighted room, the test illumination level will be approximately 50 lux, normally corresponding to a brightness of 30 candelas per square metre.
b. Visual acuity should be measured by means of a series of optotypes of Landolt, or similar optotypes at a distance of 5 or 6 metres from the candidate with the appropriate chart for the distance.

Fire crew

The following minimum standards apply:

i. Distance visual acuity should not be less than 6/12 in one eye and 6/36 in the other, with glasses if necessary, and not less than 6/18 with both eyes unaided.
ii. Where spectacles are required to achieve the above standard, for operational duties they should be of a safety type approved by the Authority.
iii. The use of contact lenses is not permitted.
iv. Colour perception should be normal on initial testing by Ishihara plates. If a defect is found

during the examination, a further test is to be carried out using a suitable lantern to demonstrate the ability to distinguish the signal colour red, green and white.

v. Where the fire-fighter's duties require the holding of a Heavy Goods Vehicle Licence (HGV), the appropriate DVLC standards and examination recommendations will apply.

Airside drivers

i. Eyesight standards required are DVLA Group 2 standard plus.
ii. Colour perception should be normal on initial testing by Ishihara plates. If a defect is found during the examination, a further test is to be carried out using a suitable lantern to demonstrate the ability to distinguish the signal colour red, green and white (Giles-Archer lantern on large aperture).

RVR observers

i. Personnel selected for RVR observer should have examination performed:

   a. Prior to acceptance for RVR duties
   b. 5-yearly up to 40, then 2-yearly to 50, then annually thereafter
   c. before return to duty following any sickness involving eyesight.

ii. Visual acuity in each eye separately must be not less than 6/9 at distance using Snellen test types. If correcting spectacles or contact lenses are worn, the refractive error should not exceed ± 5.00 dioptres of equivalent spherical error.
iii. The near vision should be N5 or equivalent at a distance between 30 and 50 cm in each eye separately. Spectacles may be worn to achieve this standard.
iv. The visual fields shall be normal as tested by the confrontation method.
v. The ocular muscle balance should be normal.
vi. Colour perception should be tested by Ishihara or other pseudo-isochromatic colour plates. Candidates who are shown to be defective by this means should be subjected to an approved lantern test, e.g. Giles-Archer or Holmes-Wright, to demonstrate that the colours signal red, signal green and white can be readily identified. Colour perception testing should not be repeated at the periodic vision testing.

Air traffic control officers, flight engineers, flight navigators

The visual requirements are as follows:

1. The function of the eyes and their adnexae shall be normal. There shall be no active pathological conditions, acute or chronic, of either eye or adnexae, which is likely to interfere with its proper function to an extent that would interfere with the safe exercise of the applicant's licence privileges.
2. The applicant shall be required to have normal fields of vision.
3. The applicant shall be required to have a distance vision of not less than 6/9 monocularly, with or without correction. Where this standard can be obtained only with the use of correcting lenses, the applicant may be assessed as fit provided that:

   a. The refractive error falls within the range ± 3.00 D. There must be no more than 2.00 D astigmatism.
   b. Such correcting lenses are worn when exercising the privileges of the licence or rating applied for or held.

4. The applicant shall have the ability to read the N5 (Times Roman print) chart or its equivalent at a distance selected by the applicant within the range of 30 to 50 cm and the ability to read the N14 chart or its equivalent at a distance of 100 cm. If this requirement is met only by the use of correcting lenses, the applicant may be assessed as fit provided that such lenses are available for immediate use when exercising the privileges of the licence. No more than one pair of correcting lenses shall be used in demonstrating compliance with this visual requirement (half eye spectacles recommended for applicants needing correction for near only).
5. An applicant shall have no abnormalities of binocular vision. If the heterophorias exceed 6 Δ esophoria, 8 Δ exophoria or 1 Δ hyperphoria, an evaluation by the CAA s consultant ophthalmologist may be necessary.
6. An applicant who has had RK or PRK will be

grounded for a minimum of 1 year and will have two assessments by a CAA ophthalmologist (at 6 and 12 months post-operative) before a medical certificate can be issued.

7. The requirements at final review (assuming stable refraction) are:

   a. Pre-operative refraction must be less than −5.00 D (correction of hypermetropia is not acceptable)
   b. VA 6/6 or better monocularly with or without correction
   c. No greater than 2.00 D astigmatism.
   d. No problems with glare.

8. There will then be an annual follow up with a CAA ophthalmologist at Gatwick.

9. Contact lens wearers should carry a pair of reserve spectacles (bifocal contacts are not permitted).

10. An applicant shall have normal perception of colours (defined as no mistakes on Ishihara plates (24-plate version) tested in daylight or in artificial light of the same colour temperature such as that provided by illuminant C or D) or be colour safe. Applicants who fail Ishihara shall be assessed as colour safe if they pass extensive testing with methods acceptable to the Aeromedical Section (Holmes–Wright lantern or anomaloscopy).

11. An applicant who fails the acceptable colour perception tests is to be considered colour unsafe and shall be assessed as unfit.

Glossary of terms

The majority of these terms are taken from **The Dictionary of Optometry and Visual Science** (4th edition), by kind permission of M. Millodot and Butterworth-Heinemann Ltd.

Accommodation
Adjustment of the dioptric power of the eye. It is generally involuntary, and is made in order to see objects clearly at any distance. In man, this adjustment is brought about by a change in the shape of the crystalline lens.

Accommodation, amplitude of
The maximum amount of accommodation that one eye can exert. It is expressed in dioptres (D), as the difference between the far point and the near point, measured with respect to the spectacle plane, the corneal apex, or some other reference point. The amplitude of accommodation declines from about 14 D at age 10 years to about 0.5 D at age 60 years (although the measured value is usually higher due to the depth of focus of the eye).

Accommodation, range of
The linear distance between the far point and the near point.

Acuity, dynamic
Capacity to see moving objects distinctly. Also referred to as kinetic acuity.

Acuity, static
Capacity for seeing the details of a stationary target distinctly.

Acuity, visual

Capacity for seeing the details of an object distinctly. Quantitatively, it is represented in two ways:

1. As the reciprocal of the minimum angle of resolution (in minutes of arc). This is the resolution visual acuity.
2. As the Snellen fraction. This is measured using letters or Landolt rings, or equivalent objects.

Average clinical visual acuity varies between 6/4 and 6/6 (or 20/15 and 20/20 in feet). Visual acuity varies with the region of the retina (being maximum at the foveola), with general illumination, contrast, colour and type of test, time of exposure, the refractive error of the eye, etc.

Adaptation, dark

Adjustment of the eye (particularly the retinal pigments but also the pupil), such that after observation in the dark the sensitivity to light is greatly increased, i.e. the threshold response to light is decreased. This is a much slower process than light adaptation.

Adaptation, light

Adjustment of the eye (particularly the retinal pigments but also the pupil), such that after observation of a bright field the sensitivity to light is diminished, i.e. the threshold of luminance is increased.

Amblyopia

A condition characterized by low visual acuity without any apparent lesion of the eye or proven disorder in the visual pathway that is not correctable by optical means.

Ametropia

Anomaly of the refractive state of the eye in which, with relaxed accommodation, the image of objects at infinity is not formed on the retina. Thus vision may be blurred. The ametropias are: astigmatism, hypermetropia and myopia. The absence of ametropia is called emmetropia.

Anisometropia

Condition in which the refractive state of a pair of eyes differs. Therefore one eye requires a lens power that is different to that of the other eye.

Asthenopia

Term used to describe any symptoms associated with the use of the eyes. The causes of asthenopia are numerous: sustained near vision, either when the accommodation amplitude is low or hypermetropia is uncorrected (accommodative asthenopia), aniseikonia (aniseikonic asthenopia), astigmatism (astigmatic asthenopia), pain in the eye (asthenopia dolens), heterophoria (heterophoric asthenopia), ocular inflammation (asthenopia irritans), hysteria (nervous asthenopia), uncorrected presbyopia (presbyopic asthenopia), improper illumination (photogenous asthenopia), or retinal disease (retinal asthenopia).

Astigmatism

A condition of refraction in which the image of a point object is not a single point but two mutually perpendicular lines at different distances from the optical system. The two focal lines are perpendicular to each other. In the eye, astigmatism is a refractive error that is generally caused by one or several toroidal shapes of the refracting surfaces, or by the obliquity of the light entering the eye, but it can also develop as a result of a subluxation of the lens or as a result of diabetes, cataract or trauma (acquired astigmatism).

Candela

A measure of luminous intensity, which is the power of a source or illuminated surface to emit light in a given direction. One candela is equal to one lumen per steradian.

Cataract

Partial or complete loss of transparency of the crystalline lens substance or its capsule. Cataract may occur as a result of age, trauma, systemic disease (e.g. diabetes), ocular disease (e.g. anterior uveitis), high myopia, long-term steroid therapy, excessive exposure to IR and UV light, heredity, and maternal infections (Down syndrome, etc.). The main symptom is a gradual loss of vision, often described as 'misty'. Some patients may also notice transient monocular diplopia, others fixed spots (not floaters) in the visual field, and others better vision in dim illumination.

Chart, Snellen

A visual acuity test using a graduated series of Snellen letters (or Snellen test types) in which the limbs and the spaces between them subtend an angle of one min of arc at specified distances. The letters are usually constructed so that they are five units high and four units wide, although some charts use letters that fit within a square subtending 5 min of arc at that distance.

CIE

Abbreviation for Commission Internationale de l'Eclairage.

Colour, confusion

Colours that are confused by a dichromat. The colours confused by a deuteranope, a protanope and a tritanope are not the same. A deuteranope will confuse reds, greens and greys, whereas a protanope will confuse reds, orange, blue–greens and greys.

Convergence

1. Movement of the eyes turning inwards or towards each other.
2. Characteristic of a pencil of light rays directed towards a real image point.

Convergence insufficiency

An inability to converge, or to maintain convergence, usually associated with a high exophoria at near and a relatively orthophoric condition at distance. It results in complaints of fatigue, or even diplopia, due to the inability to maintain (and sometimes even to obtain) adequate convergence for prolonged close work.

Convergence, near point of

The nearest point where the lines of sight intersect when the eyes converge to the maximum. This point is normally about 8 cm from the spectacle plane. If further away, the patient may have convergence insufficiency.

Depth perception

See perception, depth.

Differential threshold

The smallest difference between two stimuli presented simultaneously that gives rise to a perceived difference in sensation. The difference may be related to brightness, but also to colour and specifically to either saturation (whilst hue is kept constant) or hue (whilst saturation is kept constant). The differential

threshold of luminance is equal to about 1 per cent photopic vision.

Dioptre (D)

A unit indicating the refractive power of a lens or of an optical system. It is equal to the product of the refractive index in the image space and the reciprocal of the focal length in metres. Thus a lens with a focal length (in air) of 1 m has a power of 1 D, one with a focal length of 0.5 m has a power of 2 D, etc.

Diplopia

The condition in which a single object is seen as two rather than one. This is usually due to images not stimulating corresponding retinal areas in each of a pair of eyes.

Disability glare

See glare, disability.

Discomfort glare

See glare, discomfort.

Disparity, retinal (fixation)

Binocular vision in which the retinal image in each eye does not quite fall on corresponding retinal points. As the discrepancy is very small it is not experienced as diplopia, but in some cases it can cause symptoms of eyestrain.

Dispersion

The separation of light into its monochromatic components.

Divergence

1. Movement of the eyes turning away from each other so that the lines of sight intersect behind the eyes.
2. Characteristic of a pencil of light rays, as when emanating from a point source.

Emmetropia

Refractive condition of the eye in which distant objects are focused on the retina, when accommodation is relaxed. This is the ideal refractive state of the eye.

Esophoria
Turning of the eye inward when binocular vision is interrupted.

Esotropia (convergent strabismus)
Strabismus in which the deviating eye turns inwards. This is the most common type of strabismus in children.

Exophoria
Turning of the eye outwards when binocular vision is interrupted.

Exotropia (divergent strabismus)
Strabismus in which the deviating eye turns outwards.

Fatigue, visual
Feeling of a diminution in visual performance, which is not necessarily produced by an excessive use of the eyes. However, there does not seem to be concrete objective proof of a reduction in visual aptitude (e.g. visual acuity) accompanying visual fatigue.

Field, visual
The extent of space in which objects are visible to an eye in a given position. The visual field extends to approximately 100° temporally, 60° nasally, 65° superiorly and 75° inferiorly. The visual field can be measured either monocularly or binocularly. In the latter case its extent is much larger, especially in the horizontal plane.

Filter
See lens, absorptive.

Fusion
The process by which the retinal images from each eye are perceived as a single percept. In normal binocular vision this occurs when each eye is directed at the object and the image falls on corresponding retinal points.

Glare
A visual condition in which the observer feels discomfort and/or exhibits a lower performance in visual tests (e.g. visual acuity or contrast sensitivity). This is produced by a relatively bright source of light (called the glare source) within the visual field. A given bright light may or may not produce glare, depending upon the location, the intensity of the light source, the background luminance, the state of adaptation of the eye, and the clarity of the media of the eye.

Glare, disability
Glare that reduces visual performance without necessarily causing discomfort.

Glare, discomfort
Glare that produces discomfort without necessarily interfering with visual performance.

Heterophoria
The condition where the lines of sight of a pair of eyes do not meet at the fixation point when binocular vision is interrupted. The deviation can take various forms according to its relative direction, e.g. esophoria, exophoria, hyperphoria, hypophoria.

Heterotropia (strabismus, squint)
The condition in which the lines of sight of the two eyes are not directed towards the same fixation point when the subject is actively fixating an object. Thus, the image of the fixation point is not formed on the fovea of the deviating eye and there may be diplopia. In most cases the diplopic image is suppressed and vision is essentially monocular.

Hyper(metr)opia
Refraction condition of the eye in which distant objects are focused behind the retina when the accommodation is relaxed; thus, vision is blurred. In hypermetropia, the point conjugate with the retina, that is the far point of the eye, is located behind the eye.

Hyperphoria
The tendency for the line of sight of one eye to deviate upwards relative to that of the other eye when binocular vision is interrupted. If the deviation tends to be downwards relative to the other eye, or if the other eye in hyperphoria is used as a reference, the condition is called hypophoria.

Hypertropia
Strabismus in which one eye is directed to the fixation point whilst the other is directed upwards (right or left hypertropia). If one eye fixates whilst the other is directed downwards the condition is called hypotropia (right or left hypotropia).

Illuminants, CIE standard

The colorimetric illuminants A, B, C and D65 defined by the CIE in terms of relative spectral energy (power distribution): standard illuminant A represents the full radiator at $T = 2854$ K; standard illuminant B represents direct sunlight with a correlated colour temperature of $T = 4874$ K; standard illuminant C represents daylight with a correlated colour temperature of $T = 6774$ K; standard illuminant D represents daylight with a correlated colour temperaure of $T = 6504$ K (CIE).

Illumination

Quotient of the luminous flux incident on an element of surface by the area of that element of surface. Symbol: E. The units are lux (lx) or footcandles.

Interpupillary distance

The distance between the centres of the pupils of the eyes. It usually refers to the eyes fixating at infinity, otherwise reference must be made to the fixation distance (e.g. near interpupillary distance). The average interpupillary distance for men is about 64 mm and for women about is 62 mm.

Kelvin

The Kelvin (K) unit of thermodynamic temperature is the fraction 1/273.16 of the thermodynamic temperature of the triple point of water.

Landolt ring

A test object used for measuring visual acuity, consisting of an incomplete ring resembling the letter C. The width of the break and of the ring are each one-fifth of its overall diameter. The subject must indicate where the break is located. The minimum angle of resolution corresponds to the angular subtense of the just noticeable break, at the eye.

Laser

An intense luminous source of coherent and monochromatic light. The term is an acronym for Light Amplification by Stimulated Emission of Radiation.

Lens, absorptive

A (tinted) lens that absorbs a proportion of the incident radiation. Some lenses absorb in the infrared region of the spectrum, some in the ultra-violet region, and others absorb more or less equally throughout, or selectively in, the visible spectrum.

Lens, afocal

A lens of zero power.

Lens, laminated

A lens consisting of a thin layer of plastic (e.g. cellulose acetate) cemented between two layers of glass. Such a lens provides mechanical protection for the eye because in case of breakage the glass pieces remain attached to the plastics layer.

Lens, safety

1. A lens made of safety glass.
2. A general term referring to any lens that protects the eyes against injury due to impact. It is more resistant to fracture and less likely to splinter than an ordinary glass lens. Examples: plastics lenses (especially polycarbonate), toughened lenses, laminated lenses. Plastics lenses have the greatest impact resistance of all these lenses.

Lens, single-vision

An ophthalmic lens providing a correction for one viewing distance.

Lens, toughened

A lens made of glass that has been thermally or chemically strengthened.

Lens, trifocal

A multifocal lens consisting of three portions of different focal powers, usually for distance, intermediate and near vision.

Lens, varifocal; progressive

A spectacle lens having a gradual and progressive change in power either over the whole lens or over a region intermediate between areas of uniform power. This lens is used to correct presbyopia. There are several types, which are known by their tradenames (e.g. Progressive R, Truvision, Varilux).

Light

Electromagnetic vibration capable of stimulating the receptors of the retina and producing a visual sensation. The radiations that give rise to the sensation of vision are comprised within the wavelength band 380–760 nm. This band is called the visible spectrum. The borders of this band are not precise, but beyond these radiations the visual efficacy of any wavelength becomes very low indeed (less than 10^{-5}). For an older subject, the lower boundary of the visible spectrum is closer to 420 nm than 380 nm.

Line of sight

Line joining the point of fixation to the centre of the entrance pupil of the eye. The entrance pupil is what one sees when looking at an eye and is the image of the iris aperture formed by the cornea.

Lumen

SI unit of luminous flux. It is equal to the flux emitted within a unit solid angle of one steradian by a point source with a luminous intensity of one candela. Symbol: lm.

Luminaire

An electric light fitting that distributes, filters or transforms the light, and includes all the accessory items of the fittings.

Luminance

Photometric term characterizing the way in which a surface emits or reflects light in a given direction. It is equal to the luminous intensity measured in a given direction divided by the area of this surface projected on a perpendicular to the direction considered. Symbol: **L**. Units: candela per square metre (cd/m^2); footlambert; lambert.

Luminous intensity

Quotient of the luminous flux leaving the source, propagated in an element of solid angle containing the given direction, by the element of solid angle. Symbol: **I**. Unit: candela (cd).

Lux

SI unit of illumination. It is the illumination produced by a luminous flux of 1 lumen uniformly distributed over a surface area of 1 square metre. Symbol: lx.

Mesopic

See vision, mesopic.

Miosis

A condition in which the pupil is constricted.

Myopia

Refractive condition of the eye in which distant objects are focused in front of the retina when the accommodation is relaxed. Thus distance vision is blurred. In myopia the point conjugate with the retina, i.e. the far point of the eye, is located at some finite distance in front of the eye.

Nanometre

Unit of length equal to one-thousand-millionth of a metre (10^{-9} m). Abbreviation: nm.

Ophthalmoscopy

Method of examination of the interior of the eye with an ophthalmoscope.

Optometrist

A person licensed (or registered) to practise optometry (definition of the International Optometric and Optical League).

Perception, depth

Perception of relative or absolute differences in distance of objects from the observer. Depth perception is more precise in binocular vision, but is possible in monocular vision using the following cues: interposition, relative position, relative size, linear perspective, textual gradient, aerial perspective, light and shade, shadow, and motion parallax.

Photometer

An instrument for measuring the luminous intensity of a light source or a surface by comparing it with a standard source. The comparison can be done either with the human eye or with a photoelectric cell.

Photophobia

Ocular discomfort induced by bright lights.

Photopic

See vision, photopic.

Plastics

Various organic or synthetic materials (e.g. CR39, HEMA, polymethylmethacrylate, etc.), which can be transformed into solid shapes to make spectacle frames, contact lenses, ophthalmic lenses etc. They can be made to have good optical surfaces, high light transmission and refractive indices, and dispersions corresponding to that of crown or flint glass.

Presbyopia

A refractive condition in which the accommodative ability of the eye becomes insufficient for satisfactory near vision without the use of corrective plus lenses (called the addition). This condition generally occurs between the ages of 42 and 48 years in people living in Europe and North American countries.

Prism dioptre

A unit specifying the amount of deviation by an ophthalmic prism. One prism dioptre represents a deviation of 1 cm on a flat surface 1 m away from the prism.

Refractive error

The dioptric power of the ametropia of the eye. It is equal to the reciprocal of the distance between the far point and the eye, in metres.

Retinoscopy

The determination of the refractive state of the eye by means of a retinoscope.

Refractive index

The ratio of the speed of light in a vacuum or in air to the speed of light in a given medium (symbol: n). The speed of light in a given medium depends upon the wavelength of light, and consequently the index varies accordingly. The index of refraction forms the basis of Snell's law, which quantitatively determines the deviation of light rays traversing a surface separating two media of different refractive indices.

Scotoma

An area (of partial or complete) blindness surrounded by normal or relatively normal visual field.

Scotopic

See vision, scotopic.

SI unit

The Systeme international d'Unites.

Slit lamp

An instrument consisting of an illuminating system and a microscope. It can be used to examine the anterior segment of the eye. (Supplementary lenses are required to view the posterior segment.)

Strabismus

See heterotropia.

Threshold, absolute

The minimum luminance of a source that will produce a sensation of light. It varies with the state of dark adaptation, the retinal area stimulated, the type of stimulus, etc.

Vision, colour

Vision in which the colour sense is experienced.

Vision, mesopic

Vision at intermediate levels between photopic and scotopic vision, and corresponding to luminances ranging from 10^{-3} to $10 \, cd/m^2$.

Vision, photopic

Vision at high levels of luminance (above $10 \, cd/m^2$) and resulting from the functioning of the cones.

Vision, scotopic

Vision at low levels of luminance, below about 10^{-3}, and resulting from the functioning of the rods.

Visual acuity

See acuity, visual.

Visual fatigue

See fatigue, visual.

Visual field

See field, visual.

Index